Current Approaches to Newborn Emergencies

nova
Medicine & Health
New York

Emergency and Intensive Care Medicine

More information about this series can be found at
https://novapublishers.com/product-category/series/emergency-and-intensive-care-medicine/

Neonatology Research Developments

More information about this series can be found at
https://novapublishers.com/product-category/series/neonatology-research-developments/

Zuhal Keskin Sarılar
Serap Samut Bülbül
Editors

Current Approaches to Newborn Emergencies

nova
Medicine & Health
New York

DOI: https://doi.org/10.52305/HNHV5826

Additional color graphics may be available in the e-book version of this book.

Library of Congress Cataloging-in-Publication Data

ISBN: 979-8-89530-999-5 (Hardcover)
ISBN: 979-8-90134-073-8 (eBook)

Published by Nova Science Publishers, Inc. † New York

Contents

Preface

The neonatal period, though brief, represents one of the most critical stages of human life. Within these first 28 days, a newborn undergoes profound physiological and biological changes while making the transition to life outside the womb. Emergencies during this fragile time can alter the course of an infant's future, underscoring the importance of timely recognition and intervention.

Current Approaches to Newborn Emergencies was conceived as both a practical guide and a teaching resource, designed to assist clinicians in navigating the complex challenges of neonatal emergencies. By bringing together the expertise of dedicated authors across disciplines, this volume aims to provide clear, evidence-based insights into diagnosis, management, and treatment strategies.

It is our hope that this book not only supports physicians in their daily practice, but also contributes to advancing neonatal care worldwide. Above all, it stands as a testament to the resilience of newborns and the families who inspire us to pursue excellence in their care.

Chapter 1

Neonatal Anesthesia

Merve Bulun Yediyıldız*, MD
Department of Anesthesiology and Reanimation, University of Health Sciences, Kartal Dr. Lütfi Kırdar City Hospital, Istanbul, Turkey

Abstract

A tailored approach is required in neonatal anesthesia due to the unique anatomical and physiological characteristics of neonates. The immaturity of organ systems, limited cardiopulmonary reserves, and altered metabolism of drugs all contribute to the complexity of anesthetic care. This chapter extensively discusses perioperative management, including preoperative evaluation, operative management, pharmacology, and postoperative care. There is a special emphasis on preventing complications such as postoperative apnea, hemodynamic instability, and hypothermia using evidence-based approaches and multidisciplinary team care.

Keywords: neonatal anesthesia, perioperative management, postoperative complications

Introduction

Neonatal anesthesia is a specialized field focused on providing safe and effective anesthesia care to newborns. Newborns represent the highest-risk population for anesthesia-related complications and perioperative mortality

* Corresponding Author's Email: mervebulun@gmail.com

In: Current Approaches to Newborn Emergencies
Editors: Zuhal Keskin Sarılar and Serap Samut Bülbül
ISBN: 979-8-89530-999-5

(Bösenberg, 2014; De Graaff et al., 2021). This vulnerability is due to their unique physiology, characterized by a high metabolic rate and limited pulmonary, cardiac, and thermoregulatory reserves (Cote et al., 2024).

The administration of anesthesia to neonates poses a considerable challenge, even for experienced anesthesiologists, due to the paucity of clinical evidence supporting existing neonatal anesthesia guidelines. High-risk neonatal conditions requiring surgical intervention, such as necrotizing enterocolitis (NEC), congenital diaphragmatic hernia (CDH), and abdominal wall defects like gastroschisis and omphalocele, further underscore the need for anesthetic techniques that are physiologically informed, carefully individualized, and coordinated within multidisciplinary teams. The combination of narrow therapeutic margins and challenging airway management makes neonatal anesthesia one of the most demanding subspecialties within anesthesiology. To ensure safe and effective anesthetic management, it is essential to possess a comprehensive understanding of neonatal physiology and pharmacology. These fundamental principles exert a direct influence on the responses exhibited by neonates to anesthetic agents and perioperative interventions.

Basics of Neonatal Physiology and Pharmacology

Respiratory System Physiology

Anatomical and Developmental Characteristics

Although the airways are structurally developed by 16 weeks of gestation, the number of alveoli at birth is significantly lower than in adults. Premature infants, particularly those born between 24 and 28 weeks of gestation, are just beginning the process of alveolarization (Neumann & von Ungern-Sternberg, 2014).

The onset of surfactant production occurs at approximately 23-24 weeks of gestation, reaching maturity at around 35 weeks. This surfactant is crucial for maintaining lung compliance and preventing respiratory distress syndrome in preterm infants (Carroll & Agarwal, 2010). Preterm infants with insufficient surfactant are at high risk for respiratory distress syndrome, which may require both corticosteroid therapy (for maternal administration) and exogenous surfactant administration after birth (Ramaswamy et al., 2023).

Functional Respiratory Characteristics

Neonates exhibit double the alveolar ventilation of adults due to increased respiratory rates rather than tidal volume. This high ventilation-to-functional residual capacity (FRC) ratio leads to faster wash-in and wash-out of oxygen and anesthetic gases, making them more susceptible to rapid desaturation during apnea or hypoventilation. Their elevated oxygen consumption and low FRC make them particularly susceptible to rapid desaturation during apnea, a risk that is heightened under general anesthesia (Sinha, 2023).

It has been established that neonates exhibit underdeveloped central and peripheral chemoreceptors, resulting in a diminished response to hypoxia and hypercarbia. Both preterm and term infants initially exhibit a short period of hyperventilation followed by sustained hypoventilation when exposed to hypoxic conditions (Carroll & Agarwal, 2010).

Airway Characteristics and Challenges

Neonates represent the most vulnerable demographic with regard to respiratory and airway management complications (Disma et al., 2024). Neonatal airways are relatively narrow and compliant, making them prone to obstruction. Even minor secretions or mild inflammation can cause significant airway resistance, leading to respiratory distress. Although airway conductance is relatively high in neonates, the absolute airway diameter is small. This makes them highly sensitive to any degree of airway obstruction. Also, neonates are obligate nasal breathers, which increases their susceptibility to airway obstruction due to nasal congestion or secretions (Bang, 2015).

Pulmonary Vascular System and Risks

Neonates have high pulmonary vascular resistance (PVR) at birth, which gradually decreases with postnatal adaptation. However, factors like hypoxia, hyperoxia, acidosis, or sepsis can lead to persistent pulmonary hypertension (PPHN) that can result in significant morbidity and mortality (Ivy et al., 2024).

Neonatal lungs are particularly susceptible to oxidant injury caused by hyperoxia or inflammation, which can damage the pulmonary endothelium, lead to impaired alveolar growth, and contribute to bronchopulmonary dysplasia (BPD) in preterm infants (Ivy et al., 2024).

Cardiovascular System Physiology

Transition from Fetal to Neonatal Circulation

Neonates undergo a critical transition from fetal to extrauterine circulation immediately after birth. During fetal life, the circulatory system is distinguished by elevated PVR and diminished systemic vascular resistance, a consequence of the placenta. Blood bypasses the lungs via two key shunts: the foramen ovale (between the right and left atria) and the ductus arteriosus (connecting the pulmonary artery to the aorta). With the first breath, aeration of the lungs causes a rapid decline in PVR and a significant increase in pulmonary blood flow. This transition is facilitated by the release of endogenous nitric oxide, which promotes vasodilation of the pulmonary arteries. As the left atrial pressure rises above the right, the foramen ovale functionally closes, typically within the first hours to days of life. Anatomical closure occurs subsequently, typically between three months and one year after birth. The ductus arteriosus undergoes functional closure within the first 10 to 15 hours after birth, primarily due to increased arterial oxygen tension. Complete anatomical closure can take up to two months. However, in premature infants, this process may be delayed, increasing the risk of persistent fetal circulation (Brown et al., 2025).

Pulmonary Vascular Reactivity and Persistent Pulmonary Hypertension

Hypoxemia, hypercapnia, or acidosis can trigger vasoconstriction, leading to a reopening of fetal shunts and right-to-left shunting through the foramen ovale and ductus arteriosus. This vicious cycle can cause or exacerbate persistent pulmonary hypertension of the newborn, which is a major cause of morbidity in conditions such as diaphragmatic hernia, meconium aspiration syndrome, sepsis, and polycythemia (Singh & Lakshminrusimha, 2021).

Cardiac Structure and Function

Neonatal myocardium is structurally and functionally immature, characterized by limited contractility, decreased compliance, heart-rate dependency, and sympathetic innervation. Since stroke volume cannot be significantly increased, cardiac output in neonates is primarily heart-rate dependent. A normal neonatal heart rate is approximately 140 beats per minute (Hillier et al., 2004).

Although adrenergic receptors are mature at birth, the sympathetic nervous system is not fully developed. This incomplete innervation makes neonatal myocardium more sensitive to catecholamines like norepinephrine but less responsive to indirect inotropes like dopamine (Hillier et al., 2004).

Due to the neonate's limited cardiovascular reserve, even mild hypovolemia or negative inotropic effects of anesthetic agents can lead to significant hypotension. Neonates require precise fluid management to avoid both hypovolemia and fluid overload, which can lead to heart failure. This understanding of neonatal cardiovascular physiology is essential for optimizing perioperative management and minimizing the risk of hemodynamic instability.

Renal and Hepatic System Physiology

Neonatal renal physiology is characterized by immature and developing kidney function, which has significant implications for fluid balance, electrolyte management, and drug clearance. Neonatal kidneys exhibit a restricted capacity for tubular reabsorption and secretion, thereby impacting the excretion of electrolytes and pharmaceutical agents. Neonates have a reduced ability to conserve sodium and water, making them vulnerable to dehydration or fluid overload (Filler et al., 2015).

Neonatal hepatocytes exhibit a restricted capacity for conjugation reactions, including bilirubin conjugation via UDP-glucuronosyltransferase (UDPGT). This underdevelopment can result in jaundice due to an accumulation of unconjugated bilirubin (Beath, 2003).

Neonates are susceptible to hypoglycemia due to their limited glycogen stores and immature gluconeogenic pathways. This phenomenon is particularly evident in preterm infants, who exhibit a reduced capacity for hepatic glucose production (Beath, 2003).

Thermoregulation

Neonates are prone to rapid heat loss due to a disproportionately large surface area relative to their body weight, a paucity of subcutaneous fat, and an incapacity to generate heat through shivering. These cells rely on non-shivering thermogenesis in brown adipose tissue for heat production, a process that is activated by norepinephrine. Factors such as low operating room temperature, cold solutions, anesthesia-induced vasodilation, and dry anesthetic gases have been identified as contributing to increased heat loss (Hillier et al., 2004).

Pharmacology

Pharmacokinetics in Neonates

The pharmacokinetics of a drug in a newborn are influenced by immature organ systems, especially the liver and kidneys, which are responsible for drug metabolism and excretion. The volume of distribution is elevated due to increased total body water and extracellular fluid. A comprehensive review of the extant literature reveals several factors to be of particular relevance, including body composition, plasma protein binding, and blood-brain (Yalçin et al., 2022).

Pharmacodynamics in Neonates

Neonatal pharmacodynamics is characterized by increased variability due to the development of receptor systems and immature neural pathways. Monitoring pharmacodynamic outcomes in this population presents significant challenges due to the limited availability of neonatal-appropriate monitoring devices (Yalçin et al., 2022).

Perioperative Management

Preoperative Management

Preoperative Evaluation

A comprehensive preoperative evaluation is imperative for neonates due to their heightened physiological vulnerability and the intricacy of their conditions. The assessment commences with a comprehensive medical history, encompassing gestational age, birth weight, and notable perinatal events, such as asphyxia, meconium aspiration, sepsis, or the necessity for respiratory support. Additionally, the assessment considers any antecedents of congenital anomalies with particular emphasis on cardiac defects. A physical examination should prioritize the assessment of hydration status, which can be determined by measuring skin turgor, mucous membranes, and urine output. Additionally, respiratory function should be evaluated, noting any signs of distress such as tachypnea or retractions. A cardiovascular assessment entails auscultation for murmurs and monitoring for indications of hypovolemia, including but not limited to low blood pressure and diminished capillary refill. Airway evaluation is of the utmost importance, particularly in infants exhibiting syndromic features that may suggest the necessity for difficult airway management (Subramaniam, 2019).

Laboratory tests should be reviewed for anemia, electrolyte imbalances (hypoglycemia, hyperkalemia, and hypocalcemia), and coagulopathy, with necessary corrections made preoperatively. It is imperative to closely monitor blood glucose and calcium levels in neonates, as their metabolic reserves are significantly diminished relative to adults. Prior to undergoing a surgical procedure, it is imperative to ascertain that intravenous access is both patent and adequate for the procedure to be performed. In the context of high-risk or complex surgical procedures, it is imperative to engage in comprehensive discussions with the surgical team to formulate a meticulous postoperative care plan. Proper preparation is paramount in minimizing the risk of intraoperative complications and ensuring safe anesthetic management.

Parental communication is critical. Parents should be informed about the planned procedure, its risks, and expected outcomes. Informed consent must be obtained for anesthesia, blood transfusion, and any invasive procedures.

Preoperative Preparation

Effective preparation for neonatal anesthesia requires ensuring that all necessary equipment is readily available and functioning properly. Airway management tools should include facemasks with minimal dead space, appropriately sized oropharyngeal airways, and both conventional laryngoscopes and videolaryngoscopes, which facilitate intubation in small infants.

Maintaining normothermia is critical. The operating room should be pre-warmed to 27°C, and measures to reduce heat loss should be implemented. These measures include wrapping exposed areas with cling wrap or foil, using a warming mattress, and providing forced-air warming. Additionally, intravenous fluids and inhaled gases should be pre-warmed and humidified to prevent hypothermia (Zhang et al., 2023).

Intraoperative Management

Intraoperative management for neonatal anesthesia requires meticulous attention to monitoring, airway management, fluid therapy, and anesthetic administration. Standard monitoring includes continuous electrocardiography, blood pressure measurement, pulse oximetry, capnography, and temperature monitoring. For neonates at risk of transitional circulation issues, preductal (right hand) and postductal (foot) pulse oximetry is essential. The core body temperature is meticulously monitored using nasopharyngeal, rectal, or esophageal probes to ensure the patient's temperature remains within the normal range. In the event that an arterial line is utilized, it is imperative to ensure its patency and adequate distal perfusion (Subramaniam, 2019).

The meticulous preparation of drugs is paramount, necessitating precise calculations based on weight. In order to minimize dosing errors, drugs should be pre-drawn in syringes and labeled with the appropriate doses. A saline flush should be prepared to ensure that the entire drug is administered through the intravenous line. Syringes containing stock solutions should be kept separate to avoid accidental overdosing.

The induction of anesthesia can be achieved using inhalational agents like sevoflurane in the absence of intravenous access due to its minimal airway irritation and relative cardiovascular stability. For neonates with intravenous access, induction can be performed using agents such as ketamine or thiopental, with careful attention to airway management due to the risk of apnea. Tracheal intubation is commonly performed using muscle relaxants such as atracurium, with fentanyl or sufentanil for analgesia.

Neonatal airway management presents unique challenges due to the infant's small size, anatomical differences, and susceptibility to airway obstruction. The choice of airway management depends on the patient's condition, the surgical procedure, and the anesthesiologist's expertise. Although some minor surgeries may be performed using a face mask or laryngeal mask airway, most neonatal procedures require tracheal intubation (Sinha, 2014). Tracheal intubation can be performed using either uncuffed or cuffed tubes. For difficult airways, videolaryngoscopes or fiberoptic bronchoscopes are recommended. Ensuring proper tube placement is critical, confirmed by auscultation and end-tidal CO_2 monitoring. If using mechanical ventilation, pressure-limited or volume-limited ventilators may be applied, ensuring careful monitoring of ventilation parameters to avoid barotrauma. Management strategies such as gentle ventilation techniques, maintaining adequate positive end-expiratory pressure (PEEP), and using lung-protective ventilation have been shown to reduce the incidence of lung injury in preterm infants.

The management of fluid therapy is a critical aspect of patient care, and it is imperative that pre-warmed fluids are utilized to maintain normothermia. Fluid replacement should be based on surgical type, with estimated losses of 1-2 mL/kg/h for minor procedures, 4-7 mL/kg/h for thoracotomy, and 5-10 mL/kg/h for abdominal surgery. Third-space losses can be challenging to estimate but should be monitored through clinical signs like delayed capillary refill, tachycardia, and hypotension. Urine output should be maintained between 0.5-2 mL/kg/h as an indicator of adequate renal perfusion (Subramaniam, 2019).

Postoperative Management

Postoperative management of neonates is critical due to their high risk of complications. Common postoperative complications include hemodynamic instability, respiratory failure, multiple organ dysfunction syndrome, and metabolic disorders. A number of factors have been identified as key elements that increase the risk of complications. These factors include a post-conceptual age of less than 40 weeks, a history of cardiac malformations, hyaline membrane disease or necrotizing enterocolitis, preoperative intensive care unit (ICU) admission, and intraoperative fluid bolus administration (Michelet et al., 2017).

Postoperative monitoring should prioritize the maintenance of cardiovascular stability, ensuring adequate ventilation and the prevention of hypoglycemia or electrolyte imbalances. Postoperative apnea represents a significant concern, particularly in preterm neonates, necessitating meticulous monitoring and management. Neonates who have undergone major surgeries or exhibit any of the identified risk factors should undergo continuous monitoring in the ICU. A comprehensive management strategy encompasses the maintenance of normothermia, the optimization of fluid balance, and the assurance of adequate analgesia.

Conclusion

Neonatal anesthesia is a highly specialized and complex field that demands an in-depth understanding of the neonate's unique physiology and the interplay between immaturity of organ systems and anesthetic drug behavior. Ensuring safe anesthetic care for this population necessitates a meticulous preoperative evaluation, precise intraoperative monitoring, and vigilant postoperative management. Advancements in monitoring techniques, ventilatory strategies, and pharmacology have led to substantial improvements in patient outcomes. Nevertheless, variability in clinical practice remains a persistent challenge. Standardized protocols, ongoing education, and close interdisciplinary collaboration are critical to ensure optimal safety and improve outcomes in neonatal anesthesia.

References

Bang, S. R. (2015). Neonatal anesthesia: How we manage our most vulnerable patients. *Korean Journal of Anesthesiology, 68*(5), 434–441. https://doi.org/10.4097/kjae.2015.68.5.434.

Beath, S. V. (2003, October). Hepatic function and physiology in the newborn. *Seminars in Neonatology, 8*(5), 337–346. https://doi.org/10.1016/S1084-2756(03)00066-6.

Bösenberg, A. T. (2014). Neonatal anesthesia with limited resources. *Pediatric Anesthesia, 24*(1), 98–105. https://doi.org/10.1111/pan.12291.

Brown, D. W., Freed, M. D., & Mayer Jr, J. E. (2025). Fetal and transitional circulation. In *Nadas' pediatric cardiology* (pp. 49–54). WB Saunders.

Carroll, J. L., & Agarwal, A. (2010). Development of ventilatory control in infants. *Paediatric Respiratory Reviews, 11*(4), 199–207. https://doi.org/10.1016/j.prrv.2010.06.002.

Coté, C. J., Lerman, J., & Anderson, B. (Eds.). (2024). *A practice of anesthesia for infants and children* (E-Book).

De Graaff, J. C., Johansen, M. F., Hensgens, M., & Engelhardt, T. (2021). Best practice & research clinical anesthesiology: Safety and quality in perioperative anesthesia care. Update on safety in pediatric anesthesia. *Best Practice & Research Clinical Anaesthesiology, 35*(1), 27–39. https://doi.org/10.1016/j.bpa.2020.12.007.

Disma, N., Asai, T., Cools, E., Cronin, A., Engelhardt, T., Fiadjoe, J., & Afshari, A. (2024). Airway management in neonates and infants: European Society of Anaesthesiology and Intensive Care and British Journal of Anaesthesia joint guidelines. *European Journal of Anaesthesiology, 41*(1), 3–23. https://doi.org/10.1097/EJA.0000000000001928.

Filler, G., Lopes, L., & Awuku, M. (2015). The importance of accurately assessing renal function in the neonate and infant. *Advances in Clinical Chemistry, 71*, 141–156. https://doi.org/10.1016/bs.acc.2015.06.004.

Hillier, S. C., Krishna, G., & Brasoveanu, E. (2004, August). Neonatal anesthesia. In *Seminars in Pediatric Surgery, 13*(3), 142–151. WB Saunders.

Ivy, D., Rosenzweig, E. B., Abman, S. H., Beghetti, M., Bonnet, D., Douwes, J. M., & Berger, R. M. (2024). Embracing the challenges of neonatal and paediatric pulmonary hypertension. *European Respiratory Journal, 64*(4). https://doi.org/10.1183/13993003.01345-2024.

Michelet, D., Brasher, C., Kaddour, H. B., Diallo, T., Abdat, R., Malbezin, S., & Dahmani, S. (2017). Postoperative complications following neonatal and infant surgery: Common events and predictive factors. *Anaesthesia Critical Care & Pain Medicine, 36*(3), 163–169. https://doi.org/10.1016/j.accpm.2016.05.012.

Neumann, R. P., & von Ungern-Sternberg, B. S. (2014). The neonatal lung–physiology and ventilation. *Pediatric Anesthesia, 24*(1), 10–21.

Ramaswamy, V. V., Bandyopadhyay, T., Abiramalatha, T., Szczapa, T., Wright, C. J., & Roehr, C. C. (2023). Clinical decision thresholds for surfactant administration in preterm infants: A systematic review and network meta-analysis. *EClinicalMedicine, 62*. https://doi.org/10.1016/j.eclinm.2023.102187.

Singh, Y., & Lakshminrusimha, S. (2021). Pathophysiology and management of persistent pulmonary hypertension of the newborn. *Clinics in Perinatology, 48*(3), 595–618.

Sinha, R., Talawar, P., Ramachandran, R., Azad, R., & Mohan, V. K. (2014). Perioperative management and post-operative course in preterm infants undergoing vitreo-retinal surgery for retinopathy of prematurity: A retrospective study. *Journal of Anaesthesiology Clinical Pharmacology, 30*(2), 258–262. https://doi.org/10.4103/0970-9185.130050.

Sinha, S. K. (2023). The respiratory system: Development and physiology in the neonate. In Saha, U. (Ed.), *Clinical anesthesia for the newborn and the neonate* (pp. xx–xx). Springer, Singapore. https://doi.org/10.1007/978-981-19-5458-0_11.

Subramaniam, R. (2019). Anaesthetic concerns in preterm and term neonates. *Indian Journal of Anaesthesia, 63*(9), 771–779. https://doi.org/10.4103/ija.IJA_591_19.

Yalçin, N., Flint, R. B., van Schaik, R. H., Simons, S. H., & Allegaert, K. (2022). The impact of pharmacogenetics on pharmacokinetics and pharmacodynamics in neonates and infants: A systematic review. *Pharmacogenomics and Personalized Medicine, 15*, 675–696. https://doi.org/10.2147/PGPM.S350205.

Zhang, M. Q., Ying, P. D., Wang, Y. J., Zhao, J. L., Huang, J. J., & Gong, F. Q. (2023). Intraoperative hypothermia in the neonate population: Risk factors, outcomes, and typical patterns. *Journal of Clinical Monitoring and Computing, 37*(1), 93–102. https://doi.org/10.1007/s10877-022-00863-9.

Chapter 2

Neonatal Pneumothorax

Mustafa Şenol Akın*, MD

Department of Neonatology, Ankara Bilkent City Hospital, Ankara, Turkey

Abstract

Neonatal pneumothorax is a potentially life-threatening condition that results from air leakage into the pleural space, leading to compromised lung expansion and gas exchange. It may arise spontaneously or as a complication of an underlying lung pathology or mechanical ventilation. Prompt recognition and management are critical for achieving favorable outcomes. This chapter explores the epidemiology, pathophysiology, clinical manifestations, diagnostic approaches, and treatment strategies of neonatal pneumothorax. Prevention and prognostic factors are also discussed to provide a comprehensive understanding of neonatal emergencies.

Keywords: neonatal pneumothorax, air leak syndrome, respiratory distress, thoracentesis, neonatal critical care

Introduction

Pneumothorax is the accumulation of air between the parietal pleura of the chest wall and the visceral pleura of the lung. It is most commonly observed during the neonatal period. It is associated with increased morbidity and mortality, particularly in extremely premature infants. Additionally, patients

* Corresponding Author's Email: mustafasenolakin@gmail.com

In: Current Approaches to Newborn Emergencies
Editors: Zuhal Keskin Sarılar and Serap Samut Bülbül
ISBN: 979-8-89530-999-5

with pneumothorax have longer hospitalizations and higher mortality rates. Although antenatal steroid administration and the use of surfactants in the treatment of RDS have decreased the rate of pneumothorax, it remains an important problem in newborns. In particular, prolonged pneumothorax (>7 days) increases the risk of chronic lung diseases.

Understanding the underlying mechanisms and clinical spectrum is essential for timely diagnosis and intervention. This chapter aims to elucidate the features of neonatal pneumothorax, offering insights into its prevention, management, and outcome optimization.

Epidemiology

While spontaneous pneumothorax is seen in 1% of births in newborn term babies, this rate increases to 7-12% in newborns with a birth week of less than 29 weeks (*Avery's Diseases of the Newborn*, 2024). As can be seen from these rates, the most important risk factor for pneumothorax is prematurity. Other risk factors include male sex, low birth weight, mechanical ventilation, and underlying lung disease (e.g., RDS, pneumonia, MAS, pulmonary hypoplasia, and pulmonary interstitial emphysema). Chorioamnionitis and prolonged rupture of membranes are independent risk factors for pneumothorax in premature and very low birth weight (VLBW) infants.

When antenatal steroid therapy, surfactant administration, and mechanical ventilation are used, high-frequency positive pressure ventilation (HFO), synchronization, volume-targeted ventilation, and low tidal volume are thought to reduce the risk of pneumothorax (Duong et al., 2014).

Several epidemiological studies have highlighted the interplay between neonatal pneumothorax and socioeconomic status, emphasizing the need for equitable access to healthcare.

Pathophysiology

Pneumothorax results from alveolar overdistension and rupture, which leads to air leakage into the pleural space. This air accumulation increases the intrathoracic pressure, compressing the lungs and mediastinum. Reduced lung compliance and impaired venous return contribute to hypoxemia and hemodynamic instability. Common causes include:

- Spontaneous Pneumothorax: Often occurs in healthy term neonates because of transient overinflation during initial breaths.
- Secondary Pneumothorax: Associated with underlying conditions such as RDS, pulmonary hypoplasia, or mechanical ventilation-induced barotrauma. Other contributing mechanisms include meconium aspiration, surfactant deficiency, and prolonged labor, all of which increase alveolar stress and susceptibility to rupture.

However, the impact of CPAP use on pneumothorax rates remains controversial. Some studies, such as the COIN trial, have suggested that CPAP use may increase the risk of pneumothorax (Morley et al., 2008). In particular, this risk is more pronounced in late preterm and term neonates with increased lung elasticity, decreased chest wall elasticity, increased lung expandability, and decreased surface tension. In the COIN trial, extremely premature infants born between 25-28 weeks were randomized to CPAP (pressure 8) or intubation after birth. The incidence of pneumothorax was higher in infants who received CPAP. However, other studies, such as the SUPPORT study, did not support this association (Newman et al., 2010; Geary et al., 2008; Smithhart et al., 2019).

Clinical Presentation

The clinical manifestations of neonatal pneumothorax vary according to its severity. Common presentations include the following.

- Mild Cases: Subtle tachypnea or reduced breath sounds on the affected side. They can also be asymptomatic. Asymptomatic pneumothorax occurs in approximately 1% of newborns. It is more common in term and postmature infants. It is usually unilateral and is detected by routine chest radiography in most hospitalizations.
- Moderate Cases: Increased work of breathing, nasal flaring, and intercostal retraction.
- Severe Cases: Marked respiratory distress, cyanosis, and hemodynamic compromise
- Tension Pneumothorax: Mediastinal shift with life-threatening cardiovascular instability

Physical examination may reveal an asymmetric chest rise, diminished air entry, and hyperresonance on percussion. A high index of suspicion is necessary in neonates with abrupt respiratory deterioration, particularly those on mechanical ventilation (Lichtenstein, 2014).

The exact time of onset of pneumothorax is difficult to determine; one study suggests that there may be a delay of 1 to 10 hours between onset and diagnosis (Mcintosh et al., 2000).

Diagnosis

Therefore, it is important to identify and diagnose pneumothorax. Although completely asymptomatic in the first stage, it may progress to tension pneumothorax and cause cardiac arrest. Therefore, a timely and accurate diagnosis is very important. Key diagnostic modalities include the following.

- Clinical Assessment: Observation of respiratory distress and physical findings suggestive of pneumothorax. On blood gas assessment, infants may develop hypercarbia and hypoxemia, which are more common in premature infants.
- Transillumination: Useful in emergency settings, particularly for preterm infants. However, their accuracy and reliability are not fully understood.
- Imaging:
  - Chest X-ray: Diagnosis was confirmed by showing air in the pleural cavity and a collapsed lung. Radiographically, in the case of pneumothorax, the lung markings are asymmetric, with the affected side appearing more transparent (black) due to the accumulation of air outside the lung. The edge of the visceral pleura may be visible, and more peripheral lung markings may be reduced. In cases of tension pneumothorax, the mediastinum shifts away from the affected side. Small pneumothoraxes may be difficult to recognize on an anteroposterior chest radiograph, and detection can be improved using a lateral or lateral decubitus (suspected side up) radiograph.
  - Ultrasound: Ultrasound is increasingly used because of its safety and reliability, especially in unstable infants (Lichtenstein, 2014). The absence of sliding motion in the pleura and the presence of a

barcode sign in the M mode on lung USG are typical. In addition, mirror reflections of the costae can be observed.

- CT Scan: Rarely utilized but may offer detailed insights into complex or refractory cases.

Emerging technologies, such as artificial intelligence-based image analysis, show promise for improving diagnostic accuracy, especially in resource-constrained environments.

Management

However, there is a lack of clear guidelines for the treatment of pneumothorax in neonates. Treatment depends on the age of the infant, the degree of symptoms, the size of the pneumothorax, whether there is an ongoing air leak or tension pneumothorax, whether the infant has underlying lung disease, and ventilator use. Management strategies for neonatal pneumothorax depend on its severity and underlying etiology.

- Observation: Small asymptomatic pneumothorax often resolves spontaneously. Infants are more likely to not require treatment, especially those without underlying lung disease. Furthermore, Litmanovitz and Carlo showed that symptomatic newborns requiring respiratory support could be managed by waiting. Predictors of successful standby management include increased gestational age, low respiratory support requirements, and normal blood gas levels (Litmanovitz & Carlo, 2008).
- Needle Aspiration: Immediate relief of tension pneumothorax using a 22-gauge needle inserted into the second intercostal space at the midclavicular line (Figure 1).
- Chest Tube Placement: Required for large or recurrent pneumothorax. For optimal placement, the chest tube should be inserted in the fourth or fifth intercostal space (Figure 2), located between the anterior and midaxillary lines (referred to as the modified Buelau position). This specific site is deemed appropriate for both thoracic sides in preterm and term infants, as it only involves the lung tissue without affecting other organs. Selecting this lateral location prevents scarring in the front of the chest and nipple region. The tube

was subsequently attached to a water-sealed drainage mechanism (Gomella, Eyal, & Bany-Mohammed, 2020). When active treatment is required, there is insufficient evidence regarding whether thoracentesis or thoracostomy and chest tube placement should be performed. A review of two recent studies suggested that initial thoracentesis, especially when an angiocath is used and left in place, may eventually prevent the need for thoracostomy and chest tube placement. Supporting these findings, a more recent randomized trial showed that thoracostomy and chest tube placement could be avoided in some infants initially treated with thoracentesis, requiring only three patients to be treated (Bruschettini et al., 2019; Murphy et al., 2018). Complications of thoracostomy and chest tube placement include lung injury, infection at the insertion site and in the lung, phrenic nerve injury, chylothorax, hemorrhagic pericardial effusion, and breast deformities later in life (Reed et al., 2016; Rainer et al., 2003) (Figure 2).

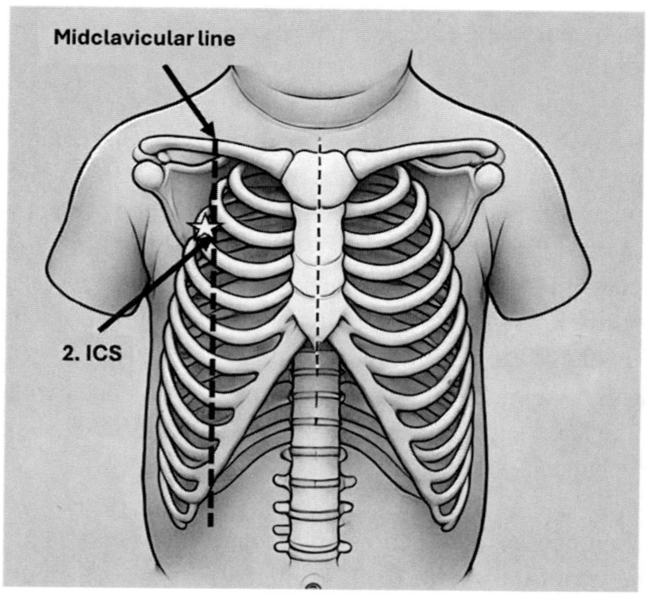

Figure 1. Midclavicular line.

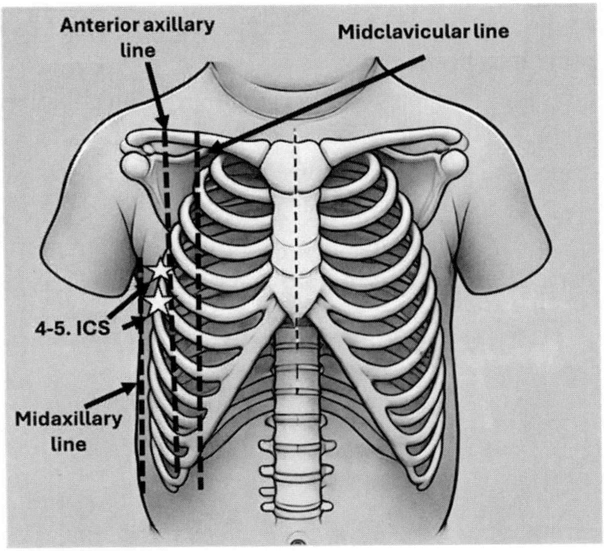

Figure 2. Midaxillary line.

- Supportive Care: Includes oxygen supplementation, mechanical ventilation adjustments, and treatment of underlying conditions such as sepsis or RDS. For hypoxic infants, supplemental oxygen is only used as needed, and sufficient oxygen is administered to maintain oxygen levels within the targeted pulse oximetry range (92–95%). The use of FiO2 at 100% has not been shown to accelerate the resorption of pneumothorax. Therefore, its use may result in unnecessary oxygen exposure (Clark et al., 2014; Shaireen et al., 2014).

Additional treatment options for difficult-to-control or persistent pneumothorax include pleurectomy, chemical pleurodesis, and selective intubation of the bronchus to bypass the lung.

Prevention and Prognosis

Preventive strategies aim to minimize the risk factors, particularly barotrauma, in ventilated neonates. Key measures include:

- Optimizing ventilator settings to avoid excessive pressures

- The use of less invasive respiratory support methods such as CPAP or nasal high-flow therapy.
- Administering antenatal steroids to improve lung maturity in preterm infants
- Ensuring timely surfactant administration in neonates with RDS.

Prognosis varies with the underlying cause and promptness of treatment. Although most cases resolve without long-term consequences, severe or delayed treatment can result in chronic lung disease or neurological impairment.

Conclusion

Neonatal pneumothorax remains a critical condition that requires prompt recognition and intervention. Advances in neonatal care have improved outcomes; however, challenges persist in prevention and early diagnosis. Multidisciplinary collaboration and adherence to evidence-based practices are essential for reducing the morbidity and mortality associated with neonatal pneumothorax.

References

Avery's Diseases of the Newborn. (2024). *Elsevier*. https://doi.org/10.1016/c2020-0-02133-x.

Bruschettini, M., Calevo, M. G., Romantsik, O., Zappettini, S., & O'Donnell, C. P. (2019). Needle aspiration versus intercostal tube drainage for pneumothorax in the newborn. *Cochrane Database of Systematic Reviews, 2*(2). https://doi.org/10.1002/14651858.cd011724.pub3.

Clark, S. D., Schneeberger, M. T., Littner, Y., Park, E., Saker, F., Sutton, D. W., … Saker, F. (2014). Administration of 100% oxygen does not hasten resolution of symptomatic spontaneous pneumothorax in neonates. *Journal of Perinatology, 34*(7), 528–531. https://doi.org/10.1038/jp.2014.55.

Duong, H. H., Yang, J., Mirea, L., Lee, S. K., Shah, P. S., & Sankaran, K. (2014). Pneumothorax in neonates: Trends, predictors and outcomes. *Journal of Neonatal-Perinatal Medicine, 7*(1), 29–38. https://doi.org/10.3233/npm-1473813.

Geary, C., Caskey, M., Fonseca, R., & Malloy, M. (2008). Decreased incidence of bronchopulmonary dysplasia after early management changes, including surfactant and nasal continuous positive airway pressure treatment at delivery, lowered oxygen saturation goals, and early amino acid administration: A historical cohort study. *Pediatrics, 121*(1), 89–96. https://doi.org/10.1542/peds.2007-0225.

Gomella, T. L., Eyal, F. G., & Bany-Mohammed, F. (Eds.). (2020). *Gomella's neonatology: Management, procedures, on-call problems, diseases, and drugs* (8th ed.). McGraw-Hill Education. https://accesspediatrics.mhmedical.com/book.aspx?bookid=2762.

Lichtenstein, D. A. (2014). Lung ultrasound in the critically ill. *Annals of Intensive Care, 4*(1), 1. https://doi.org/10.1186/2110-5820-4-1.

Litmanovitz, I., & Carlo, W. A. (2008). Expectant management of pneumothorax in ventilated neonates. *Pediatrics, 122*(5), e975–e979. https://doi.org/10.1542/peds.2008-1269.

McIntosh, N., Badger, P., Stenson, B., Lyon, A. J., Becher, J.-C., Cunningham, S., & Laing, I. A. (2000). Clinical diagnosis of pneumothorax is late: Use of trend data and decision support might allow preclinical detection. *Pediatric Research, 48*(3), 408–415. https://doi.org/10.1203/00006450-200009000-00025.

Morley, C. J., Doyle, L. W., Brion, L. P., Davis, P. G., Carlin, J. B., & Hascoet, J.-M. (2008). Nasal CPAP or intubation at birth for very preterm infants. *New England Journal of Medicine, 358*(7), 700–708. https://doi.org/10.1056/nejmoa072788.

Murphy, M. C., Blennow, M., O'Donnell, C. P. F., Doglioni, N., Heiring, C., Lista, G., Trevisanuto, D., Bohlin, K., & Stucchi, I. (2018). Effect of needle aspiration of pneumothorax on subsequent chest drain insertion in newborns. *JAMA Pediatrics, 172*(7), 664. https://doi.org/10.1001/jamapediatrics.2018.0623.

Newman, N., Bell, E., Buchter, S., Ambalavanan, N., Walsh, M., Meurs, K., Sood, B., Watterberg, K., Yoder, B., Frantz, I., Cotten, C., Gantz, M., Poole, W., Narendran, V., Das, A., Rich, W., Duara, S., O'Shea, T., Faix, R., … Higgins, R. (2010). Early CPAP versus surfactant in extremely preterm infants. *New England Journal of Medicine, 362*(21), 1970–1979. https://doi.org/10.1056/nejmoa0911783.

Rainer, C., Frühwirth, M., Fritsch, H., Meirer, R., Gardetto, A., Trawöger, R., & Piza-Katzer, H. (2003). Breast deformity in adolescence as a result of pneumothorax drainage during neonatal intensive care. *Pediatrics, 111*(1), 80–86. https://doi.org/10.1542/peds.111.1.80.

Reed, R. C., Waters, B. L., & Siebert, J. R. (2016). Complications of percutaneous thoracostomy in neonates and infants. *Journal of Perinatology, 36*(4), 296–299. https://doi.org/10.1038/jp.2015.190.

Shaireen, H., Metcalfe, A., Kamaluddeen, M., Lodha, A., Rabi, Y., Akierman, A., & Amin, H. (2014). Impact of oxygen concentration on time to resolution of spontaneous pneumothorax in term infants: A population-based cohort study. *BMC Pediatrics, 14*(1). https://doi.org/10.1186/1471-2431-14-208.

Smithhart, W., Wyckoff, M. H., Jaleel, M., Kakkilaya, V., Brion, L. P., Nelson, D. B., Kapadia, V., & Brown, L. S. (2019). Delivery room continuous positive airway pressure and pneumothorax. *Pediatrics, 144*(3). https://doi.org/10.1542/peds.2019-0756.

Chapter 3

Congenital Diaphragmatic Hernias

Aytaç Taşcı[1], MD

Department of Pediatric Surgery, Sinop Atatürk State Hospital, Sinop, Turkey

Abstract

Congenital diaphragmatic hernia (CDH), one of the most common anomalies observed in newborns, is characterized by the passage of intra-abdominal organs into the thorax due to a developmental defect in the diaphragm (Soyer, 2019). The clinical presentation of CDH varies depending on the degree of pulmonary hypoplasia and pulmonary hypertension, ranging from asymptomatic cases to severe mortality (Moyer et al., 2002; Wilson et al., 1997). Despite advances in antenatal diagnostic methods, surgical techniques, and neonatal intensive care, mortality and morbidity rates for CDH remain high (Moyer et al., 2002; Wilson et al., 1997; Bohn et al., 1996; Stoll et al., 2008). CDH has been the subject of numerous studies and books.

Keywords: congenital diaphragmatic hernia, bochdalek hernia, morgagni hernia

Introduction

Congenital Diaphragmatic Hernia (CDH) is an anomaly that can occur in 1-4 cases per 10,000 live births, usually accompanied by cardiac, genitourinary, gastrointestinal, respiratory, and central nervous system anomalies, and can

---

[1] Corresponding Author's Email: dr_aytactasci@hotmail.com

In: Current Approaches to Newborn Emergencies
Editors: Zuhal Keskin Sarılar and Serap Samut Bülbül
ISBN: 979-8-89530-999-5

very often lead to deaths in the intrauterine and early neonatal period. Diaphragmatic hernias are divided into two main groups: congenital and acquired. Acquired diaphragmatic hernias are classified as traumatic and iatrogenic hernias. Congenital diaphragmatic hernias are classified as left posterior lateral defect (Bochdalek), anterior defect (Morgagni), peritoneopericardial central growth hernia (septum transverse type), diaphragm eventration, hiatal hernia, paraesophageal hernia, and other rare forms (Skandalakis, 2004). Among congenital hernias, Bochdalek and Morgagni types constitute 95-98% of CDH. Left CDH (Bochdalek) is seen in 80-85% and usually herniates into the bowel loops, spleen, stomach, liver, and rarely the kidneys and adrenal thorax. Left diaphragmatic hernia is usually seen in 80%; 20% is on the right side, and it is very rarely bilateral. Bilateral CDH is seen in 5%, and most result in death due to lung hypoplasia. Since it is the most common type seen in the clinic, the term congenital diaphragmatic hernia (CDH) will be used for Bochdalek hernia in the rest of the article.

Etiology and Pathophysiology

The etiology of CDH, typically sporadic, is not fully understood. The existence of a wide variety of hernia types has led to the emergence of many theories. The most emphasized of these theories is that the abdominal internal organs herniate from the diaphragm to the thorax as a result of inadequate closure of the pleuroperitoneal canal, resulting in pulmonary hypoplasia due to compression of the organs in the thorax, while the other most advocated view claims that diaphragmatic hernia results from the developmental insufficiency of the lung bud due to various embryological accidents (Bremer, 1943; Greer et al., 2000). It is suggested that parenchymal deficiency due to pulmonary hypoplasia leads to failure of diaphragm fusion/contraction, and intestinal organs migrate to the thorax to fill this deficiency (Iritani, 1984). However, there is no complete theory explaining the etiology of CDH. Recent studies have identified teratogenic substances like 2,4-dichloro-phenyl-p-nitrophenyl (Nifedipine), which prevent the conversion of retinoic acid to retinaldehyde, as factors contributing to the formation of posterolateral CDH formation, and this situation is beginning to suggest vitamin A deficiencies in the etiology (Mey et al., 2003). Although the exact cause of CDH is unknown, its consequences on lung development are well known. During the early development of the diaphragm, the midgut herniates into the tuber sac. If the pleuroperitoneal canal does not close when the midgut returns to the abdomen at 9–10 weeks of gestation, the abdominal viscera herniate into the ipsilateral thoracic cavity through the lumbocostal trigone. The resulting abnormal position of the bowel prevents its normal counterclockwise rotation and fixation. If the event occurs before complete closure of the pleuroperitoneal canal, a hernia sac does not form, but a nonmuscular membrane may form a hernia sac in 10-15% of patients with CDH, and CDH is usually noticeable after the first 12 weeks of gestation (Stolar & Dillon, 2012). Pulmonary development and parallel pulmonary vascular development are disrupted in the later weeks of gestation. The herniation process usually coincides with the time of bronchial subdivision, and the number of bronchiole branches and the number and development of alveoli decrease bilaterally, with the number and development of bronchioles being greater on the affected side (Stolar & Dillon, 2012; Dibbins, 1978). Abnormal septae are observed in the alveoli and terminal sacs, disrupting the air-capillary interface that limits gas exchange (Suen et al., 1993). In addition, these alveoli have increased glycogen content, leading to thickened secretions that further limit gas exchange. This results in fewer alveoli, thickened alveolar walls, increased interstitial tissue, and a markedly reduced alveolar airspace and gas exchange area in CDH patients. CDH infants have significantly fewer pulmonary parenchymal arterioles, and significant adventitial and medial wall thickening has been noted in the pulmonary arteries, with abnormal muscularization of the small preacinar and intraacinar arterioles and decreased endogenous surfactant synthesis (Suen et al., 1993; Moya et al., 1995). The physiological consequence of this abnormal arterial muscularization may be an increased susceptibility to the development of fixed and persistent pulmonary hypertension.

The permanent increase in pulmonary vascular resistance at the end of the fetal circulation with birth causes an increase in pulmonary artery pressures and a decrease in pulmonary vascular blood flow. The increased vascular resistance causes right-to-left shunting of blood at the atrial or ductal levels, together with the delivery of unsaturated blood to the systemic circulation. As blood flow in the shunt increases, oxygen saturation in the systemic circulation decreases further, and mixed venous blood returning to the right side of the heart becomes increasingly desaturated. Hypoxia with the first breath due to pulmonary hypoplasia deepens, further increasing pulmonary vascular resistance and compromising pulmonary blood flow, increasing right-to-left shunt flow. Severe and progressive respiratory failure occurs due to pulmonary vascular changes and is induced by known stimuli of pulmonary hypertension, including hypoxia, acidosis, hypothermia, and stress. Recent studies have also shown that various prostaglandins, leukotrienes, and catecholamines are secreted by pulmonary vascular structures in CDH infants, triggering persistent pulmonary hypertension (Stolar & Dillon, 2012; Kobayashi & Puri, 1994; Taira et al., 1998).

Diagnosis

CDH can be diagnosed in up to 90% of cases using antenatal ultrasonography (US) today, and furthermore, the prognosis is determined with US, guiding the delivery to be carried out in a hospital where there are teams specialized in newborns that provide appropriate intervention conditions for the baby (Stolar & Dillon, 2012). CDH is usually diagnosed with US performed in the 2nd trimester, and the earliest case diagnosed is at the 11th week in the literature (Stolar & Dillon, 2012). CDH in US is interpreted as a sign of poor prognosis if it is noticed in early pregnancy weeks, lung-to-head ratio (LHR) is below 1 between the 24th and 26th gestational weeks, presence of more than 50% liver in the thorax in right hernias, presence of any of the liver, stomach, and spleen in the thorax in left hernias, absence of a hernia sac, small fetal lung in 3D US and magnetic resonance (MR) imaging. The antenatal differential diagnosis for CDH includes congenital pulmonary airway malformations (CPAM), other pulmonary anomalies such as bronchogenic cysts, and mediastinal lesions such as neuroenteric or thymic cysts (Jeanty et al., 2007; Kosiński & Wielgoś, 2017). In these cases, normal intra-abdominal anatomy is not disrupted. On US, the presence of abdominal organs in the thorax, polyhydramnios, and mediastinal shift to the right may be among the findings of CDH. However, US may not provide clear information due to reasons such as lack of experience of the person performing the positioning of the fetus, and in these cases, antenatal MRI may be needed. MRI, which is thought to be more useful, especially in terms of prognosis, is superior to prenatal USG by being more specific in terms of liver herniation and being able to clearly measure fetal lung volume (Taira et al., 1998; Kosiński &Wielgoś, 2017).

CDH should be suspected in newborns with severe respiratory distress after birth, retraction of accessory respiratory muscles, a scaphoid abdomen due to herniation of intra-abdominal organs into the thorax, and an increased chest-anterior-arc diameter. Diagnosis is supported by decreased or absent lung sounds on the side with herniation during auscultation, bowel sounds being heard, and the heartbeat being heard on the opposite side (Figure 1, Bochdalek type diaphragmatic hernia in which the stomach and intestinal loops are located in the thorax along with cardiac shift). Respiratory distress due to pulmonary hypoplasia and displacement of the large main vessels and trachea may disrupt venous return and lead to hypotension and cyanosis. These babies can be diagnosed very easily with a radiograph (Figure 2, Bochdalek-type diaphragmatic hernia). However, in newborns with CDH of 2-20%, there is no clinical finding at the time of birth, and respiratory distress may begin within 24-48 hours, while some CDH cases may be diagnosed later in life with milder respiratory symptoms, chronic pulmonary infections, pleural effusions, pneumonias, feeding intolerance, or gastric volvulus. The clinical course is generally much better in cases without respiratory distress at birth (Manning et al., 1992; Paut et al., 1996).

Although many factors related to the anatomical and physiological postnatal period have been presented to determine the prognosis in CDH, no factor is sufficient to determine the mortality rate. Diagnosis before the 24th week of intrauterine life, especially the location of the liver and the lung-to-head ratio (LHR<1 indicates poor prognosis, LHR > 1.4 indicates good prognosis), low cardioventricular and cardiovascular indices, a McGoon index below 1.3, accompanying additional anomalies, right-sided CDH, the presence of polyhydramnios and stomach herniation have been associated with poor prognosis (Stolar & Dillon, 2012; Kobayashi & Puri, 1994; Kosiński & Wielgoś, 2017; Manning et al., 1992; Paut et al., 1996). In a study conducted by the CDH Study Group, low birth weight, low 5th minute APGAR score, the presence of chromosomal or major cardiac anomalies, and the presence of suprasystemic pulmonary hypertension have been interpreted in favor of poor prognosis (Brindle et al., 2014). It is recommended that all newborns with CDH be investigated for additional cardiac, urinary, neurological, and chromosomal anomalies after birth.

Treatment

Presurgical Management

Advances in obstetric methods have led to an increase in antenatal CDH diagnoses, allowing families to receive prenatal counseling. Since respiratory distress may begin at birth in newborns with CDH, it is recommended that all CDH patients be directed to centers with prenatal and advanced neonatal critical care facilities.

Medical methods such as steroids and thyrotropin-releasing hormones and surgical methods such as fetal tracheal occlusion have been tried to positively affect intrauterine prognosis, but there is no data on the positive contribution of these methods to prognosis, and their routine use is not recommended (Lally et al., 2006; Liao et al., 2000).

The main goal in patients with CDH is to maintain cardiopulmonary stabilization after birth, to prevent hypoxia with hypercapnia, and to avoid expansion of abdominal organs located in the thorax (Reiss et al., 2010). For this purpose, newborns with CDH should be intubated very gently and then decompressed with a nasogastric tube. During intubation, barotrauma and hyperinsufflation that may develop in the hypoplastic lung should be avoided, and ventilation should never be done with a mask, as this will cause air to enter the stomach. Sedation can be applied during intubation, but there is no need to use muscle relaxants (Reiss et al., 2010). Preductal and umbilical catheterizations are recommended for monitoring acid-base balance, oxygenation level, and metabolic levels such as lactate.

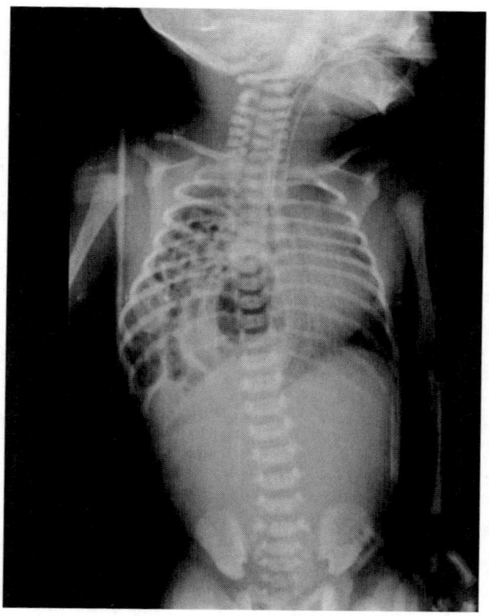

Figure 1. Bochdalek-type diaphragmatic hernia in which the stomach and intestinal loops are located in the thorax, along with cardiac shift.

As a result of increasing scientific data on the pathophysiology of CDH, emergency surgery to reposition the intra-abdominal organs in the thorax and repair the hernia sac has been moved away from the practice of surgery and directed towards delayed surgical repair after cardiorespiratory and hemodynamic stability.

Ventilation strategies in infants with CDH vary from patient to patient, but the aim should be to avoid mechanical ventilator-related lung injury while providing oxygenation. It should not be forgotten that inadequate ventilation will exacerbate pulmonary hypertension, increase pulmonary vascular resistance, and lead to deepening hypoxia and acidosis. In particular, to protect cerebral perfusion, preductal saturation should be maintained above 85%, CO2 pressure should be kept below 60 mmHg, and moderate hypercapnia should be acceptable as long as blood gas pH is > 7.2. For this purpose, higher respiratory rates and lower peak airway pressures (18-22 cm H2O) are generally used (Reiss et al., 2010). Tidal volume increases are inversely proportional to frequency and should be performed with caution because they may cause hyperinflation and compromise venous return. Optimal lung volume can be roughly measured by the expansion of the eighth rib in the contralateral hemithorax as a guide in the clinic (Reyes et al., 1998). Continuous assessment of acid-base status and end-organ perfusion is necessary because lung compliance may change before and after CDH repair.

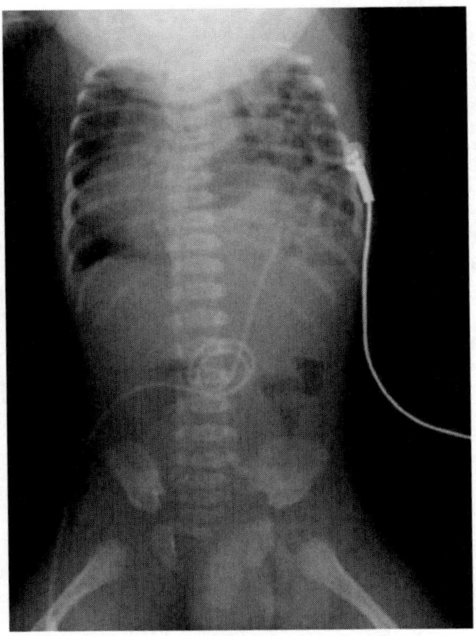

Figure 2. Bochdalek-type diaphragmatic hernia.

Despite appropriate ventilation therapy in CDH newborns, the major cause of mortality is pulmonary hypertension, and the aim should be to reduce pulmonary vascular resistance in these infants. For this purpose, iNO, a powerful vasodilator, has been used; although it has reduced respiratory failure and increased oxygenation, studies have shown that it is not effective in the treatment of mortality and pulmonary hypertension (Oliveira et al., 2000; Neonatal Inhaled Nitric Oxide Study Group [NINOS], 1997). For this purpose, new agents such as calcium channel blockers, phosphodiesterase inhibitor (PDE) 5 inhibitor sildenafil, PDE 3 inhibitor milrinone, prostaglandins or endothelin-1 receptor antagonists, L-citrulline, and Rho-kinase inhibitors, or proliferator-activated receptor-γ agonists are currently being investigated (Lakshminrusimha et al., 2016).

There are publications showing that surfactant has no mortality benefit in the treatment of CDH and that it increases chronic lung damage and the need for extracorporeal membrane oxygenation (Lally et al., 2016). If persistent pulmonary hypertension continues in newborns with CDH despite appropriate medical treatment and maximum mechanical ventilation, ECMO treatment has been increasingly used as a part of stabilization since 1977 (Morini et al., 2006; Puligandla et al., 2015). Although the success rate varies between 40 and 80% in different centers, there are also studies claiming that ECMO has no effect on survival (Morini et al., 2006).

In the treatment of CDH, appropriate fluid management and the use of inotropic agents such as dopamine, dobutamine, and epinephrine in patients who require it, and bicarbonate support for metabolic acidosis are of vital importance. Adequate sedation and pain management should be used without muscle relaxants. Surgery should not be performed until the baby is stable in terms of ventilation and circulation, and for this purpose, blood gas values and diuresis of the baby should be closely monitored (Puligandla et al., 2015).

Surgery and Postoperative Management and Long-Term Problems

Since the first surgical repair by Gros in 1948, there have been significant advancements in the surgical approach to CDH (Soyer, 2020). Emergency surgical repair has given way to delayed surgical repair, and in recent years there has been a shift from open surgery to minimally invasive surgery, especially in patients with late diagnoses. The surgical method to be applied varies according to the experience of the surgeon, the characteristics of the patient, and the location and size of the hernia sac, and in recent years the number of centers reporting minimally invasive repair has increased considerably. Laparotomy has the advantages of easy reduction of the abdominal organs with good visibility and the recognition and correction of associated gastrointestinal anomalies. The intestines and colon should be gently reduced to the abdomen first, followed by the spleen in left-sided hernias and the liver in right-sided hernias. After reduction, the hernia should be clearly defined, and the hernia sac, if any, should be removed and then repaired with primary sutures, or if it is too large to be closed primarily, with absorbable or non-absorbable patches, natural or synthetic, planned for this purpose, without any intervention for other accompanying pathologies such as malrotation. The application of tube thoracostomy after repair is a controversial issue.

The first laparoscopic CDH repair was performed in 1995 and thoracoscopically in 2001 (Soyer, 2020). Although right CDH and large hernia sac cases were not initially considered suitable for minimally invasive repair, successful case results have recently been reported in these patients. Minimally invasive techniques, which provide less postoperative pain, less surgical stress, and a better cosmetic appearance, may also carry the risks of hypercapnia-related acidosis and increased pulmonary shunting due to CO2 insufflation (Bliss et al., 2009). In addition, meta-analysis studies indicate that recurrences are higher after repair with minimally invasive techniques, but it is hoped that this situation will decrease with the development of techniques (Lansdale et al., 2010).

In CDH cases that survive the neonatal period and cling to life, chronic pulmonary changes secondary to pulmonary hypoplasia and pulmonary hypertension can be observed more frequently in later periods of life, especially in patients with frequently recurring respiratory tract infections, obstructive or restrictive lung diseases, and in patients who undergo surgical repair with ECMO and patches (Tsao & Lally, 2019). In addition, neurologically, delays in neuromotor development, learning difficulties, EEG abnormalities, visual loss, sensorineural hearing loss, and, rarely, cerebral palsy and intraventricular hemorrhages can be observed in these patients. Again, gastroesophageal reflux and dysmotility problems in the gastrointestinal system and chest wall anomalies and scoliosis in the skeletal system are frequently observed in these patients (Soyer, 2020; Tsao & Lally, 2019).

Anterior Diaphragm Hernia (Morgagni Hernia)

It constitutes 2% of all diaphragmatic hernias, and the defect is between the septum transversum, which is the passage route of the superior epigastric artery known as Larrey space, and the chest wall. In Morgagni hernia, which is usually diagnosed at a later age, the defect is on the right side in 90% of cases and bilateral in 8% (Corbett & Losty, 2009). The small intestines, colon, omentum, and right lobe of the liver can be found in the most commonly observed sac. Chromosomal anomalies, cardiac anomalies, and midline defects can often accompany it. Although it varies clinically, epigastric discomfort, intermittent vomiting, recurrent respiratory tract infections, abdominal pain, and, very rarely, volvulus can be encountered (Tsao & Lally, 2019; Corbett & Losty, 2009). As seen in the graphs below (Figure 3 and Figure 4), although chest radiography is usually sufficient for diagnosis, sometimes contrast-enhanced chest radiography or, usually, computed tomography imaging may be required for small hernias. Surgical repair is recommended since it can rarely lead to volvulus.

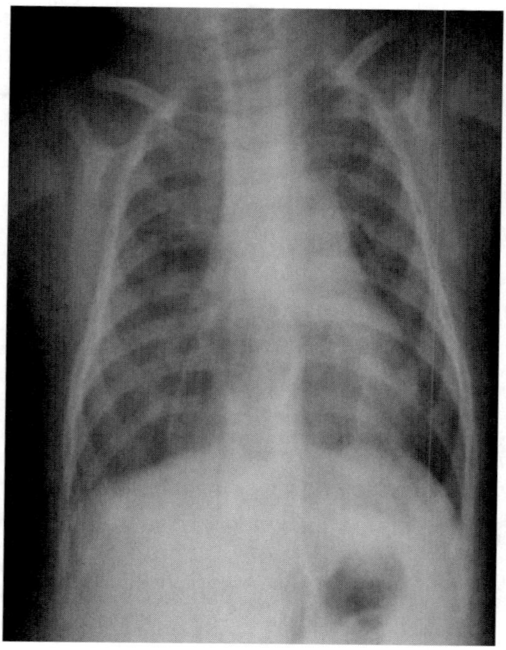

Figure 3. Morgagni hernia in chest radiography.

Diaphragm Eventration

Diaphragm eventration, which causes a paradoxical respiratory movement, describes the abnormal elevation of the diaphragm. It can occur congenitally due to intrauterine nerve and muscle development anomalies, or it can be acquired as a result of phrenic nerve damage caused by various reasons, especially cardiac surgery and brachial plexus injuries (Yazıcı et al., 2003; Akay et al., 2006). Although it is usually diagnosed with chest radiography, fluoroscopy and US may be required for diagnosis in order to see the paradoxical condition. Even though it is mostly asymptomatic, surgical treatment is rarely required in its congenital form, which causes functional pulmonary disorders or recurrent respiratory tract infections. In its acquired form, surgery is often required because extubation cannot be achieved.

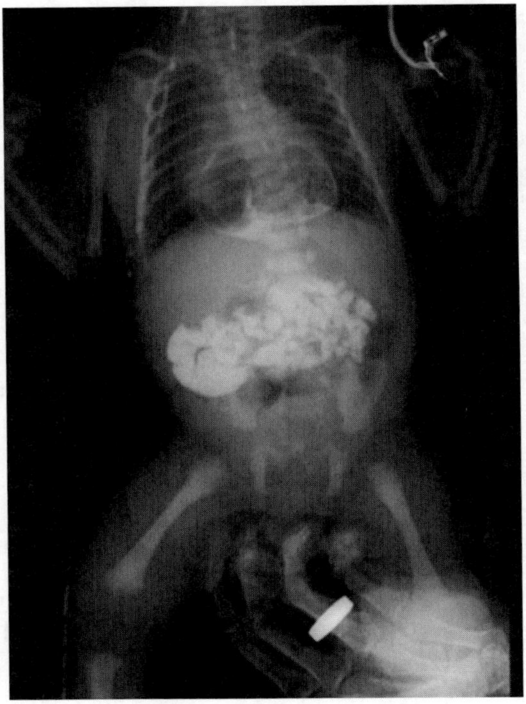

Figure 4. Contrast radiography of a patient.

Conclusion

Despite increasing knowledge and expertise in managing CDH, mortality and morbidity rates remain high. The unknown fetal mortality rate associated with CDH conceals the actual number of cases. It is hoped that the mortality and morbidity rates, which have already been reduced due to advances in ECMO, neonatal intensive care units, newly developed medications, and improvements in surgical techniques, will continue to decrease further.

References

Akay, T. H., Özkan, S., Gültekin, B., Uguz, E., Varan, B., Sezgin, A., Tokel, K., & Aslamacı, S. (2006). Diaphragmatic paralysis after cardiac surgery in children: Incidence, prognosis, and surgical management. *Pediatric Surgery International, 22*(4), 341–346. https://doi.org/10.1007/s00383-006-1704-0.

Bliss, D., Matar, M., & Krishnaswami, S. (2009). Should intraoperative hypercapnea or hypercarbia raise concern in neonates undergoing thoracoscopic repair of diaphragmatic hernia of Bochdalek? *Journal of Laparoendoscopic & Advanced Surgical Techniques, 19*(Suppl. 1), S55–S58.

Bohn, D. J., Pearl, R., Irish, M. S., Schreiber, R., Harrison, M., Finley, R., & Moes, C. (1996). Postnatal management of congenital diaphragmatic hernia. *Clinical Perinatology, 23*(6), 843–872.

Bremer, J. L. (1943). The diaphragm and diaphragmatic hernia. *Archives of Pathology, 36*(5), 539.

Brindle, M. E., Cook, E. F., Tibboel, D., Lally, P. A., & Lally, K. P. (2014). A clinical prediction rule for the severity of congenital diaphragmatic hernias in newborns. *Pediatrics, 134*(3), e413–e419.

Corbett, H. J., & Losty, P. D. (2009). Congenital diaphragmatic hernia. In D. K. Parikh, D. C. G. Crabbe, A. W. Auldist, & S. Rothenberg (Eds.), *Pediatric thoracic surgery* (pp. 483–500). Springer.

Dibbins, A. W. (1978). Congenital diaphragmatic hernia: Hypoplastic lung and pulmonary vasoconstriction. *Clinical Perinatology, 5*(1), 93–104.

Greer, J. J., Allan, D. W., Babiuk, R. P., Beasley, C. R., McElroy, S. J., McMillin, R. D., & Mitchell, J. D. (2000). Recent advances in understanding the pathogenesis of nitrofen-induced congenital diaphragmatic hernia. *Pediatric Pulmonology, 29*(5), 394–399.

Iritani, I. (1984). Experimental study on embryogenesis of congenital diaphragmatic hernia. *Anatomy and Embryology, 169*(2), 133–139.

Jeanty, C., Nien, J. K., Espinoza, J., Kageyama, T., & Gonçalves, L. F. (2007). Pleural and pericardial effusion: A potential ultrasonographic marker for the prenatal differential diagnosis between congenital diaphragmatic eventration and congenital diaphragmatic hernia. *Ultrasound in Obstetrics & Gynecology, 29*(3), 378–387.

Kobayashi, H., & Puri, P. (1994). Plasma endothelin levels in congenital diaphragmatic hernia. *Journal of Pediatric Surgery, 29*(9), 1258–1261.

Kosiński, P., & Wielgoś, M. (2017). Congenital diaphragmatic hernia: Pathogenesis, prenatal diagnosis and management. Literature review. *Ginekologia Polska, 88*(1), 24–30.

Lakshminrusimha, S., Mathew, B., & Leach, C. L. (2016). Pharmacologic strategies in neonatal pulmonary hypertension other than nitric oxide. *Seminars in Perinatology*.

Lally, K. P., Bagolan, P., Hosie, S., Lally, K. P. Jr., Anselmo, M., & Bizzarri, C. (2006). Corticosteroids for fetuses with congenital diaphragmatic hernia: Can we show benefit? *Journal of Pediatric Surgery, 41*(5), 668–674.

Lally, K. P., Lally, P. A., Langham, M. R., Rellinger, E. J., Lally, K. P. Jr., & Lee, H. K. (2004). Surfactant does not improve survival rate in preterm infants with congenital diaphragmatic hernia. *Journal of Pediatric Surgery, 39*(6), 829–833.

Lansdale, N., Alam, S., Losty, P. D., & Jesudason, E. C. (2010). Neonatal endosurgical congenital diaphragmatic hernia repair: A systematic review and meta-analysis. *Annals of Surgery, 252*(1), 20–26.

Liao, L. S., Luks, F. I., Piasecki, G. J., Wild, Y. K., Papadakis, K., & Paepe, M. E. de. (2000). Late gestation tracheal occlusion in the fetal lamb causes rapid lung growth with type II cell preservation. *Journal of Surgical Research, 92*(1), 64–70.

Manning, P. B., Murphy, J. P., Raynor, S. C., Wesson, D. E., & Reisch, J. A. (1992). Congenital diaphragmatic hernia presenting due to gastrointestinal complications. *Journal of Pediatric Surgery, 27*(9), 1225–1228.

Mey, J., Babiuk, R. P., Clugston, R., Houghton, R., Greer, J. J., & Allan, D. W. (2003). Retinal dehydrogenase-2 is inhibited by compounds that induce congenital diaphragmatic hernias in rodents. *American Journal of Pathology, 162*(3), 673–679.

Morini, F., Goldman, A., & Pierro, A. (2006). Extracorporeal membrane oxygenation in infants with congenital diaphragmatic hernia: A systematic review of the evidence. *European Journal of Pediatric Surgery, 16*(6), 385–391.

Moya, F. R., Thomas, V. L., Romaguera, J., Lee, H., Castaneda, P. A., & Sweet, D. (1995). Fetal lung maturation in congenital diaphragmatic hernia. *American Journal of Obstetrics and Gynecology, 173*(5), 1401–1405.

Moyer, V., Moya, F., Tibboel, R., Gischler, S., Lally, K. P., & Lally, P. A. (2002). Late versus early surgical correction for congenital diaphragmatic hernia in newborn infants. *Cochrane Database of Systematic Reviews*, CD001695.

Oliveira, C. A., Troster, E. J., & Pereira, C. R. (2000). Inhaled nitric oxide in the management of persistent pulmonary hypertension of the newborn: A meta-analysis. *Revista do Hospital das Clínicas da Faculdade de Medicina da Universidade de São Paulo, 55*(2), 145–154.

Paut, O., Mely, L., Viard, L., Dufresne, L., Dufresne, A., & Pujol, A. (1996). Acute presentation of congenital diaphragmatic hernia past the neonatal period: A life-threatening emergency. *Canadian Journal of Anesthesia, 43*(7), 621–625.

Puligandla, P. S., Grabowski, J., Austin, M., Hedrick, H., Renaud, E., Arnold, M., Fonkalsrud, E., Lally, K. P., Lally, P. A., & DeUgarte, D. A. (2015). Management of congenital diaphragmatic hernia: A systematic review from the APSA outcomes and evidence-based practice committee. *Journal of Pediatric Surgery, 50*(12), 1958–1970.

Reiss, I., Schaible, T., van den Hout, L., Capolupo, I., Allegaert, K., van Heijst, A., DeKoninck, P., Zimmermann, L. J., Jory, A., Perri, T., Diez, M. H., Iacobelli, S., & de Cunto, L. (2010). Standardized postnatal management of infants with congenital diaphragmatic hernia in Europe: The CDH EURO Consortium consensus. *Neonatology, 98*(4), 354–364.

Reyes, C., Chang, L. K., Waffarn, F., Ho, S. B., Hackel, J. A., & Fisher, J. A. (1998). Delayed repair of congenital diaphragmatic hernia with early high frequency oscillatory ventilation during preoperative stabilization. *Journal of Pediatric Surgery, 33*(8), 1010–1016.

Skandalakis, J. (2004). Diaphragm. In *Surgical anatomy: The embryologic and anatomic basis of modern surgery* (pp. 353–392). Paschalidis Medical Publications.

Soyer, T. (2019). Konjenital diyafram hernisi. In E. A. Balcı & M. Özyüksel (Eds.), *Pediatric thoracic surgery* (pp. 297–313). Akademisyen Kitapevi.

Soyer, T. (2020). Doğumsal diyafram hernisi. In İ. H. Ulukaya Durakbaşa & T. Soyer (Eds.), *Çocuklarda cerrahi göğüs hastalıkları* (pp. 363–380). Akademisyen Kitapevi.

Stolar, C. J. H., & Dillon, P. W. (2012). Congenital diaphragmatic hernia and eventration. In A. G. Coran (Ed.), *Pediatric surgery* (7th ed., pp. 809–824). Mosby.

Stoll, C., Alembik, Y., Dott, B., Roth, M. P., & David, E. (2008). Associated malformations in cases with congenital diaphragmatic hernia. *Genetic Counseling, 19*(4), 331–339.

Suen, H. C., Catlin, E. A., Ryan, D. P., Rosenberg, M. I., & Green, J. A. (1993). Biochemical immaturity of lungs in congenital diaphragmatic hernia. *Journal of Pediatric Surgery, 28*(5), 471–475.

Taira, Y., Yamataka, T., Miyazaki, E., & Puri, P. (1998). Adventitial changes in pulmonary vasculature in congenital diaphragmatic hernia complicated by pulmonary hypertension. *Journal of Pediatric Surgery, 33*(4), 382–387.

The Neonatal Inhaled Nitric Oxide Study Group (NINOS). (1997). Inhaled nitric oxide and hypoxic respiratory failure in infants with congenital diaphragmatic hernia. *Pediatrics, 99*(6), 838–845.

Tsao, K., & Lally, K. P. (2016). Congenital diaphragmatic hernia and eventration. In G. W. Holcomb, J. P. Murphy, & D. J. Ostlie (Eds.), *Ashcraft's pediatric surgery* (6th ed., pp. 320–340). W. B. Saunders.

Wilson, J. M., Lund, D. P., Lillehei, C. W., Ricketts, R. R., & Morrow, W. R. (1997). Congenital diaphragmatic hernia–A tale of two cities: The Boston experience. *Journal of Pediatric Surgery, 32*(3), 401–405.

Yazıcı, M., Karaca, I., Arıkan, A., Şahin, A., Bozkurt, A., & Özgür, F. (2003). Congenital eventration of the diaphragm in children: 25 years' experience in three pediatric surgery centers. *European Journal of Pediatric Surgery, 13*(5), 298–301.

Chapter 4

Esophageal Atresia and Tracheoesophageal Fistula

Sema Tural Bozoğlu, MD
Department of Pediatric Surgery, Sinop Atatürk State Hospital, Sinop, Turkey

Abstract

Esophageal atresia (EA) is a congenital anomaly of the esophagus, often associated with a tracheoesophageal fistula (TEF). The incidence of EA varies globally, but it is generally reported as one case per 3000-4500 live births (Alberti et al., 2011). It is the most common congenital anomaly of the esophagus. Approximately 30-60% of infants with EA have accompanying anomalies in the cardiovascular, genitourinary, gastrointestinal, vertebral-skeletal, and nervous systems (Coran et al., 2013). These additional anomalies are important in terms of morbidity and mortality. There are five types of EA, classified based on their anatomical features, with the most common being EA/distal TEF (Holcomb et al., 2020). Antenatal diagnosis can be made in 20-31% of cases (Hunt et al., 2016). Infants without antenatal screening or a prenatal diagnosis typically receive a postnatal diagnosis within the first 24 hours. Excessive secretions are often one of the first signs in these infants. In cases suspected of EA either antenatally or postnatally, the first step is the insertion of an orogastric (OG) catheter and obtaining a posteroanterior (PA) babygram. The sight of the OG catheter tip curled in the proximal esophageal pouch on the radiograph is a key diagnostic sign. Once the diagnosis is confirmed, a catheter should be placed in the upper esophageal pouch for continuous aspiration of secretions, and plans for surgical intervention should be made (Hunt et al., 2016; Spitz, 2007).

In: Current Approaches to Newborn Emergencies
Editors: Zuhal Keskin Sarılar and Serap Samut Bülbül
ISBN: 979-8-89530-999-5

Keywords: esophageal atresia, tracheoesophageal fistula, congenital anomalies

Introduction

Esophageal atresia (EA) is characterized by the absence of continuity in the esophagus and is the most common congenital anomaly of the esophagus (Conforti et al., 2014). It was first described in 1670 by William Durston in the twin of a patient. The classic proximal EA and distal tracheoesophageal fistula (TEF) were first defined by Thomas Gibson in 1696. Over the years, various surgical approaches have been attempted, and in 1939, N.L. Leven and W.T. Ladd, working at two separate centers, diagnosed EA and performed staged surgical procedures, successfully saving their patients (Holder & Ashcraft, 1966). However, the true revolution in the treatment of EA occurred in 1941, when Cameron Haight performed a primary anastomosis with extrapleural intervention in a patient with EA and distal TEF. Although a fistula developed initially, it closed spontaneously, and the patient survived for many years (Muensterer & Berdon, 2015). As a result, today, with a multidisciplinary approach including advancements in surgery, anesthesia, and neonatal care, mortality rates for these conditions have significantly decreased. In fact, survival rates approaching 100% have been achieved in infants weighing over 1500 grams and without major cardiac issues (Alberti et al., 2011).

Epidemiology and Etiology

Although there is no clear information regarding the incidence of EA, it is generally accepted that one case occurs for every 3000-4500 live births (Alberti et al., 2011). The male-to-female ratio has been found to be 1.3 (Sfeir et al., 2013). The risk is higher in first pregnancies. If one of the parents was born with EA, the likelihood of their child having the same condition is increased (Pletcher, 1991). In patients without chromosomal anomalies, it has been shown that advanced maternal age is not associated with EA (Shaw-Smith, 2006). Additionally, EA is more common in twins, with the rate being 2-3 times higher (Orford et al., 2000).

The presence of vertebral defects, anorectal malformations, cardiac anomalies, extremity anomalies, and renal anomalies in conjunction with EA suggests a general disruption in embryogenesis. However, the exact cause of this disruption is not yet known. In cases where a baby with EA also has many additional anomalies, the etiology is not expected to be the same. Therefore, it is believed that multiple external factors may negatively impact the process during the critical period of embryogenesis.

In monozygotic twins, cases where both babies have EA/TEF have been reported. However, in most cases, one twin has EA/TEF while the other is normal. This suggests that developmental events are more significant than genetic factors in the etiology (German et al., 1979).

In the 1990s, pregnant rats were exposed to doxorubicin (adriamycin) to create an experimental EA/TEF model. However, the etiology of this experimental model is not completely clear in comparison to the etiology of EA/TEF in humans (Diez-Pardo et al., 1996).

Embryology

The embryopathogenesis of EA/TEF is not yet fully understood, but it is related to the common embryological development of the esophagus and trachea. The esophagus and trachea, which develop from the foregut region, undergo two different developmental processes during organogenesis: elongation and separation. In the normal embryological development process, by the 32nd day of gestation, the formation of the tracheoesophageal septum is completed, and the trachea and esophagus become separate structures in the fetus. Therefore, any developmental error that might occur in the esophagus or trachea before the 32nd day of gestation can lead to tracheoesophageal anomalies (Skandalakis et al., 1994; Smith, 1957; Crisera et al., 1999; Crisera et al., 2000).

Several theories have been proposed regarding the development of esophageal atresia and tracheoesophageal fistula. These include:

Intraembryonic Pressure Theory: This theory suggests that intraembryonic pressure during the embryonic period can lead to developmental errors. It proposes that pressure changes may prevent the separation of the esophagus and trachea (Crisera et al., 1999; Crisera et al., 2000; Qi & Beasley, 1999).

Epithelial Obstruction Theory: This theory attributes developmental disruptions in the esophagus and trachea to problems in the epithelial tissue. It argues that these issues obstruct normal organ development (Qi et al., 2001).

Altered Growth Theory: This theory suggests that changes in the growth phases of the organs prevent the proper development of the esophagus and trachea (Crisera et al., 1999; Crisera et al., 2000; Orford et al., 2001; Williams et al., 2000; Zhou et al., 1999; Xia et al., 1999).

Vascular Theory: This theory proposes that insufficient blood flow or abnormal vascular development could lead to tracheoesophageal anomalies (Qi & Beasley, 1999).

However, none of these theories have been able to explain all the variations of congenital anomalies. Therefore, it is accepted that the development of EA and TEF is shaped by the influence of multiple factors, and this remains an unresolved issue.

Associated Anomalies

The negative effects of the development and separation processes of the esophagus and trachea during fetal development can cause issues across all systems, leading to additional anomalies in patients with EA. The frequency of associated anomalies in patients diagnosed with EA ranges between 30-60%. It is lowest in isolated TEF cases (27%) and highest in isolated EA cases (60%) (Coran et al., 2013). Therefore, every baby diagnosed with EA should be carefully examined for associated anomalies. The reason for the importance of these additional anomalies is that they are the most significant factors determining mortality and morbidity in these patients.

Associated anomalies can be classified into minor and major anomalies. Minor anomalies are those that do not threaten life and do not require urgent intervention. Examples include hypertrophic pyloric stenosis, Meckel's diverticulum, cleft lip and palate, aberrant right subclavian vein, vertebral anomalies, and limb anomalies. Major anomalies, on the other hand, are life-threatening and require urgent medical intervention. These anomalies include duodenal atresia, anal atresia, polycystic kidney disease, hydrocephalus, and congenital heart diseases requiring emergency treatment (George et al., 2020).

The most common associated anomalies in babies with EA are cardiovascular anomalies. The most frequently observed cardiac anomaly is ventricular septal defect (VSD). Other cardiac anomalies include atrial septal defect (ASD), patent ductus arteriosus (PDA), tetralogy of Fallot, vascular rings, and aortic coarctation. The presence of these cardiac anomalies is responsible for much of the mortality. Other associated anomalies include those in the genitourinary system, gastrointestinal system, vertebral-skeletal system, and nervous system. Genitourinary anomalies include transient hydronephrosis, ureteropelvic junction obstruction, vesicoureteral reflux, renal agenesis, horseshoe kidney, undescended testis, and hypospadias. The most common gastrointestinal anomaly is anal atresia. Other gastrointestinal anomalies include duodenal, jejunal, and ileal atresia; hypertrophic pyloric stenosis; rotation anomalies; and annular pancreas. Vertebral-skeletal anomalies include hemivertebrae, sacral agenesis, polydactyly, and absence of the radius. Rib anomalies are also quite common and usually occur alongside vertebral anomalies. The presence of 13 pairs of ribs is a sign of long-gap EA. Long-gap EA is also associated with aortic arch and major vessel anomalies. Central nervous system malformations are relatively rare compared to other systems (Stoll et al., 2009; Stoll et al., 2009).

The VACTERL association (V: Vertebral anomalies, A: Anal atresia, C: Cardiac anomalies, TE: Tracheoesophageal fistula and esophageal atresia, R: Renal anomalies, L: Limb anomalies) is named after the initials of the anomalies commonly seen together. It is not a syndrome, as no specific gene has been identified to explain the combination of these anomalies. They are simply named for their frequent occurrence together. Publications indicate that 52-82% of patients with VACTERL have EA/TEF (Solomon et al., 2010).

Another association related to EA is CHARGE syndrome (C: Coloboma, H: Heart defects, A: Choanal atresia, R: Mental retardation, G: Genital hypoplasia, E: Ear anomalies). This condition is considered a syndrome because a defect has been identified in the CHD7 gene. EA/TEF is not part of the acronym, but 10% of patients with CHARGE syndrome have EA (Tellier et al., 1998).

Additionally, EA may be associated with Down syndrome, DiGeorge syndrome, Pierre Robin sequence, Holt-Oram syndrome, Feingold syndrome, Townes-Brocks syndrome, Bartsocas-Papas syndrome, McKusick-Kaufman syndrome, and Schisis association (Ein et al., 1989; Chittmittrapap et al., 1989).

Classification

EA is anatomically classified based on the location of the atresia and the presence or absence of a fistula with the trachea. The first classification was introduced by the radiologist Vogt in 1929 (Vogt, 1929). This classification was later modified by Ladd in 1944, Gross in 1953, Roberts in 1955, Swenson in 1962, and Holder in 1966. In 1976, Kluth published the "Atlas of Esophageal Atresia," which provided the most detailed classification, with 96 subtypes expressed using letters and numbers (Kluth, 1976). Due to its practicality and usefulness, the classification most commonly used today is Gross's classification. It divides esophageal atresia into 5 groups (Figure 1) (George et al., 2020).

Gross Classification of Esophageal Atresia Types:

A. *Isolated EA:* Also called esophageal atresia without tracheoesophageal fistula. It is seen in about 7% of cases. The proximal esophageal segment is thickened and dilated, while the distal segment is usually very short. The distance between the two segments is typically very long, often preventing anastomosis.
B. *EA with Proximal TEF:* Found in 2% of cases. Similar to isolated EA, the distal segment is very short, and the proximal TEF is short and narrow, opening directly into the trachea.
C. *EA with Distal TEF:* The most common type, seen in 86% of cases. The proximal esophagus is thickened and dilated, typically ending at the level of the 3rd thoracic vertebra. The distal esophagus is narrow with a thin wall and usually enters the trachea posteriorly at the carina or about 1-2 cm above it. The distance between the two esophageal segments is generally short.
D. *EA with Proximal and Distal TEF*: It is thought to have an incidence of less than 1%. The distance between the segments is not expected to be long. Proximal fistulas are often discovered either during a preoperative bronchoscopy or incidentally during the dissection of the proximal segment during surgery.
E. *Isolated TEF:* Also known as H-type TEF. It occurs in about 4% of cases. The fistulas are very short, with a diameter of 2-4 mm, and are

usually located just proximal to the thoracic inlet (George et al., 2020).

In addition to the anatomical classification, in 1962, D.J. Waterston and colleagues developed a classification system to predict the prognosis of patients with esophageal atresia based on risk factors. Birth weight, pneumonia, and the presence of associated congenital anomalies form the basis of this classification (Table 1) (Waterston et al., 1962).

However, improvements in preoperative care, early diagnosis, diagnosis and treatment of associated anomalies, and advancements in neonatal intensive care conditions have led to an increase in the survival rates of EA patients, which has caused Waterston's classification to lose its validity. This has led to the need for a new classification. The new classification was introduced by Spitz and later modified by Okamoto. This classification is based on birth weight and the presence of major cardiac anomalies (Table 2 and Table 3) (Spitz et al., 1994; Okamoto et al., 2009).

Table 1. Waterston risk groups

Group	Classification
A	Birth weight above 2500g with no associated anomalies.
B	Birth weight between 2000g and 2500g with no associated anomalies, or a higher birth weight with moderate pneumonia and associated anomalies
C	Birth weight below 2000g, or a higher birth weight with severe pneumonia and serious associated anomalies.

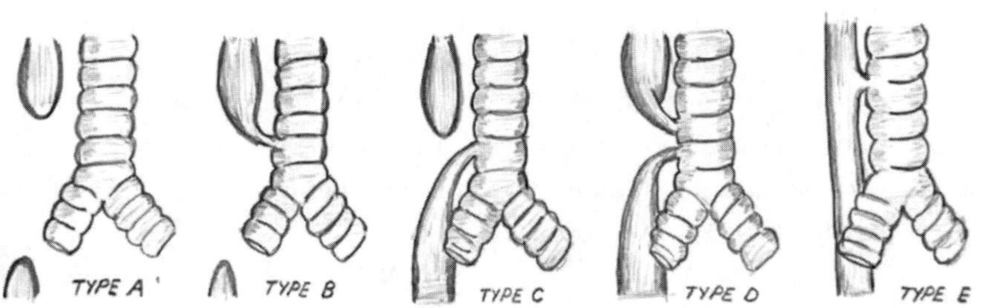

Figure 1. Gross classification of esophageal atresia.

Table 2. Spitz risk classification

Group	Classification
I	Birth weight of 1500g or less with no major cardiac anomalies
II	Birth weight of less than 1500g or with major cardiac anomalies
III	Birth weight of less than 1500g and with major cardiac anomalies

Table 3. Okamoto modification of the spitz classification

Class	Survival %	Risk	
Group 1	100	Low	Birth weight ≥ 2000 grams, no major cardiac anomalies.
Group 2	81	Moderate	Birth weight < 2000 grams, no major cardiac anomalies.
Group 3	72	Relatively High	Birth weight ≥ 2000 grams, has major cardiac anomalies.
Group 4	27	High	Birth weight < 2000 grams, has major cardiac anomalies.

Diagnosis and Clinical Management

Antenatal diagnosis plays a crucial role in shaping treatment plans before birth and in ensuring more effective management of the patient after birth. Additionally, it allows the family to be informed about the potential situations they will face post-delivery, enabling them to psychologically prepare for the process.

EA/TEF can be diagnosed antenatally in 20-31% of cases (Hunt et al., 2016). Important findings on antenatal ultrasound (USG) include polyhydramnios, a small or absent stomach bubble, and dilation of the proximal esophageal pouch. The presence of associated anomalies, such as cardiac and genitourinary anomalies, further increases suspicion of EA (Shulman et al., 2002).

In recent years, studies have been exploring how fetal magnetic resonance imaging (MRI) and amniotic fluid analysis may assist in antenatal diagnosis of EA/TEF cases. Fetal MRI is commonly used to evaluate anatomical abnormalities. In congenital structural anomalies like EA/TEF, MRI allows for more detailed examination of the development of the esophagus and its connections with the trachea (Langer et al., 2001). Amniotic fluid analysis, a prenatal diagnostic method through the measurement of biochemical markers, has been studied for its potential to predict EA. Specifically, studies suggest that elevated levels of gamma-glutamyl transpeptidase (GGTP) and alpha-fetoprotein (AFP) may aid in antenatal diagnosis (Czerkiewicz et al., 2011). The use of these imaging and biochemical markers may enhance the accuracy of antenatal USG, but more comprehensive tests and imaging techniques are required for a definitive diagnosis and management.

In cases without any antenatal follow-up, diagnosis is typically made in the first 24 hours postnatally. These infants often present with excessive secretions as they are unable to swallow their saliva. Aspiration of these secretions from the TEF or proximal pouch may result in coughing, tachypnea, and cyanosis. Early diagnosis at this stage is critical, as feeding the infant could likely lead to aspiration of milk into the lungs, causing aspiration pneumonia, which significantly affects morbidity and mortality. Therefore, in newborns presenting with excessive secretions, difficulty swallowing, cyanosis during feeding, or respiratory distress, EA should be suspected, and diagnostic tests should be promptly planned.

For suspected antenatal or postnatal cases, an orogastric (OG) catheter is typically inserted through the mouth. The catheter is advanced 9-11 cm and then placed. A postero-anterior (PA) babygram (a radiograph showing the infant's neck, chest, abdomen, and pelvis in a single film) is then taken. If the catheter tip is seen to curl in the proximal esophageal pouch, it is a significant diagnostic sign. The upper pouch typically ends at the T2-T4 vertebral level (Hunt et al., 2016; Spitz, 2007). Although injecting contrast material into the OG catheter for imaging the upper pouch may seem like a definitive diagnosis, it should be avoided due to the risk of aspiration. Contrast agents can be fatal in these patients (Gopal & Woodward, 2007). The abdomen should also be examined on the radiograph, and the absence of gas suggests the absence of a fistula. However, it should be kept in mind that a distal fistula could appear similar due to blockage by a mucus plug (Gedicke et al., 2007).

Furthermore, the patient should be evaluated for VACTERL association. Anomalies in the vertebrae and extremities should be assessed through the babygram. An echocardiogram (ECHO) should be requested to check for cardiac anomalies. The ECHO is important both for detecting any cardiac anomalies and for determining the direction of the aortic arch. Abdominal and urinary ultrasound (USG) should also be performed to assess for any additional intra-abdominal pathologies (Spitz et al., 1993).

Preoperative Preparation

In reducing the mortality and morbidity associated with EA, preoperative preparation and postoperative care are just as crucial as early diagnosis. The infant with EA should have their mouth kept closed, and intravenous fluids and antibiotic treatment should be started promptly. Since the mouth will remain closed for several weeks, it would be more reasonable to initiate total parenteral nutrition (TPN). The patient should be positioned in the right lateral position with the head slightly elevated. Continuous aspiration of secretions should be ensured with a catheter placed in the upper esophageal pouch.

In cases where the infant requires intubation due to respiratory distress, the endotracheal tube should be inserted so that its tip passes beyond the distal fistula, and ventilation should be performed with low pressure. Otherwise, air will pass from the fistula into the stomach, potentially causing gastric distention and later perforation (Spitz, 2007).

Surgery

In order to assess the presence of TEF, its location, and the status of tracheomalacia, bronchoscopy can be performed just before starting surgery. Although some centers have made preoperative bronchoscopy routine, many centers do not perform it (Dingemann et al., 2020). The surgical options for the repair of EA/TEF include open thoracotomy or video-assisted thoracoscopic surgery (VATS) (Patkowski et al., 2009) (Figure 2).

Repair with Thoracotomy

The patient is prepared in the left lateral position, with the right arm elevated (Lillehei & Shamberger, 2003). A right posterolateral thoracotomy is planned for the repair. However, in rare cases, when the arch of the aorta is found on the right side on ECHO, a left thoracotomy is preferred (Mortell & Azizkhan, 2009). After passing through the skin and subcutaneous tissue, the latissimus dorsi muscle is cut, and the serratus anterior muscle is retracted to the side. The thorax is accessed through the 4th or 5th intercostal space. Care should be taken to avoid damaging the long thoracic nerve, which runs along the mid-axillary line and innervates the serratus anterior muscle. It is recommended to use an extrapleural approach if possible, as this reduces the risk of postoperative empyema in cases of anastomotic leak. Starting from the posterior, blunt dissection is continued until the pleura is freed from the chest wall. The dissection continues until the azygos vein is visible, at which point it is ligated and cut (Spitz, 2007). In some cases, the operation can be completed without cutting the azygos vein. Preserving the azygos vein can help prevent respiratory complications during the postoperative period (Soyer et al., 2021). If the azygos vein is not cut, it is lifted with a vessel loop for protection. The distal portion of the esophagus is then dissected medially to the vagus nerve. The vagus is preserved, and the distal esophagus is mobilized to the site of the fistula, after which it is tied off. Care must be taken to leave the right amount of tissue at the site of the fistula; leaving too much can result in diverticulum formation, and pulling it too tightly can cause stenosis. Since the blood supply to the distal esophagus is weak, dissection should be minimized.

Next, with the help of the OG tube moved back and forth by the anesthesiologist, the proximal pouch is located. The proximal esophagus is then mobilized, and an end-to-end anastomosis is performed between the proximal and distal esophagus. Care should be taken to leave the knots outside. During the anastomosis, the OG tube is advanced into the stomach, and the anesthesiologist is asked to secure its position. A chest tube is placed, and the incision is closed in layers (Spitz, 2006; Gupta & Sharma, 2008; Mortell & Azizkhan, 2009).

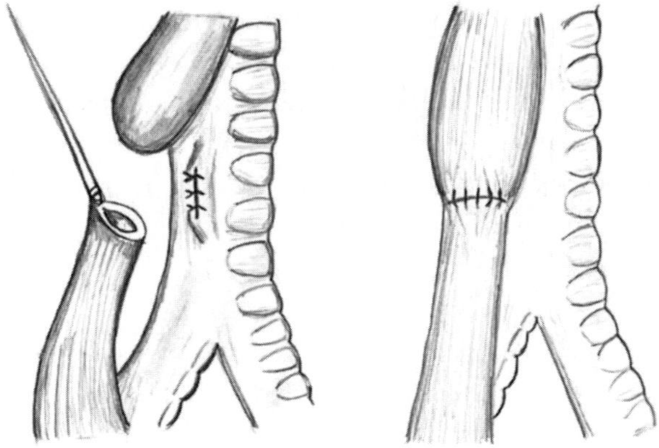

Figure 2. Primary repair of EA with distal TEF.

Repair with Thoracoscopy

In thoracoscopic repair, 3 or 4 trocars of 2.5-5 mm in size are inserted into the thorax. A 30-degree angled optical scope is used for viewing, and instruments such as dissectors, needle holders, hook cauters, and bipolar forceps are used for manipulation. The hemithorax is insufflated with carbon dioxide (CO2), and lung collapse is induced before starting the same procedures as those in thoracotomy. The azygos vein is cauterized, the fistula is ligated, and the proximal and distal pouches are mobilized to perform the anastomosis between the esophageal ends. After the anastomosis is completed, a chest tube is placed through the lower trocar site (Fonte et al., 2017).

Thoracoscopy has several advantages, including better cosmetic outcomes, the absence of scoliosis and asymmetric chest wall problems caused by thoracotomy, and less postoperative pain and respiratory distress. However, there is no difference in complications and outcomes between open and thoracoscopic repairs (Holcomb et al., 2005).

Long Gap

During surgery, when the distal and proximal segments of the esophagus are mobilized, if the gap between the two segments is ≥2 cm or spans more than two thoracic vertebrae, the condition is referred to as “long gap” esophageal atresia (von Allmen & Wijnen, 2015). A long gap occurs in approximately 7-10% of children born with esophageal atresia (Jensen et al., 2020). With the development of surgical techniques in recent years, primary anastomosis is attempted regardless of the distance between the esophageal ends, and interposition is avoided as much as possible. However, when primary anastomosis is not feasible, there is still no standard surgical approach (Stadil et al., 2019; Bagolan et al., 2004).

Postoperative Care

After surgery, the patient should be closely monitored in the neonatal intensive care unit (NICU). If the respiratory status is adequate, blood gas values are within normal limits, and there are no additional cardiac anomalies, the patient may be followed without the need for intubation. However, even without respiratory issues, if there is a tense anastomosis, mechanical ventilation may be required to keep the patient immobile during the follow-up period.

Postoperative chest X-rays should be performed and repeated after 4-5 days. The antibiotic therapy and TPN initiated before surgery should be continued postoperatively. Additionally, careful aspiration of secretions during the postoperative period helps prevent respiratory complications. In cases of tense anastomosis, the head should not be excessively hyperextended, and excessive rotational movements should be avoided (Gupta & Sharma, 2008).

The chest tube should only be removed after ensuring that there is no anastomotic leakage. In the early postoperative period, the patient can be fed via a transanastomotic catheter (OG tube). On the 5th postoperative day, a contrast study is performed. Once it is confirmed that there is no leak or stricture, the catheter can be removed, and the baby can begin oral feeding (Holcomb, 1993).

The discharged infant should be scheduled for frequent follow-up visits. During these visits, weight gain and development should be assessed, as well as potential complications such as gastroesophageal reflux (GER), TEF recurrence, respiratory issues, and anastomotic stricture.

Complications

Early Complications

Anastomotic Leak

Anastomotic leak is an early complication. It can result from factors such as a tense anastomosis, insufficient surgical technique, the type of suture material used, and ischemia due to excessive dissection of the esophageal ends (Chittmittrapap et al., 1992). This complication occurs in 14-16% of patients (Harmon & Coran, 2006). Minor leaks are more common and are typically detected in routine contrast studies performed between 5 and 7 days postoperatively. They usually resolve with conservative management. Major leaks, however, occur in the early postoperative period and present with tachypnea, tachycardia, and a worsening general condition. Secretions, formula, or breast milk may be observed coming from the chest tube. The prognosis is generally worse in these cases, and gastrostomy or cervical esophagostomy may be required (Spitz, 2006).

Anastomotic Stricture

Almost all cases of esophageal atresia will encounter some degree of anastomotic stricture (Ten Kate, 2020). Factors like excessive mobilization of the distal esophagus leading to impaired blood flow, long-gap esophageal atresia, and the presence of gastroesophageal reflux (GER) increase the risk of stricture development. Treatment typically involves bougie or balloon dilation. In cases of recurrent strictures, GER should be suspected and treated accordingly (Engum et al., 1995).

Recurrent TEF

Recurrent TEF occurs in 5-10% of patients (Touloukian & Seashore, 2004). The risk is higher in cases where an anastomotic leak has occurred, due to secondary inflammation. While it can occur early in the postoperative period, diagnosis can take months. Recurrent TEF should be suspected in cases of coughing, cyanosis, and apnea during feeding or recurrent respiratory infections. Diagnosis can be confirmed using contrast esophagography, but if the fistula cannot be demonstrated, bronchoscopy is recommended. Once diagnosed, the fistula can be closed orally, and nasogastric (NG) or orogastric (OG) tubes should be placed for further management, followed by reoperation (Spitz, 2007).

Late Complications

Gastroesophageal Reflux (GER)

The incidence of GER in patients who have undergone surgery for esophageal atresia is approximately 43% (Tovar & Fragoso, 2013). GER can lead to anastomotic stricture and chronic aspiration pneumonia. It may also result in esophageal metaplasia, which can progress to adenocarcinoma later in life. GER must be treated to prevent these complications. Diagnosis can be made via contrast upper GI studies, 24-hour pH monitoring, and endoscopy (Lopez & Lemberg, 2020). Treatment options include feeding the baby in an upright position, placing the baby at a 30-degree angle, thickening feeds, and using H2 receptor blockers and proton pump inhibitors. In cases that do not respond to medical therapy, fundoplication may be indicated (Jönsson, 2019).

Tracheomalacia

Tracheomalacia refers to the weakness of the anterior and posterior walls of the trachea, which can be either partial or complete. After coughing or exhalation, the trachea may collapse (Felix et al., 2004). It is a significant cause of respiratory distress following TEF repair. In infants with tracheomalacia, wheezing, coughing, and apnea episodes are common. Diagnosis is made through bronchoscopy. In these cases, compression by large vessels may contribute to the apnea, and aortopexy may be performed to relieve the pressure (Van der Zee & Klaas, 2007; Pinheiro, 2012). In severe symptomatic cases, tracheostomy may be indicated.

Growth and Developmental Delay

Feeding difficulties, nutritional deficiencies, recurrent respiratory infections, and GER can result in growth retardation in the early years. However, most children with esophageal atresia will catch up to normal growth curves as they get older (Patria, 2017).

Chest Deformities

In patients who undergo thoracotomy, late complications such as scoliosis, shoulder girdle muscle weakness, and chest wall deformities may occur. However, these complications are significantly reduced with the use of a thoracoscopic approach (Rothenberg, 2013).

Conclusion

EA and TEF are congenital conditions that are often life-threatening and require timely intervention in newborns. Early diagnosis and appropriate surgical management are crucial in improving the survival rates of these patients. Antenatal diagnosis enables a faster and more effective treatment process after birth. This is particularly important for surgical planning and preventing complications.

The success of surgery, as well as preoperative and postoperative management, plays a significant role in survival. The treatment of these patients should not be limited to surgery alone; a multidisciplinary approach is essential, which includes nutritional support, respiratory assistance, and psychosocial care.

In recent years, advancements in surgical techniques and improvements in postoperative care have allowed for significant progress in enhancing the quality of life for these patients. However, further research into genetic factors, environmental influences, and organogenesis processes will help improve the understanding of the disease and enhance treatment options. The genetic mutations, environmental factors, and disruptions in organogenesis involved in EA and TEF may be better understood through future studies, which will further refine treatment strategies.

Additionally, the frequent presence of associated anomalies in these patients can complicate the treatment process and make postoperative monitoring more challenging. This highlights the importance of a multidisciplinary approach. Monitoring these patients should not only focus on EA but also include the management of any associated systemic anomalies. Furthermore, when these anomalies are identified early, the treatment process can be better planned, minimizing complications and optimizing outcomes.

In conclusion, complex congenital anomalies like EA and TEF can be managed effectively with early diagnosis, appropriate surgical intervention, and long-term follow-up. However, the presence of associated anomalies is a critical factor that can affect the treatment process, underscoring the necessity of a multidisciplinary approach. Ongoing developments in medical strategies are improving the quality of life for these patients, and future research will bring even greater success in the management of these conditions.

References

Alberti, D., Boroni, G., Corasaniti, L., & Torri, F. (2011). Esophageal atresia: Pre and post-operative management. *Journal of Maternity, Fetal & Neonatal Medicine, 24*(suppl 1), 4-6. https://doi.org/10.3109/14767058.2011.607558.

Bagolan, P., Iacobelli, B. D. B., De Angelis, P., Federici di Abriola, G., Laviani, R., Trucchi, A., Orzalesi, M., & Dall'Oglio, L. (2004). Long gap esophageal atresia and esophageal replacement: Moving toward a separation? *Journal of Pediatric Surgery, 39*(7), 1084-1090. https://doi.org/10.1016/j.jpedsurg.2004.03.036.

Chittmittrapap, S., Spitz, L., Kiely, E. M., & Brereton, R. J. (1989). Oesophageal atresia and associated anomalies. *Archives of Disease in Childhood, 64*(3), 364-368. https://doi.org/10.1136/adc.64.3.364.

Chittmittrapap, S., Spitz, L., Kiely, E. M., & Brereton, R. J. (1992). Anastomotic leakage following surgery for esophageal atresia. *Journal of Pediatric Surgery, 27*(1), 29-32. https://doi.org/10.1016/0022-3468(92)90139-Q.

Conforti, A., Morini, F., & Bagolan, P. (2014). Difficult esophageal atresia: Trick and treat. *Seminars in Pediatric Surgery, 23*(5), 261-269. https://doi.org/10.1053/j.sempedsurg.2014.09.006.

Coran, A. G., Caldamone, A., Adzick, N. S., Krummel, T. M., Laberge, J.-M., & Shamberger, R. (2012). Pediatric surgery e-book (pp. 893-918). Elsevier Health Sciences.

Crisera, C. A., Connelly, P. R., Marmureanu, A. R., Colen, K. L., Rose, M. I., Li, M., Longaker, M. T., & Gittes, G. K. (1999). Esophageal atresia with tracheoesophageal fistula: Suggested mechanism in faulty organogenesis. *Journal of Pediatric Surgery, 1*, 204–208. https://doi.org/10.1016/S0022-3468(99)90054-6.

Crisera, C. A., Grau, J. B., Maldonado, T. S., Kadison, A. S., Longaker, M. T., & Gittes, G. K. (2000). Defective epithelial- mesenchymal interactions dictate the organogenesis of tracheoesophageal fistula. *Pediatric Surgery International, 4*, 256-261. https://doi.org/10.1007/s003830050314.

Czerkiewicz, I., Dreux, S., Beckmezian, A., Benachi, A., Salomon, L. J., Schmitz, T., de Saint Blanquat, P., Oury, J. F., & Dumez, Y. (2011). Biochemical amniotic fluid pattern for prenatal diagnosis of esophageal atresia. *Pediatric Research, 70*(2), 199-202. https://doi.org/10.1203/PDR.0b013e31822198f3.

Diez-Pardo, J. A., Baoquan, Q., Navarro, C., & Tovar, J. A. (1996). A new rodent experimental model of esophageal atresia nd tracheoesophageal fistula. *Journal of Pediatric Surgery, 31*(4), 498-502. https://doi.org/10.1016/S0022-3468(96)90202-2.

Dingemann, C., Eaton, S., Aksnes, G., et al., (2020). ERNICA Consensus Conference on the management of patients with esophageal atresia and tracheoesophageal fistula: Diagnostics, preoperative, operative, and postoperative management. *European Journal of Pediatric Surgery, 30*, 326–336. https://doi.org/10.1055/s-0039-3407962.

Ein, S. H., Shandling, B., Wesson, D., & Filler, R. M. (1989). Esophageal atresia with distal tracheoesophageal fistula: Associated anomalies and prognosis in the 1980s. *Journal of Pediatric Surgery, 24*(10), 1055-1059. https://doi.org/10.1016/S0022-3468(89)80405-9.

Engum, S. A., Grosfeld, J. L., West, K. W., Rescorla, F. J., Scherer, L. R., 3rd. (1995). Analysis of morbidity and mortality in 227 cases of esophageal atresia and/or tracheoesophageal fistula over two decades. *Archives of Surgery, 130*(5), 502-508. https://doi.org/10.1001/archsurg.1995.01430170010004003.

Felix, J. F., Keijzer, R., van Dooren, M. F., Rottier, R. J., & Tibboel, D. (2004). Genetics and developmental biology of oesophageal atresia and tracheo-oesophageal fistula: Lessons from mice relevant for paediatric surgeons. *Pediatric Surgery International, 20*(10), 731-736. https://doi.org/10.1007/s00383-004-1189-3.

Fonte, J., Barroso, C., Lamas-Pinheiro, R., Silva, A. R., & Correia-Pinto, J. (2016). Anatomic thoracoscopic repair of esophageal atresia. *Frontiers in Pediatrics, 4*, 142. https://doi.org/10.3389/fped.2016.00142.

German, J. C., Mahour, G. H., & Woolley, M. M. (1979). The twin with esophageal atresia. *Journal of Pediatric Surgery, 14*(4), 432-435. https://doi.org/10.1016/s0022-3468(79)80008-1.

Gedicke, M. M., Gopal, M., & Spicer, R. (2007). A gasless abdomen does not exclude distal tracheoesophageal fistula: The value of a repeat x-ray. *Journal of Pediatric Surgery, 42*, 576-577. https://doi.org/10.1016/j.jpedsurg.2006.11.021.

Gopal, M., & Woodward, M. (2007). Potential hazards of contrast study diagnosis of esophageal atresia. *Journal of Pediatric Surgery, 42*, E9-E10. https://doi.org/10.1016/j.jpedsurg.2007.04.031.

Gupta, D. K., & Sharma, S. (2008). Esophageal atresia: The total care in a high-risk population. *Seminars in Pediatric Surgery, 17*, 236-243. https://doi.org/10.1053/j.sempedsurg.2008.06.005.

Harmon, C. M., & Coran, A. G. (2006). Congenital anomalies of the esophagus. In J. L. Grosfeld, E. W. Fonkalsrud, & A. G. Coran (Eds.), *Pediatric surgery* (Vol. 1, pp. 1051-1081). Mosby Elsevier.

Holcomb, G. W., 3rd. (1993). Survival after gastrointestinal perforation from esophageal atresia and tracheoesophageal fistula. *Journal of Pediatric Surgery, 28*(12), 1532-1535. https://doi.org/10.1016/S0022-3468(05)80437-0.

Holcomb, G. W., 3rd, Rothenberg, S. S., Bax, K. M. A., Martinez-Ferro, M., Albanese, C. T., Ostlie, D. J., van Der Zee, D. C., & Yeung, C. K. (2005). Thoracoscopic repair of esophageal atresia and tracheoesophageal fistula: A multi-institutional analysis. *Annals of Surgery, 242*(3), 422-428; discussion 428-430. https://doi.org/10.1097/01.sla.0000185332.79592.82.

Holcomb, G. W. III, St. Peter, S. D., & Ashcraft, K. W. (2020). Holcomb and Ashcraft's Pediatric Surgery (7th ed.). Elsevier.

Holder, T. M., & Ashcraft, K. W. (1966). Esophageal atresia and tracheo-esophageal fistula. *Current Problems in Surgery, 3*(8), 1-68. https://doi.org/10.1016/S0011-3840(66)80017-5.

Hunt, R. W., Perkins, E. J., & King, S. (2016). Peri-operative management of neonates with esophageal atresia and tracheoesophageal fistula. *Pediatric Respiratory Reviews, 19*, 3-9. https://doi.org/10.1016/j.prrv.2015.11.001.

Jensen, A. R., McDuffie, L. A., Groh, E. M., & Rescorla, F. J. (2020). Outcomes for correction of long-gap esophageal atresia: A 22-year experience. *The Journal of Surgical Research, 251*, 47–52. https://doi.org/10.1016/j.jss.2020.02.035.

Jönsson, L., Dellenmark-Blom, M., Enoksson, O., Friberg, L. G., Gatzinsky, V., Sandin, A., Bache, J., Linde, J., Berg, A., & Garp, C. (2019). Long-term effectiveness of antireflux surgery in esophageal atresia patients. *European Journal of Pediatric Surgery: Official Journal of the Austrian Association of Pediatric Surgery, 29*(6), 521–527. https://doi.org/10.1055/s-0038-1678497.

Kluth, D. (1976). Atlas of esophageal atresia. *Journal of Pediatric Surgery, 11*, 901-919. https://doi.org/10.1016/S0022-3468(76)80243-7.

Langer, J. C., Hussain, H., Khan, A., Minkes, R. K., Gray, D., Siegel, M., Glick, P., & Levey, J. A. (2001). Prenatal diagnosis of esophageal atresia using sonography and magnetic resonance imaging. *Journal of Pediatric Surgery, 36*(5), 804-807. https://doi.org/10.1053/jpsu.2001.23294.

Lillehei, C. W., & Shamberger, R. C. (2003). Reoperative esophageal surgery. *Seminars in Pediatric Surgery, 12*, 100-106. https://doi.org/10.1053/j.sempedsurg.2003.04.002.

Lopez, R. N., & Lemberg, D. A. (2020). Gastro-oesophageal reflux disease in infancy: A review based on international guidelines. *The Medical Journal of Australia, 212*(1), 40–44. https://doi.org/10.5694/mja2.50567.

Mortell, A. E., & Azizkhan, R. G. (2009). Esophageal atresia repair with thoracotomy: The Cincinnati contemporary experience. *Seminars in Pediatric Surgery, 18*, 12-19. https://doi.org/10.1053/j.sempedsurg.2008.12.003.

Muensterer, O. J., & Berdon, W. E. (2015). From Vogt to Haight and Holt to now: The history of esophageal atresia over the last century. *Pediatric Radiology, 45*(8), 1230-1235. https://doi.org/10.1007/s00247-015-3276-1.

Okamoto, T., Takamizawa, S., Arai, H., Bitoh, Y., Nakao, M., Yokoi, A., Yokoyama, T., Sumi, S., Oka, S., & Kato, Y. (2009). Esophageal atresia: Prognostic classification revisited. *Surgery, 145*(6), 675-681. https://doi.org/10.1016/j.surg.2008.12.027.

Orford, J., Glasson, M., Beasley, S., Shi, E., Myers, N., & Cass, D. (2000). Oesophageal atresia in twins. *Pediatric Surgery International, 16*(8), 541-545. https://doi.org/10.1007/s003830000435.

Orford, J., Manglick, P., Cass, D. T., & Tam, P. P. (2001). Mechanisms for the development of esophageal atresia. *Journal of Pediatric Surgery, 36*, 985-994. https://doi.org/10.1053/jpsu.2001.25286.

Patkowski, D., Rysiakiewicz, K., Jaworski, W., Zielinska, M., Siejka, G., Konsur, K., & Czernik, J. (2009). Thoracoscopic repair of tracheoesophageal fistula and esophageal atresia. *Journal of Laparoendoscopic & Advanced Surgical Techniques A, 19*(Suppl 1), S19-S22. https://doi.org/10.1089/lap.2008.0412.

Pletcher, B. A., Friedes, J. S., Breg, W. R., & Touloukian, R. J. (1991). Familial occurrence of esophageal atresia with and without tracheoesophageal fistula: Report of two unusual kindreds. *American Journal of Medical Genetics, 39*(4), 380-384. https://doi.org/10.1002/ajmg.1320390403.

Patria, M. F., Ghislanzoni, S., Macchini, F., Lelii, M., Mori, A., Leva, E., Principi, N., & Esposito, S. (2017). Respiratory morbidity in children with repaired congenital esophageal atresia with or without tracheoesophageal fistula. *International Journal of Environmental Research and Public Health, 14*(10), 1202. https://doi.org/10.3390/ijerph14101202.

Pinheiro, P. F. M., e Silva, A. C. S., & Pereira, R. M. (2012). Current knowledge on esophageal atresia. *World Journal of Gastroenterology, 18*, 3662–3672. https://doi.org/10.3748/wjg.v18.i27.3662.

Qi, B. Q., & Beasley, S. W. (1999). Communicating bronchopulmonary foregut malformations in the adriamycin-induced rat model of esophageal atresia. *Australian and New Zealand Journal of Surgery, 1*, 56-59. https://doi.org/10.1046/j.1440-1622.1999.01884.x.

Qi, B. Q., & Beasley, S. W. (1999). Relationship of the notochord to foregut development in the fetal rat model of esophageal atresia. *Journal of Pediatric Surgery, 11*, 1593-1598. https://doi.org/10.1016/S0022-3468(99)90262-7.

Qi, B. Q., Beasley, S. W., & Williams, A. K. (2001). Evidence of a common pathogenesis for foregut duplications and esophageal atresia with tracheoesophageal fistula. *Journal of Pediatric Surgery, 36*(7), 985-994. https://doi.org/10.1053/jpsu.2001.25285.

Rothenberg, S. S. (2013). Thoracoscopic repair of esophageal atresia and tracheoesophageal fistula in neonates, first decade's experience. *Diseases of the Esophagus: Official Journal of the International Society for Diseases of the Esophagus, 26*(4), 359–364. https://doi.org/10.1111/dote.12038.

Shaw-Smith, C. (2006). Oesophageal atresia, tracheo-oesophageal fistula, and the VACTERL association: Review of genetics and epidemiology. *Journal of Medical Genetics, 43*(7), 545-554. https://doi.org/10.1136/jmg.2005.038158.

Sfeir, R., Bonnard, A., Khen-Dunlop, N., Auber, F., Gelas, T., Michaud, L., Podevin, G., Breton, A., Fouquet, V., Piolat, C., Lemelle, J. L., Petit, T., Lavrand, F., Becmeur, F., Polimerol, M. L., Michel, J. L., Elbaz, F., Habonimana, E., Allal, H., Lopez, E., Lardy, H., Morineau, M., Pelatan, C., Merrot, T., Delagausie, P., Vries, P., Levard, G., Buisson, P., Sapin, E., Jaby, O., Borderon, C., Weil, D., Gueiss, S., Aubert, D., Echaieb, A., Fourcade, L., Breaud, J., Laplace, C., Pouzac, M., Duhamel, A., & Gottrand, F. (2013). Esophageal atresia: Data from a national cohort. *Journal of Pediatric Surgery, 48*(8), 1664–1669. https://doi.org/10.1016/j.jpedsurg.2013.03.075.

Smith, E. I. (1957). The early development of the trachea and esophagus in relation to atresia of the esophagus and tracheoesophageal fistula. *Contributions to Embryology, 245*, 42-57. https://doi.org/10.2307/25726655.

Skandalakis, J. E., Gray, S. W., & Ricketts, R. (1994). The esophagus. In J. E. Skandalakis & S. W. Gray (Eds.), *Embryology for surgeons* (2nd ed., pp. 245-270). Williams & Wilkins.

Shulman, A., Mazkereth, R., Zalel, Y., Kuint, J., Lipitz, S., Avigad, I., Ben-Rafael, Z., & Achiron, R. (2002). Prenatal identification of esophageal atresia: The role of ultrasonography for evaluation of functional anatomy. *Prenatal Diagnosis, 22*, 669-674. https://doi.org/10.1002/pd.351.

Solomon, B. D., Pineda-Alvarez, D. E., Raam, M. S., Bous, S. M., Keaton, A. A., Vélez, J. I., & Cummings, D. A. T. (2010). Analysis of component findings in 79 patients diagnosed with VACTERL association. *American Journal of Medical Genetics Part A, 152*(9), 2236–2244. https://doi.org/10.1002/ajmg.a.33592.

Spitz, L. (2006). Esophageal atresia: Lessons I have learned in a 40-year experience. *Journal of Pediatric Surgery, 41*(10), 1635-1640. https://doi.org/10.1016/j.jpedsurg.2006.02.011.

Spitz, L. (2007). Oesophageal atresia. *Orphanet Journal of Rare Diseases, 2*, 24. https://doi.org/10.1186/1750-1172-2-24.

Spitz, L., Kiely, E., Brereton, R. J., & Drake, D. (1993). Management of esophageal atresia. *World Journal of Surgery, 17*(3), 296-300. https://doi.org/10.1007/BF01655838.

Spitz, L., Kiely, E. M., Morecroft, J. A., & Drake, D. P. (1994). Oesophageal atresia: At risk groups for the 1990s. *Journal of Pediatric Surgery, 29*(6), 723-725. https://doi.org/10.1016/0022-3468(94)90056-2.

Soyer, T., Oztorun, C. I., & Fırıncı, B. (2021). The effect of azygos vein preservation on postoperative complications after esophageal atresia repair: Results from the Turkish Esophageal Atresia Registry. *Journal of Pediatric Surgery, 56*, 1940-1943. https://doi.org/10.1016/j.jpedsurg.2021.01.038.

Stadil, T., Koivusalo, A., Pakarinen, M., Mikkelsen, A., Emblem, R., Svensson, J. F., Ehrén, H., Jönsson, L., Bäckstrand, J., Engstrand Lilja, H., Donoso, F., Thorup, J. M.,

Sæter, T., Rasmussen, L., Pedersen, R. N., Stenström, P., Arnbjörnsson, E., Óskarsson, K., & Qvist, N. (2019). Surgical repair of long-gap esophageal atresia: A retrospective study comparing the management of long-gap esophageal atresia in the Nordic countries. *Journal of Pediatric Surgery, 54*(3), 423-428. https://doi.org/10.1016/j.jpedsurg.2018.09.019.

Stoll, C., Alembik, Y., Dott, B., & Roth, M.-P. (2009). Associated malformations in patients with esophageal atresia. *European Journal of Medical Genetics, 52*(5), 287–290. https://doi.org/10.1016/j.ejmg.2009.01.008.

Tellier, A. L., Cormier-Daire, V., Abadie, V., Amiel, J., Sigaudy, S., Bonnet, D., de Lonlay-Debeney, P., Morrisseau-Durand, M. P., Hubert, P., Michel, J. L., Jan, D., Dollfus, H., Baumann, C., Labrune, P., Lacombe, D., Philip, N., LeMerrer, M., Briard, M. L., Munnich, A., & Lyonnet, S. (1998). CHARGE syndrome: Report of 47 cases and review. *American Journal of Medical Genetics, 76*, 402-409. https://doi.org/10.1002/(SICI)1096-8628(19980413)76:5<402::AID-AJMG7>3.0.CO;2-O.

Ten Kate, C. A., Tambucci, R., Vlot, J., Spaander, M. C. W., Gottrand, F., Wijnen, R. M. H., & Dall'Oglio, L. (2020). An international survey on anastomotic stricture management after esophageal atresia repair: Considerations and advisory statements. *Surgical Endoscopy, 34*(10), 4329–4336. https://doi.org/10.1007/s00464-020-07844-6.

Touloukian, R. J., & Seashore, J. H. (2004). Thirty-five-year institutional experience with end-to-side repair for esophageal atresia. *Archives of Surgery, 139*(4), 371-374. https://doi.org/10.1001/archsurg.139.4.371.

Tovar, J. A., & Fragoso, A. C. (2013). Gastroesophageal reflux after repair of esophageal atresia. *European Journal of Pediatric Surgery, 23*(3), 175–181. https://doi.org/10.1055/s-0033-1342476.

Van der Zee, D. C., & Klaas, M. A. (2007). Thoracoscopic treatment of esophageal atresia with distal fistula and of tracheomalacia. *Seminars in Pediatric Surgery, 16*, 224–230. https://doi.org/10.1053/j.sempedsurg.2007.06.010.

Vogt, E. C. (1929). Congenital esophageal atresia. *American Journal of Roentgenology, 22*, 463-465.

von Allmen, D., & Wijnen, R. M. (2015). Bridging the gap in the repair of long-gap esophageal atresia: Still questions on diagnostics and treatment. *European Journal of Pediatric Surgery: Official Journal of the Austrian Association of Pediatric Surgery, 25*(4), 312–317. https://doi.org/10.1055/s-0035-1551453.

Waterston, D. J., Carter, R. E., & Aberdeen, E. (1962). Oesophageal atresia: Tracheo-oesophageal fistula. A study of survival in 218 infants. *Lancet,* 1(7234), 819-822. https://doi.org/10.1016/S0140-6736(62)92206-7.

Williams, A. K., Qi, B. Q., & Beasley, S. W. (2000). Temporospatial aberrations of apoptosis in the rat embryo developing esophageal atresia. *Journal of Pediatric Surgery, 11*, 1617-1620. https://doi.org/10.1016/S0022-3468(00)90098-6.

Xia, H., Otten, C., Migliazza, L., Diez-Pardo, J. A., & Tovar, J. A. (1999). Tracheobronchial malformations in experimental esophageal atresia. *Journal of Pediatric Surgery, 4*, 536-539. https://doi.org/10.1016/S0022-3468(99)90103-4.

Zhou, B., Hutson, J. M., Farmer, P. J., Hasthorpe, S., Myers, N. A., & Liu, M. (1999). Apoptosis in tracheoesophageal embryogenesis in rat embryos with or without adriamycin treatment. *Journal of Pediatric Surgery, 5*, 872-875. https://doi.org/10.1016/S0022-3468(99)90063-0.

Chapter 5

Gastric Outlet Obstructions

Hüseyin Şimşek*, MD
Neonatology Clinic, Mersin City Training and Research Hospital, Mersin, Turkey

Abstract

Gastric outlet obstruction (GOO) is a clinical condition that prevents the passage of gastric contents into the intestine. Complete or partial obstructions of the stomach, pylorus, or proximal duodenum are known as gastric outlet obstructions. Mechanical obstruction usually involves the pylorus itself in the prepyloric area of the stomach or the first parts of the duodenum. Gastric outlet obstructions are one of the pathologies requiring surgery in the neonatal period. Obstructions can be seen not only in the stomach but also at any point, especially in the duodenum. While vomiting is common in the neonatal period due to diseases such as sepsis, nutritional intolerance, metabolic disease, necrotizing enterocolitis, and endocrine disorders, we should also consider gastrointestinal diseases that require surgery. They can be confused with many clinical conditions in the neonatal period and should be managed by pediatric surgeons and neonatologists acting together in the diagnosis and treatment process. There are many pathologies in the differential diagnosis, and sometimes it may be difficult to reach a definitive diagnosis and can only be diagnosed at the time of operation.

Keywords: gastric outlet obstructions, newborn, vomiting

---

* Corresponding Author's Email: drhuseyinsmsk84@hotmail.com

In: Current Approaches to Newborn Emergencies
Editors: Zuhal Keskin Sarılar and Serap Samut Bülbül
ISBN: 979-8-89530-999-5

Introduction

GOO is the clinical and pathophysiologic consequence of any disease process that creates a mechanical barrier to the transfer of gastric contents to the intestine and prevents gastric contents from passing distal to the proximal duodenum. Mechanical obstructions or, very rarely, motility disorders can cause gastric outlet obstruction. GOO is one of the pathologies requiring frequent surgical intervention in the neonatal period (Saha et al., 2012; Seth et al., 2015). It is vital that the cases are recognized by neonatologists during neonatal follow-up and referred to pediatric surgeons appropriately. Babies with a prenatal diagnosis are naturally more fortunate than patients without a diagnosis. They should be managed in coordination with pediatric surgery after birth. While some patients without prenatal diagnosis can be easily and rapidly recognized with rapid clinical presentation after birth, some patients may experience delays in diagnosis (Stanescu et al., 2017; Vinocur et al., 2012). In infants with delayed diagnosis, aspiration due to recurrent vomiting and associated infections may occur, and in even more delayed cases, it may lead to serious consequences up to perforation. Therefore, it is very important to recognize these patients and plan their treatment quickly. Nausea and abdominal distension, especially vomiting without bile, are signs of GOO. The pattern and color of vomiting are important in diagnosing the disease and ruling out other conditions. While these symptoms may be vague in the early stages of the disease, they become more prominent as the disease progresses. Other symptoms include epigastric discomfort, weight loss, and early satiety (Saha et al., 2012). In infants with complete obstruction, nutritional inadequacy and dehydration develop as a result of increased severity of vomiting, leading to electrolyte imbalance. Hypochloromia and hypokalemia are observed in these patients. Metabolic alkalosis develops due to acid loss (Saha et al., 2012). In this article, an overview of the importance, diagnosis, and treatment of gastric outlet obstruction, which is one of the important emergencies of the neonatal period and infancy, will be presented.

There are many causes of gastric outlet obstruction in the neonatal period. The incidence of gastric outlet obstructions is difficult to estimate. Especially when infantile hypertrophic pyloric stenosis (IHPS) is considered as gastric outlet obstruction, it appears to be one of the relatively common surgical causes, with a frequency of 1.5-3/1000. When IHPS is not included, it becomes a very rare pathology with a rate of 1/100,000. Gastric outlet obstruction was classified by Sharma et al., in 2008 and divided into three main groups: congenital causes, acquired causes, and IHPS (Table 1) (Sharma et al., 2008). In this article, we will discuss the common gastric outlet obstructions.

Infantile Hypertrophic Pyloric Stenosis

Infantile hypertrophic pyloric stenosis (IHPS) is a disorder of newborns or infants caused by pyloric hypertrophy that almost completely blocks the gastric outflow tract, causing severe vomiting in infants. IHPS is usually diagnosed when the baby is between three and five weeks old and very rarely can be diagnosed after 12 weeks of age. Although the diagnosis was made at a later period in the previous studies, recently, the age of diagnosis can be made at an earlier period (Papadakis et al., 1999). The mean age at presentation was significantly younger in recent years (Demian et al., 2009). Early diagnosis of IHPS has recently become easier due to advances in technology, improved quality of imaging modalities, and good agreement between clinicians. Although IHPS shows geographical regional differences, it is seen in approximately 1 to 3.5 per 1000 live births (To et al., 2005). Studies from economically better countries have recently shown that the incidence has decreased (Hedbäck et al., 2001; Kapoor et al., 2019).

The etiology of IHPS has not been fully elucidated. Environmental and genetic predisposition have been implicated (MacMahon, 2006). The risk of IHPS has been shown to increase when erythromycin and azithromycin are administered, especially in infants younger than two weeks of age (Eberly et al., 2015).

Maternal smoking during pregnancy has also been shown to increase the risk of IHPS approximately 2-fold (Krogh et al., 2012; Svenningsson et al., 2014). A study on bottle use found that the risk of IHPS was more than four times higher in infants who used a bottle than in infants who never used a bottle (Krogh et al., 2012).

Table 1. Sharma's classification of gastric outlet obstruction

Group	Reason
Congenital intrinsic obstructions of the antrum and pylorus	Aplasia, atresia, diaphragm or web, luminal obstructions
IHPS	
Acquired causes	Peptic diseases, neoplasia, corrosive injuries

IHPS usually presents with vomiting after feeding. The vomiting is usually bilious and gushing, and as symptoms progress, problems with weight gain may occur (Aboagye et al., 2014). Infants with delayed treatment develop electrolyte imbalances, especially hypochloremia, due to loss of hydrochloric acid from the stomach. Hypokalemia is especially common in infants with prolonged vomiting, although it may not be seen in the early period of symptoms (Nmadu, 1992). In the early phase of IHPS, an olive-like mass in the right upper quadrant, which is typically palpable on examination, is often absent (Taylor et al., 2013). In general, an olive-like mass is often palpable late in the course of IHPS in infants with IHPS and is almost pathognomonic for the diagnosis of the disease when it is definitively detected (White et al., 1998). IHPS is usually symptomatic in infants between three and six weeks of age but can sometimes be symptomatic after three months (Demian et al., 2009). Hyperbilirubinemia, especially elevated unconjugated bilirubin, is one of the common clinical pathologies in IHPS. This is usually associated with inadequate nutritional intake and dehydration of the infant. This condition tends to normalize in the short term after surgical treatment (Hua et al., 2005). The association with esophageal atresia in infants with IHPS has been shown in many studies (Applegate & Druschel, 1995; Van Beelen et al., 2014).

Radiologic examination may start with a simple direct radiograph, and a distended stomach appearance is expected. However, direct radiography may also be completely normal. Ultrasound is the preferred imaging modality for suspected IHPS in contrast to radiography. Direct ultrasound visualization of the pyloric muscle and canal approaches 100% sensitivity and specificity for the diagnosis of IHPS, especially when performed by experienced radiologists (Sivitz et al., 2013; Niedzielski et al., 2011).

Cases with a wall thickness of more than 4 mm and a length of more than 16 mm are evaluated in favor of pyloric stenosis (Schwartz, 2012). Opaque passage radiographs have become less common in diagnostic use due to improved USG quality and the ability to provide many diagnostic findings. On opaque radiographs, delayed gastric emptying, a highly narrowed pylorus (rope sign), and the appearance of a wide duodenum after this narrow pylorus (shoulder sign) are pathognomonic (Otjen et al., 2012). However, the use of opaque radiographs has decreased due to the ease of access to USG, ease of application, and avoidance of radiation (Stanescu et al., 2017).

Pyloric Atresia

Pyloric atresia is a rare anomaly compared to pyloric stenosis. Although its etiology has not been clearly elucidated, it has been suggested that it is related to a dysfunction of the duct system or a vascular defect. Hypertrophic pyloric stenosis may take up to two to three weeks to become symptomatic in the postnatal period, whereas infants with pyloric atresia present with vomiting without bile from the first day of life in the postnatal period. While IHPS is difficult to recognize in the antenatal period, polyhydramnios and single bubble sign are suspicious in patients with pyloric atresia (Prasad et al., 2021). Fetal distended stomach in the last trimester may be diagnostic (Schwartz, 2012). In a series of 11 patients presented by Prasad et al., it was reported that 7 patients were symptomatic within the first 12 hours, and all patients were symptomatic within the first 24 hours (Prasad et al., 2021). Delays in diagnosis may be detected with excessive distension and ultimately gastric perforation (Schwartz, 2012). It should be kept in mind that association with epidermolysis bullosa is common. Skin findings may be helpful in the diagnostic process, and planning of preventive measures is also important (Prasad et al., 2021).

Patient Management and Treatment

Treatment of IHPS is a medical emergency, as it requires surgical treatment. First of all, the general condition of the patients should be carefully examined, and appropriate hydration support, electrolyte imbalances, and metabolic control should be ensured. In patients with low potassium, potassium replacement should be planned if necessary if urine output is normal (Emil, 2020). Surgical planning should be started after the patient's urine output and biochemical and metabolic imbalances are normalized. Ramstedt pyloromyotomy is used in the surgical treatment of hypertrophic pyloric stenosis. Depending on the preference of the surgeon and the patient's condition, pyloromyotomy can be performed by laparotomy or laparoscopy. In a meta-analysis by Sathya et al., no statistically significant difference was found in the length of hospital stay and complication rate between patients who underwent laparotomy and laparoscopy (Sathya et al., 2017). In cases of pyloric atresia, the surgical method varies according to the type of atresia (Prasad et al., 2021).

Annular Pancreas

As a consequence of the fact that a significant proportion of patients with annular pancreas present no symptoms, the precise prevalence of this condition remains uncertain. The prevalence of annular pancreas in autopsy cases of adults with duodenal dissection has been reported to range from 5 to 15 per 100,000 (Ravitch, 1975; Ravitch & Woods, 1950). Annular pancreas has been documented in conjunction with a range of congenital anomalies, including esophageal and duodenal atresia, Meckel's diverticulum, and imperforate anus. The incidence is increased in infants with Down syndrome and in cases where maternal polyhydramnios is present (Sencan et al., 2002; Zyromski et al., 2008). In individuals with a ring pancreas, the ring typically comprises a band of pancreatic tissue surrounding the second part of the duodenum. The band of pancreatic tissue is typically fused with the duodenal muscularis, although it may also be independent of the duodenum. Approximately two-thirds of patients with a ring pancreas are asymptomatic (Cunha et al., 2005). The age of onset of symptoms is dependent on the severity of duodenal obstruction. In children, more than two-thirds present in the neonatal period with feeding intolerance, vomiting, and abdominal distension (Kiernan et al., 1980). As the ring pancreas is usually located in a proximal position to the major papilla, vomiting is typically bile-free (Jimenez et al., 2004).

Radiological findings suggestive of a ring pancreas include narrowing of the duodenum, with narrowing of the second part of the duodenum, and symmetric dilation of the proximal duodenum. Additionally, reverse peristalsis of the duodenal segment proximal to the ring and dilatation of the duodenum distal to the ring may be observed (Urayama et al., 1995; Maker et al., 2003). Diagnosis can be achieved through the use of ultrasound, abdominal CT, and cholangiopancreatogram (Urayama et al., 1995; Choi et al., 2004).

Treatment

The majority of patients with annular pancreas are asymptomatic, and thus the presence of a ring pancreas does not necessarily indicate that symptoms are attributable to it. Although endoscopic treatment has been described, surgery remains the procedure of choice in patients whose symptoms are attributable to the annular pancreas (Gromski et al., 2019). The objective of surgical intervention is to circumvent the ring and alleviate duodenal or gastric outlet obstruction (Maker et al., 2003). In neonates, obstruction is relieved by means of a duodenoduodenostomy. In adults, a duodenojejunostomy or gastrojejunostomy is the recommended surgical procedure due to the reduced mobility of the duodenum (De Ugarte et al., 2006; Thomford et al., 1972).

Prognosis

The prognosis of patients with a ring pancreas is largely dependent on the age of onset of symptoms. In infants and children, the prognosis is largely dependent on associated congenital abnormalities (Hill & Lebenthal, 1993). Most adults with a ring pancreas have a favorable prognosis and do not require treatment. In adults, morbidity and mortality are mainly associated with surgical complications of bypass procedures (Zyromski et al., 2008; Hill & Lebenthal, 1993).

Antral Web

The antral web, also referred to as the mucosal diaphragm of the pyloric antrum or prepyloric diaphragm, represents a rare etiology for congenital gastric outlet obstruction. The antral web is situated at a distance of approximately 1-5 cm from the pylorus, with a typical thickness of 2-4 cm (Hait et al., 1972). The etiology of webs remains unclear, although excessive endodermal proliferation during early gastric development may be a contributing factor (Hait et al., 1972; Bell et al., 1977). The incidence is estimated to be approximately 1 in 100,000 births (Lui et al., 2000). Although antral curtain may manifest symptoms during early infancy, it can also be observed in adults (Bell et al., 1977).

Ultrasonography is an invaluable diagnostic tool. An upper gastrointestinal (UGI) series may reveal a persistent, sharp, band-like linear defect in the antrum, as well as a "double bulb sign." One is the normal duodenal bulb, and the other is the proximal antral chamber, situated between the web and the pylorus (Tiao, 2005). Conditions that may result in gastric obstruction include prepyloric antral web, pyloric stenosis, pylorospasm, excess or hypertrophic mucosal folds, perigastric adhesions, or heterotopic pancreatic tissue. Prior to the UGI series findings, multiple hypertrophic excess mucosal folds are typically more irregular than antral webs and do not circumferentially surround the stomach (Lui et al., 2000).

Treatment

In cases where the antral web is causing symptoms, surgical correction is the recommended course of action (Lui et al., 2000). Surgical options include the excision of the anomaly, either alone or in conjunction with pyloroplasty, and the replacement of the affected area with a prosthetic. The prognosis following surgical correction is favorable. Endoscopic treatment represents an additional option for the antral web, contingent upon the feasibility of endoscopic intervention. Endoscopic transection is feasible when the mucosal structure is smooth, devoid of substantial vessels or muscular or serosal layers, and the membrane is taut and amenable to vertical insertion (Berr et al., 1985).

Conclusion

In the neonatal period, vomiting has many non-biliary causes, such as feeding intolerance, pyloric stenosis, metabolic disorders, increased intracranial pressure, sepsis, milk allergy, necrotizing enterocolitis, or adrenal insufficiency. Non-biliary vomiting, even in the absence of abdominal distension, should alert us to congenital gastric outlet obstruction. Gastric outlet obstruction is one of the pathologies requiring surgery in the neonatal period. Obstructions can be seen not only in the stomach but also at any point, especially in the duodenum. They can be confused with many clinical conditions in the neonatal period and should be managed by pediatric surgeons and neonatologists acting together in the diagnosis and treatment process. Direct radiography, ultrasound, tomography, barium radiography, endoscopy, and MRI may be required in the diagnosis. There are many pathologies in the differential diagnosis, and sometimes it may be difficult to reach a definitive diagnosis and can only be diagnosed at the time of operation.

References

Aboagye, J., Goldstein, S. D., Salazar, J. H., Papandria, D., Okoye, M. T., Al-Omar, K., Stewart, D., Lukish, J., & Abdullah, F. (2014). Age at presentation of common pediatric surgical conditions: Reexamining dogma. *Journal of Pediatric Surgery, 49*(6), 995–999. https://doi.org/10.1016/j.jpedsurg.2014.01.039.

Applegate, M. S., & Druschel, C. M. (1995). The epidemiology of infantile hypertrophic pyloric stenosis in New York State, 1983 to 1990. *Archives of Pediatrics & Adolescent Medicine, 149*(10), 1123–1129. https://doi.org/10.1001/archpedi.1995.02170230077011.

Bell, M. J., Ternberg, J. L., McAlister, W., Keating, J. P., & Tedesco, F. J. (1977). Antral diaphragm—A cause of gastric outlet obstruction in infants and children. *Journal of Pediatrics, 90*(2), 196–202. https://doi.org/10.1016/S0022-3476(77)80629-X.

Berr, F., Rienmueller, R., & Sauerbruch, T. (1985). Successful endoscopic transection of a partially obstructing antral diaphragm. *Gastroenterology, 89*(5), 1147–1151. https://doi.org/10.1016/0016-5085(85)90222-7.

Choi, J. Y., Kim, M. J., Kim, J. H., Lim, S. K., Oh, Y. T., Chung, J. J., Song, S. Y., Chung, J. B., Yoo, H. S., Lee, J. T., & Kim, K. W. (2004). Annular pancreas: Emphasis on magnetic resonance cholangiopancreatography findings. *Journal of Computer Assisted Tomography, 28*(4), 528–532. https://doi.org/10.1097/00004728-200407000-00015.

Cunha, J. E., de Lima, M. S., Jukemura, J., Penteado, S., Jureidini, J., Patzina, R. A., & Siqueira, S. A. C. (2005). Unusual clinical presentation of annular pancreas in the adult. *Pancreatology, 5*(1), 81–85. https://doi.org/10.1159/000084493.

De Ugarte, D. A., Dutson, E. P., & Hiyama, D. T. (2006). Annular pancreas in the adult: Management with laparoscopic gastrojejunostomy. *American Surgeon, 72*(1), 71–73. https://pubmed.ncbi.nlm.nih.gov/16494188/.

Demian, M., Nguyen, S., & Emil, S. (2009). Early pyloric stenosis: A case control study. *Pediatric Surgery International, 25*(12), 1053–1057. https://doi.org/10.1007/s00383-009-2463-2.

Eberly, M. D., Eide, M. B., Thompson, J. L., & Nylund, C. M. (2015). Azithromycin in early infancy and pyloric stenosis. *Pediatrics, 135*(3), 483–488. https://doi.org/10.1542/peds.2014-2026.

Emil, S. (2020). Pyloric stenosis. In *Clinical pediatric surgery: A case-based interactive approach* (1st ed., pp. 249–257). CRC Press.

Gromski, M. A., Lehman, G. A., Zyromski, N. J., Watkins, J. L., El Hajj, I., Tan, T., McHenry, L., Easler, J. J., Tirkes, T., Sherman, S., & Fogel, E. L. (2019). Annular pancreas: Endoscopic and pancreatographic findings from a tertiary referral ERCP center. *Gastrointestinal Endoscopy, 89*(2), 322–328. https://doi.org/10.1016/j.gie.2018.09.008.

Hait, G., Esselstyn, C. B. Jr., & Rankin, G. B. (1972). Prepyloric mucosal diaphragm (antral web): Report of a case and review of the literature. *Archives of Surgery, 105*(3), 486–490. https://doi.org/10.1001/archsurg.1972.04180090089021.

Hedbäck, G., Abrahamsson, K., Husberg, B., Granholm, T., & Oden'e, L. (2001). The epidemiology of infantile hypertrophic pyloric stenosis in Sweden 1987–96. *Archives of Disease in Childhood, 85*(5), 379–381. https://doi.org/10.1136/adc.85.5.379.

Hill, I. D., & Lebenthal, E. (1993). Congenital abnormalities of the exocrine pancreas. In V. L. Go, E. P. DiMagno, J. D. Gardner, et al., (Eds.), *Pancreas: Pathology, pathobiology and disease* (2nd ed., p. 1029). Raven Press. https://www.uptodate.com/contents/annular-pancreas/abstract/12,13.

Hua, L., Shi, D., Bishop, P. R., Gosche, J., May, V. L., & Nowicki, M. J. (2005). The role of UGT1A1*28 mutation in jaundiced infants with hypertrophic pyloric stenosis. *Pediatric Research, 58*(5), 881–884. https://doi.org/10.1203/01.pdr.0000183372.23726.ca.

Jimenez, J. C., Emil, S., Podnos, Y., & Nguyen, N. (2014). Annular pancreas in children: A recent decade's experience. *Journal of Pediatric Surgery, 39*(11), 1654–1657. https://doi.org/10.1016/j.jpedsurg.2004.07.003.

Kapoor, R., Kancherla, V., Cao, Y., Oleson, J., Suhl, J., Canfield, M. A., Druschel, C. M., Kirby, R. S., Meyer, R. E., & Romitti, P. A. (2019). Prevalence and descriptive epidemiology of infantile hypertrophic pyloric stenosis in the United States: A multistate, population-based retrospective study, 1999–2010. *Birth Defects Research, 111*(3), 159–169. https://doi.org/10.1002/bdr2.1439.

Kiernan, P. D., ReMine, S. G., Kiernan, P. C., & ReMine, W. H. (1980). Annular pancreas: Mayo Clinic experience from 1957 to 1976 with review of the literature. *Archives of Surgery, 115*(1), 46–50. https://doi.org/10.1001/archsurg.1980.01380010038007.

Krogh, C., Biggar, R. J., Fischer, T. K., Lindholm, M., Wohlfahrt, J., & Melbye, M. (2012). Bottle-feeding and the risk of pyloric stenosis. *Pediatrics, 130*(4), e943–e949. https://doi.org/10.1542/peds.2011-2785.

Krogh, C., Gørtz, S., Wohlfahrt, J., Biggar, R. J., Melbye, M., & Fischer, T. K. (2012). Pre- and perinatal risk factors for pyloric stenosis and their influence on the male predominance. *American Journal of Epidemiology, 176*(1), 24–31. https://doi.org/10.1093/aje/kwr493.

Lui, K. W., Wong, H. F., Wan, Y. L., Hung, C. F., & Ng, K. K. (2000). Antral web—a rare cause of vomiting in children. *Pediatric Surgery International, 16*(5–6), 424–425. https://doi.org/10.1007/s003839900317.

MacMahon, B. (2006). The continuing enigma of pyloric stenosis of infancy: A review. *Epidemiology, 17*(2), 195–201. https://doi.org/10.1097/01.ede.0000192032.83843.c9.

Maker, V., Gerzenshtein, J., & Lerner, T. (2003). Annular pancreas in the adult: Two case reports and review of more than a century of literature. *American Surgeon, 69*(5), 404–410. https://pubmed.ncbi.nlm.nih.gov/12769212/.

Niedzielski, J., Kobielski, A., Sokal, J., & Krakós, M. (2011). Accuracy of sonographic criteria in the decision for surgical treatment in infantile hypertrophic pyloric stenosis. *Archives of Medical Science, 7*(3), 508–511. https://doi.org/10.5114/aoms.2011.23419.

Nmadu, P. T. (1992). Alterations in serum electrolytes in congenital hypertrophic pyloric stenosis: A study in Nigerian children. *Annals of Tropical Paediatrics, 12*(2), 169–172. https://doi.org/10.1080/02724936.1992.11747564.

Otjen, J. P., Iyer, R. S., Phillips, G. S., & Parisi, M. T. (2012). Usual and unusual causes of pediatric gastric outlet obstruction. *Pediatric Radiology, 42*(6), 728–737. https://doi.org/10.1007/s00247-012-2375-5.

Papadakis, K., Chen, E. A., Luks, F. I., Lessin, M. S., Wesselhoeft, C. W. Jr., & DeLuca, F. G. (1999). The changing presentation of pyloric stenosis. *American Journal of Emergency Medicine, 17*(1), 67–69. https://doi.org/10.1016/s0735-6757(99)90020-7.

Prasad, G. R., Rao, J. V. S., Fatima, F., & Anjum, F. (2021). Congenital pyloric atresia: Experience with a series of 11 cases and collective review. *Journal of Indian Association of Pediatric Surgeons, 26*(6), 416–420. https://doi.org/10.4103/jiaps.jIAPS_295_20.

Ravitch, M. M. (1975). The pancreas in infants and children. *Surgical Clinics of North America, 55*(2), 377–385. https://doi.org/10.1016/s0039-6109(16)40587-6.

Ravitch, M. M., & Woods, A. C. Jr. (1950). Annular pancreas. *Annals of Surgery, 132*(6), 1116–1127. https://doi.org/10.1097/00000658-195012000-00011.

Saha, A. K., Ali, M. B., Biswas, S. K., Sharif, H. M. Z., & Azim, A. (2012). Neonatal intestinal obstruction: Patterns, problems and outcome. *Bangladesh Medical Journal, 45*(1–2), 6–10. https://doi.org/10.3329/bmjk.v45i1-2.13638.

Sathya, C., Wayne, C., Gotsch, A., Vincent, J., Sullivan, K. J., & Nasr, A. (2017). Laparoscopic versus open pyloromyotomy in infants: A systematic review and meta-analysis. *Pediatric Surgery International, 33*(3), 325–333. https://doi.org/10.1007/s00383-016-4030-y.

Schwartz, M. S. (2012). Hypertrophic pyloric stenosis. In A. G. Coran, N. S. Adzick, T. M. Krummel, J. M. Leberge, R. Shamberger, & A. Caldamone (Eds.), *Pediatric surgery* (7th ed., pp. 1021–1029). Elsevier.

Sencan, A., Mir, E., Günsar, C., & Akcora, B. (2002). Symptomatic annular pancreas in newborns. *Medical Science Monitor, 8*(6), CR434–CR437. https://pubmed.ncbi.nlm.nih.gov/12070435/.

Seth, A., Chanchlani, R., & Rakhonde, A. K. (2015). Neonatal gastrointestinal emergencies in a tertiary care center in Bhopal, India: A prospective study. *IJSS Journal of Surgery.* https://www.semanticscholar.org/paper/736d13f15e3ddb9309444977edecc26c34e6aee8.

Sharma, K. K., Ranka, P., Goyal, P., & Dabi, D. R. (2008). Gastric outlet obstruction in children: An overview with report of Jodhpur disease and Sharma's classification. *Journal of Pediatric Surgery, 43*(10), 1891–1897. https://doi.org/10.1016/j.jpedsurg.2008.07.001.

Sivitz, A. B., Tejani, C., & Cohen, S. G. (2013). Evaluation of hypertrophic pyloric stenosis by pediatric emergency physician sonography. *Academic Emergency Medicine, 20*(7), 646–651. https://doi.org/10.1111/acem.12163.

Stanescu, A. L., Liszewski, M. C., Lee, E. Y., & Phillips, G. S. (2017). Neonatal gastrointestinal emergencies: Step-by-step approach. *Radiologic Clinics of North America, 55*(4), 717–739. https://doi.org/10.1016/j.rcl.2017.02.010.

Svenningsson, A., Svensson, T., Akre, O., & Nordenskjöld, A. (2014). Maternal and pregnancy characteristics and risk of infantile hypertrophic pyloric stenosis. *Journal of Pediatric Surgery, 49*(8), 1226–1231. https://doi.org/10.1016/j.jpedsurg.2014.01.053.

Taylor, N. D., Cass, D. T., & Holland, A. J. (2013). Infantile hypertrophic pyloric stenosis: Has anything changed? *Journal of Paediatrics and Child Health, 49*(1), 33–37. https://doi.org/10.1111/jpc.12027.

Thomford, N. R., Knight, P. R., Pace, W. G., & Madura, J. A. (1972). Annular pancreas in the adult: Selection of operation. *Annals of Surgery, 76*(2), 159–162. https://doi.org/10.1097/00000658-197208000-00007.

Tiao, M. M., Ko, S. F., Hsieh, C. S., Ng, S. H., Liang, C. D., Sheen-Chen, S. M., Chuang, J. H., & Huang, H. Y. (2005). Antral web associated with distal antral hypertrophy and prepyloric stenosis mimicking hypertrophic pyloric stenosis. *World Journal of Gastroenterology, 11*(4), 609–611. https://doi.org/10.3748/wjg.v11.i4.609.

To, T., Wajja, A., Wales, P. W., & Langer, J. C. (2005). Population demographic indicators associated with incidence of pyloric stenosis. *Archives of Pediatrics & Adolescent Medicine, 159*(6), 520–525. https://doi.org/10.1001/archpedi.159.6.520.

Urayama, S., Kozarek, R., Ball, T., Brandabur, J., Traverso, L., Ryan, J., & Wechter, D. (1995). Presentation and treatment of annular pancreas in an adult population. *American Journal of Gastroenterology, 90*(6), 995–999. https://pubmed.ncbi.nlm.nih.gov/7771437/.

Van Beelen, N. W., Mous, D. S., Brosens, E., de Klein, A., Van de Ven, C. P., Vlot, J., Ijsselstijn, H., & Wijnen, R. (2014). Increased incidence of hypertrophic pyloric stenosis in esophageal atresia patients. *European Journal of Pediatric Surgery, 24*(1), 20–24. https://doi.org/10.1055/s-0033-1352527.

Vinocur, D. N., Lee, E. Y., & Eisenberg, R. L. (2012). Neonatal intestinal obstruction. *AJR American Journal of Roentgenology, 198*(1), W1–W10. https://doi.org/10.2214/AJR.11.6931.

White, M. C., Langer, J. C., Don, S., & DeBaun, M. R. (1998). Sensitivity and cost minimization analysis of radiology versus olive palpation for the diagnosis of hypertrophic pyloric stenosis. *Journal of Pediatric Surgery, 33*(6), 913–917. https://doi.org/10.1016/S0022-3468(98)90673-X.

Zyromski, N. J., Sandoval, J. A., Pitt, H. A., Ladd, A. P., Fogel, E. L., Mattar, W. E., Sandrasegaran, K., Amrhein, D. W., Rescorla, F. J., Howard, T. J., Lillemoe, K. D., & Grosfeld, J. L. (2008). Annular pancreas: Dramatic differences between children and adults. *Journal of the American College of Surgeons, 206*(5), 1019–1025. https://doi.org/10.1016/j.jamcollsurg.2007.12.009.

Chapter 6

Congenital Duodonal Obstructions

Aybegüm Kalyoncu Aycenk*, MD
Department of Pediatric Surgery, Ordu University, Ordu, Turkey

Abstract

Congenital duodenal obstructions are a group of anomalies that result in partial or complete blockage of the duodenum, leading to significant clinical symptoms in neonates and infants. This chapter provides a comprehensive overview of the etiology, classification, and embryological basis of these conditions, including duodenal atresia, stenosis, and annular pancreas. Diagnostic approaches, including prenatal ultrasonography and postnatal imaging techniques, are discussed alongside typical clinical presentations. Additionally, the chapter explores current surgical and non-surgical treatment options, postoperative outcomes, and long-term considerations for patients affected by congenital duodenal obstructions.

Keywords: congenital, duodenal obstruction, duodenal atresia, newborn, ileus

Introduction

Congenital duodenal atresia (CDO) is an intestinal obstruction that begins during antenatal development. It is a condition where the preliminary diagnosis is made in the hours following birth when the baby begins to have bilious or non-bilious vomiting, provided there is no antenatal diagnosis, and

---

* Corresponding Author's Email: aybegumkalyoncu@gmail.com

In: Current Approaches to Newborn Emergencies
Editors: Zuhal Keskin Sarılar and Serap Samut Bülbül
ISBN: 979-8-89530-999-5

the diagnosis is confirmed through contrast imaging. CDO is the most common cause of intestinal obstruction in the neonatal period, occurring in 1 per 5000–10,000 live births (Morris et al., 2018; Akhtar& Guiney, 1992). Duodenal atresia is frequently suspected before birth when findings such as polyhydramnios or a distended stomach are noted. A prenatal ultrasound may identify the "double bubble" sign, seen in approximately 80% of cases, which consists of a large gastric bubble alongside a smaller bubble in the proximal duodenum (Bora et al., 2024).

CDO occurs due to intrinsic lesions, extrinsic lesions, or a combination of both. These pathological changes lead to obstruction, which is complete in 81% of cases and incomplete in 19%.

Intrinsic causes of CDO include conditions such as duodenal atresia, stenosis, diaphragmatic obstruction, a perforated diaphragm, or a "windsock" web. A windsock web refers to a duodenal membrane that becomes distally ballooned as a result of peristaltic pressure from the proximal side.

Extrinsic CDO may be caused by annular pancreas, malrotation, or preduodenal portal vein.

Embryology and Etiology

Gastrulation begins in the third week of embryonic development. The surface of the embryo facing the yolk sac forms the endoderm, while the surface facing the amniotic sac forms the ectoderm, and the middle portion forms the mesoderm. By the sixth week, intestinal epithelial proliferation begins, and recanalization occurs 1–2 weeks later. Defects in this recanalization process are thought to lead to intestinal stenosis or atresia. The pathogenesis of duodenal atresia is explained by an embryological theory proposing the persistence of physiologic epithelial occlusion (the "epithelial plug"), first described in 1900. Tandler's theory of developmental arrest remains widely accepted in most contemporary authoritative textbooks (Tandler, 1902).

The pancreas develops from the endodermal layer of the duodenum during the fourth week of gestation. It subsequently forms two buds: a larger dorsal pancreatic primordium and a smaller ventral one. The ventral bud rotates toward the dorsal bud in the eighth week, fusing with it. If the ventral bud fails to complete its rotation, it remains anterior to the duodenum and forms a pancreatic ring around the duodenum upon fusing with the dorsal pancreatic primordium. This results in the formation of an annular pancreas, leading to partial or complete obstruction (Sadler, 2003).

Epidemiology

Duodenal atresia is a congenital anomaly of the foregut, occurring in approximately 1 in 5,000 to 10,000 live births (Escobar et al., 2004). This rate has been gradually increasing in studies conducted in recent years (Morris et al., 2018). Duodenal atresia is frequently associated with other anomalies. The most significant link in this chain is its association with Down syndrome. The incidence of Down syndrome in infants born with congenital duodenal obstruction (CDO) ranges between 28% and 40%. It is followed by annular pancreas (23.1%), congenital cardiac malformations (22%), malrotation (19%), esophageal atresia/tracheoesophageal fistula (8.5%), genitourinary malformations (8%), and anorectal malformations (4%).

The early survival rate in the postoperative period increased from 60% to 90%. Mortality rates are gradually decreasing as neonatal intensive care improves (5%). The presence of associated anomalies, especially congenital cardiac malformations, increases mortality.

Classification

Congenital duodenal obstruction (CDO) is classified into two main categories: duodenal stenosis and duodenal atresia. Under duodenal stenosis, incomplete obstructions such as fenestrated webs or diaphragms are observed. These web formations are typically perforated, although imperforate webs may also be rarely seen. Duodenal stenosis usually occurs in the third or fourth part of the duodenum.

Duodenal atresia, on the other hand, is a complete obstruction. Gray and Scandalakis classified duodenal atresia into three types (Gray & Scandalakis, 1986). Type 1 is the most common form (92%) and is specifically referred to as the 'windsock' deformity. In this type, the duodenal wall integrity is preserved, and the obstruction is caused by an imperforate web in the duodenum. However, it appears as a balloon-like structure stretching downward within the lumen. Type II atresias (1%) are characterized by a dilated proximal segment and a collapsed distal segment, which are linked by a slender fibrous band. In Type III atresias (7%), there is a complete separation between the proximal and distal segments of the duodenum, creating a distinct V-shaped defect (Figure 1).

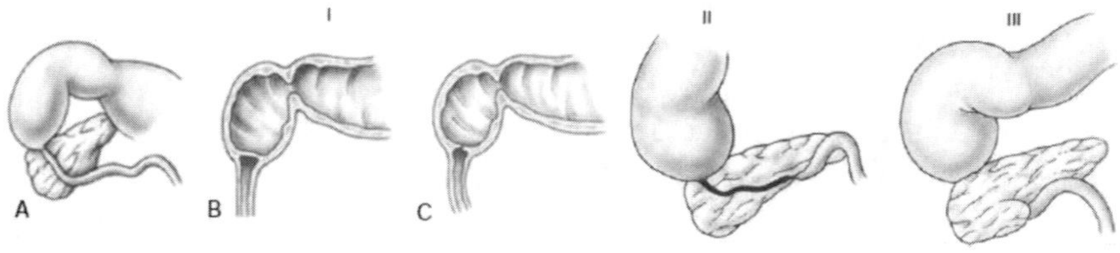

Figure 1. CDO, Gray, and Scandalakis classifications. Type I: either a membrane (B) or web (C) causes the intrinsic obstruction. Type 1B, "windsock deformity" type, in which the web is prolonged like a balloon to the distal portion. In this condition, there is no fibrous cord, and the duodenum remains continuous. Type II is defined by the complete obliteration of a segment of the duodenum, where the proximal and distal portions are connected by a fibrous cord. In Type III, the dilated proximal duodenum is entirely separated from the collapsed distal duodenum. (Aguayo et al., 2010).

The extrinsic type of duodenal obstruction arises from developmental abnormalities in adjacent structures, including the pancreas or a preduodenal portal vein, or as a result of conditions like malrotation and Ladd's bands. Annular pancreas is one of the most common extrinsic causes associated with congenital duodenal obstruction (CDO). It occurs due to a defect in the fusion of the ventral and dorsal buds during the eighth week of antenatal development, resulting in a ring-like structure encircling the duodenum. Variations in bile ducts are frequently associated with this type of obstruction. The location of the ampulla of Vater may be unusual, and the distal bile duct may divide into proximal and distal branches before joining the duodenum.

Diagnosis

Infants born with CDO typically present within the first 24 hours after birth with bilious or non-bilious vomiting. The clinical presentation may often deviate from the standard symptomatology. This variation is determined by the type and location of the defect as well as the associated anomalies. If the defect is an incomplete obstruction, findings may include a partial passage of abdominal gas to the distal segments, a confusing duodenal passage on contrast imaging, the presence of meconium, and the infant's ability to feed partially, though never effectively. If the defect is a complete obstruction, the standard symptomatology may include a 'double-bubble' sign on an abdominal X-ray, absence of meconium passage, lack of duodenal passage on contrast imaging, and bilious vomiting. In rare cases, non-bilious vomiting may be observed if the defect is located in the first or second part of the duodenum (Table 1).

The first step in diagnosis begins during the antenatal period. In antenatal sonographic evaluation, polyhydramnios is detected in the mother. Polyhydramnios is observed in 50% of pregnancies beyond 24 weeks of gestation, accompanied by the appearance of an enlarged stomach and duodenum, known as the 'double-bubble' sign (Figure 2).

Table 1. Symptoms of CDO

CONGENITAL DUODENAL OBSTRUCTIONS	
Symptom	Incidence (%)
Maternal polyhydramnios	*30-65*
Small for gestational age	*30-60*
Prematurity	*30-40*
Double bubble	*40-50*
Bilious vomiting	*90*
Non-bilious vomiting	*10*

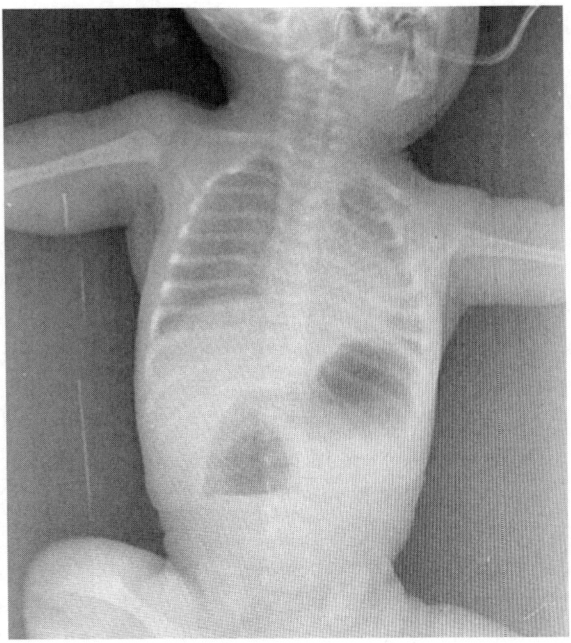

Figure 2. Neonatal erect X-ray, "double-bubble" sign.

In antenatally monitored or postnatally suspected newborns, the first recommended diagnostic test is an erect X-ray imaging. This imaging typically reveals signs of proximal obstruction. A specific finding for duodenal atresia is the 'double-bubble' sign. On the left side of the radiograph, a significantly dilated, air-filled gastric pouch can be observed, while on the right side, a smaller duodenal air bubble is noted (Koberlein & DiSantis, 2016).

Another alternative diagnostic technique is upper gastrointestinal contrast studies. Water-soluble contrast agents (such as urografin or gastrografin) administered via a nasogastric tube can be introduced into the stomach under fluoroscopic guidance to clarify the presence and level of obstruction.

Postnatal ultrasound can be used as an auxiliary diagnostic tool to understand the anomaly, evaluate the biliary tree, and distinguish associated anomalies such as malrotation.

Management

In neonates diagnosed with CDO, initial treatment begins with the placement of a nasogastric or orogastric tube to reduce the risk of aspiration. Simultaneously, resuscitation is initiated. Fluid and electrolyte imbalances caused by vomiting and the use of the gastric tube should be rapidly corrected. Following emergency management, preoperative preparation should commence. The primary focus of this preparation is the screening for associated anomalies. Initial investigations should include a biochemical metabolic blood panel, complete blood count, coagulation parameters, abdominal and spinal ultrasound, whole spine X-ray, and echocardiography. Given the need for fluid replacement and the potential for prolonged fasting during the postoperative period, the placement of an umbilical catheter immediately after birth is recommended.

Surgical treatment of CDO is not urgent once midgut volvulus is ruled out. The operation is planned at an appropriate time after fluid replacement and screening for associated anomalies.

The standard technique in surgical treatment is duodenoduodenostomy. Rarely, duodenojejunostomy, web excision, or gastrojejunostomy may be preferred. The approach can be either open or laparoscopic. In open surgical repair, a right upper quadrant transverse incision is made. After abdominal exploration, the right colon and hepatic flexure are mobilized to the left to access the duodenum and pancreas area. The proximal pouch is identified, and peritoneal dissection is performed carefully to avoid injury to the pancreas and the superior mesenteric artery and vein. Dissection of the distal pouch is carried out in the same area, during which subtypes such as type 1, 2, 3, and annular pancreas are distinguished. Once the distal pouch is identified and dissection is completed, the standard technique for anastomosis is the side-to-side, diamond-shaped anastomosis (Kimura et al., 1977). In cases where the diamond-shaped anastomosis, considered the ideal method among anastomosis alternatives, cannot be performed or is deemed unsuitable, a side-to-side anastomosis, with or without tapering duodenoplasty, can be performed. However, in cases where a duodenojejunostomy and gastrojejunostomy are deemed appropriate, the high risk of blind loop syndrome should be taken into account (Salonen & Mäkinen, 1976).

In the presence of an annular pancreas, pancreatic-duodenal dissection should never be performed. The main pancreatic ducts can be damaged during dissection. Therefore, bypassing the annular portion and opting for an anastomosis is recommended.

In the postoperative period, nasogastric tube output and total parenteral nutrition are preferred. As the color of the content from the nasogastric tube lightens and the volume decreases, initiating minimal enteral feeding should be considered. Prolonged fasting periods should be avoided, taking into account the risks of malnutrition and potential infectious complications they may cause. Rapid increases in feeding can trigger complications such as gastroesophageal reflux and megaduodenum; therefore, a gradual progression in the feeding process is recommended.

Complications

The complications associated with CDH can be evaluated under two main categories. Firstly, when assessing intraoperative complications, the most common issue encountered is incorrect anastomosis location. This is particularly true in cases of type 1 windsock deformity, where a long, floppy web is present, and if proper dissection of the web is not performed prior to anastomosis, there is a risk of performing the anastomosis proximal to the web. Additionally, the possibility of a second web should always be kept in mind. To prevent such situations, the distal and proximal lumens should be checked with the help of balloon catheters. Another intraoperative complication is anastomotic stricture and anastomotic leakage. Those incidences are below 1% overall.

When evaluating late postoperative complications, delayed gastric emptying, gastroesophageal reflux, peptic ulcer, megaduodenum, duodenogastric reflux, gastritis, blind-loop syndrome, and intestinal obstruction due to adhesions may be observed. Association with gastroesophageal reflux disease is observed in 7-10% of patients. More than half of these patients undergo surgical antireflux procedures. Therefore, close postoperative follow-up is recommended.

The most significant factors increasing the risk of complications are birth before <34 weeks of gestation, a birth weight <1500 grams, and associated anomalies (Deguchi et al., 2022).

Conclusion

CDO is the most commonly observed pathology among intestinal atresias. In recent years, the overall survival rate for CDO has exceeded 90%. Evaluation of associated anomalies is highly important and is one of the key factors influencing the development of complications. There is no well-established algorithm for postoperative management approaches. However, when postoperative complications are evaluated, it has been observed that long-term monitoring and treatment of gastroesophageal reflux disease are often necessary in the follow-up of CDO.

References

Aguayo, P., & Ostlie, D. (2010). Duodenal and intestinal atresia and stenosis. In G. W. Holcomb, J. P. Murphy, & D. J. Ostlie (Eds.), *Ashcraft's pediatric surgery* (pp. 400–415). Elsevier. https://doi.org/10.1016/B978-1-4160-6127-4.00031-8.

Akhtar, J., & Guiney, E. J. (1992). Congenital duodenal obstruction. *British Journal of Surgery, 79*(2), 133–135. https://doi.org/10.1002/bjs.1800790212.

Bora, N., Parihar, P., Raj, N., & Shetty, N. D. (2024). Imaging the double bubble: A case of duodenal atresia detected in late pregnancy. *Cureus, 16*(9), e68759. https://doi.org/10.7759/cureus.68759.

Deguchi, K., Tazuke, Y., Matsuura, R., Nomura, M., Yamanaka, H., Soh, H., & Yoneda, A. (2022). Factors associated with adverse outcomes following duodenal atresia surgery in neonates: A retrospective study. *Cureus, 14*(2), e22349. https://doi.org/10.7759/cureus.22349.

Escobar, M. A., Ladd, A. P., Grosfeld, J. L., West, K. W., Rescorla, F. J., & Scherer, L. R. (2004). Duodenal atresia and stenosis: Long-term follow-up over 30 years. *Journal of Pediatric Surgery, 39*, 867–871. https://doi.org/10.1016/j.jpedsurg.2004.02.025.

Gray, S. W., & Skandalakis, J. E. (1986). *Embryology for surgeons: The embryologic basis for the treatment of congenital defects*. WB Saunders.

Kimura, K., Tsugawa, C., Ogawa, K., Matsumoto, Y., Yamamoto, T., & Asada, S. (1977). Diamond-shaped anastomosis for congenital duodenal obstruction. *Archives of Surgery, 112*(10), 1262–1263. https://doi.org/10.1001/archsurg.1977.01370100116026.

Koberlein, G., & DiSantis, D. (2016). The "double bubble" sign. *Abdominal Radiology (New York), 41*(2), 334–335.

Morris, J. K., Springett, A. L., Greenlees, R., Loane, M., Addor, M. C., Arriola, L., Barisic, I., Bergman, J. E. H., Csaky-Szunyogh, M., Dias, C., Draper, E. S., Garne, E., Gatt, M., Khoshnood, B., Klungsoyr, K., Lynch, C., McDonnell, R., Nelen, V., Neville, A. J., ... Dolk, H. (2018). Trends in congenital anomalies in Europe from 1980 to 2012. *PLOS ONE, 13*(4), e0194986. https://doi.org/10.1371/journal.pone.0194986.

Sadler, T. W. (2003). *Langman's medical embryology* (15th ed.). Lippincott Williams & Wilkins.

Salonen, I. S., & Mäkinen, E. (1976). Intestinal blind pouch- and blind loop- syndrome in children operated previously for congenital duodenal obstruction. *Annales Chirurgiae et Gynaecologiae, 65*(1), 38–45.

Tandler, J. (1902). Zur Entwicklungsgeschichte des menschlichen Duodenum in frühen Embryonalstadien. *Morphologisches Jahrbuch, 29*, 187–216.

Chapter 7

Intestinal Atresia

Gül Şalcı*, MD
Department of Pediatric Surgery, Karadeniz Technical University, Trabzon, Turkey

Abstract

Intestinal atresia is the most common congenital malformation requiring urgent surgical intervention in newborns, characterized by bilious vomiting, abdominal distension, and failure to pass meconium. Infants with congenital colonic stenosis usually manifest most of the clinical and laboratory findings of sepsis. The incidence of gastrointestinal system malformations in infants of mothers with polyhydramnios has been reported as 27% (Başaklar, 2006). In the diagnosis, multiple different air-fluid levels are observed on the abdominal radiograph depending on the level of colonic stenosis. Lateral radiographs are useful in distinguishing low-type small bowel atresia from colonic atresia. Opaque upper gastrointestinal (GI) tract radiographs are not useful in the diagnosis, but they can be helpful in case of suspicious diagnosis or incomplete obstruction. In infants with distal obstruction, differential diagnosis can be made based on the detection of diseases such as congenital megacolon, meconium ileus, and small left colon on lower GI tract radiography. Surgery is the mainstay treatment of intestinal atresia. Fluid-electrolyte imbalance should be regulated before surgery. Nasogastric decompression is essential. Recently, mortality and morbidity rates have decreased remarkably due to the advancements in intensive care conditions and parenteral nutrition techniques.

---

* Corresponding Author's Email: gul_salci@hotmail.com

In: Current Approaches to Newborn Emergencies
Editors: Zuhal Keskin Sarılar and Serap Samut Bülbül
ISBN: 979-8-89530-999-5

Keywords: jejunal, ileal, colonic, rectal, atresia

Introduction

Intestinal atresia is a congenital condition in which the intestinal lumen is closed completely, preventing food and fluids from passing through the digestive system. The initial medical reports on intestinal atresia date back to the 15th century. The first enterostomy for intestinal atresia was performed by Voisin in 1804, and the first successful resection-anastomosis was performed by Fockens in 1911 (Grosfeld, 1998). To date, numerous theories have been suggested regarding its embryopathogenesis, while the most commonly accepted theory is that it is caused by vascular accidents. Although a definite genetic transmission has not been demonstrated, it is postulated that autosomal recessive inheritance may occur, particularly in the presence of multiple atresia.

Jejunoileal Atresia

Thromboembolic events, vascular accidents, and intraluminal inflammatory changes are considered to play a role in the embryopathogenesis of jejunoileal atresia (Coran, 2012). Its reported incidence is 1 in 5,000 live births (Dalla Vecchia et al., 1998). It is equally prevalent in boys and girls (Başaklar, 2006). Atresia is seen in the jejunum in 51% and in the ileum in 49% of the cases (Coran, 2012). Multiple atresia is detected in 10% of cases (Raffensperger 1990). Although it is mostly sporadic, familial transmission can also be observed (Kumaran et al., 2002). Less than 1% of the cases are accompanied by chromosomal abnormalities (Holcomb et al., 2019). In contrast to duodenal atresia, the overall incidence of additional abnormalities in jejunoileal atresia is relatively low, and commonly seen additional abnormalities include Hirschsprung's disease, cystic fibrosis, malrotation, Down syndrome, anorectal malformations, vertebral anomalies, neural tube defects, congenital heart defects, and other types of gastrointestinal atresia (Sweeney et al., 2001). Typically, the intestinal segment proximal to the atresia is dilated, and the bowel wall is hypertrophic and edematous. The smooth muscle cells in the proximal bowel wall are hypertrophic and hyperplastic (Cloutier, 1975), while there is insufficient peristalsis. Intestinal villi are hypertrophic due to compensatory response (Touloukian, 1978). There is also mucosal hypertrophy in the distal bowel wall. Muscle hyperplasia returns to normal within two to three weeks postoperatively (Cloutier, 1975).

According to the Grosfeld Classification, jejunoileal atresia is of four types (Figure 1) (Grosfeld, et al., 1979):

Type I: It accounts for 19% of the cases (Başaklar, 2006). Atresia is present without a mesenteric defect. The length of the small bowel is normal. Ballooning of the distal bowel with increased intraluminal pressure in the proximal portion may exhibit a 'windsock' sign.

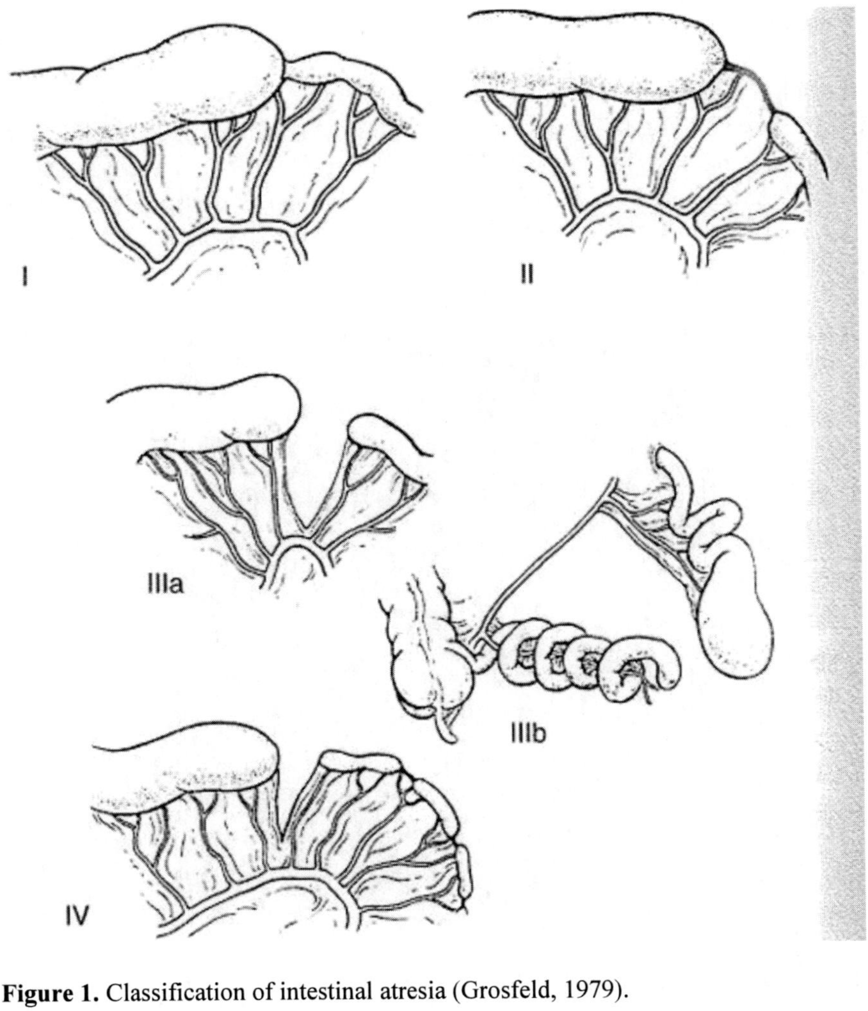

Figure 1. Classification of intestinal atresia (Grosfeld, 1979).

Type II: It constitutes 31% of the cases (Başaklar, 2006). It is characterized by a fibrous band between the two atretic ends. There is no mesenteric defect. The length of the small bowel is usually normal.

Type IIIA: It comprises 46% of the cases. It is the most common type (Başaklar, 2006). There is no band between the atretic ends. It presents with a 'V-shaped' mesenteric defect. The length of the small bowel is shorter than normal.

Type IIIB: It is also known as Christmas tree, apple-peel, or maypole intestinal atresia. It is the rarest type, constituting 11% of all cases of jejunoileal atresia (Başaklar, 2006). It is considered to result from obstruction in the superior mesenteric artery, and it is characterized by jejunal atresia very close to the ligament of Treitz. The distal portions of the bowels are wrapped in a spiral manner (Figure 2). There is no mesentery of the ileum. The length of the bowel is remarkably short. Of all infants with this type, 70% are premature and have low birth weight (Başaklar, 2006), 54% have malrotation (Coran, 2012), and 75% have short bowel syndrome (Holcomb et al., 2019). The risk of congenital anomalies is high. Almost 60% of them have a mortal course.

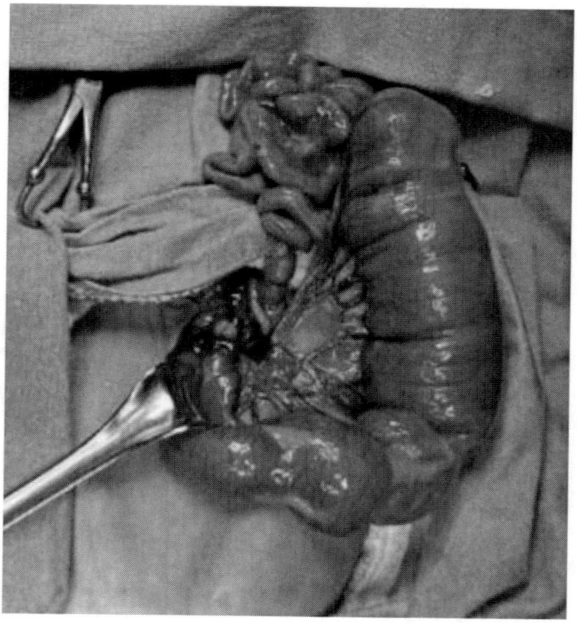

Figure 2. Apple-peel atresia (type 3b).

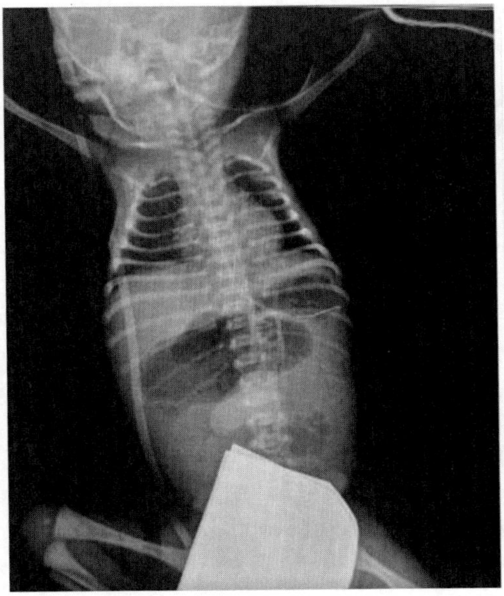

Figure 3. Abdominal radiograph demonstrating multiple air-fluid levels, with absence of distal bowel gas, consistent with intestinal obstruction.

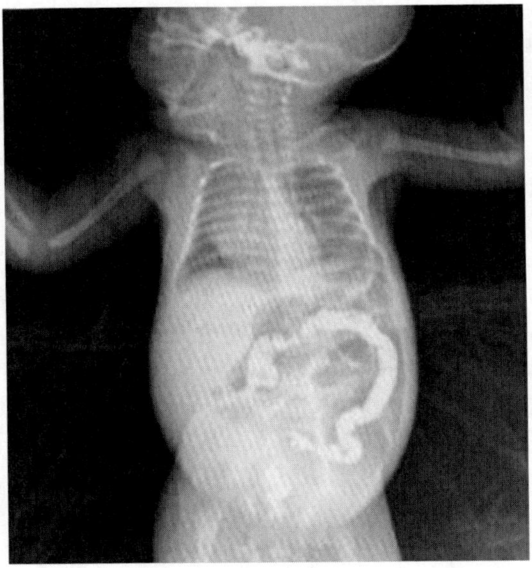

Figure 4. Contrast study of the lower gastrointestinal tract showing an unused colon, indicating the level of atresia.

Type IV: It is a combination of multiple atresias. It has a prevalence of 18% (Başaklar, 2006). Its etiology is characterized by multiple ischemic infarcts and intrauterine inflammation. Although it is considered to be inherited in an autosomal recessive manner, the responsible gene mutation has not yet been identified (Holcomb et al., 2019).

Today, most cases are diagnosed by antenatal USG. Polyhydramnios is detected in 24% of all cases of jejunoileal atresia (Grosfeld, et al., 1979). Bilious vomiting is usually the first symptom. Depending on the level of atresia, varying degrees of abdominal distension are seen. In high-type atresia, although the infants are able to pass distal meconium stools, most do not. Indirect hyperbilirubinemia can be observed. In late cases, if bowel necrosis and perforation develop, findings of abdominal sepsis can be seen. In the diagnosis, multiple different air-fluid levels can be detected on the abdominal radiography depending on the level of atresia (Figure 3). No gas is seen distal to the atresia. Following the development of intrauterine perforation, meconium pseudocysts and calcifications may be seen on the abdominal radiography due to meconium peritonitis (Grosfeld, 1986). Opaque upper gastrointestinal (GI) tract radiographs do not provide additional information in the diagnosis, but they can be useful in case of suspicious diagnosis or incomplete obstruction. Differential diagnosis should include malrotation, volvulus, meconium ileus, intestinal duplication, internal hernia, colonic atresia, and total colonic aganglionosis. In patients with suspected jejunoileal atresia, lower GI tract radiography should be used for investigating the presence of unused colon and accompanying colonic atresia, and malrotation should be explored by determining the location of the cecum (Figure 4).

In cases of jejunoileal atresia, surgery is performed after achieving decompression with a nasogastric tube and the regulation of fluid-electrolyte imbalance. In the supine position, the abdomen is entered through a transverse or circumumbilical incision above the umbilicus (Banieghbal & Beale, 2007). All bowels are carefully examined by inspection. The presence of a possible volvulus or malrotation is investigated. In case of volvulus, the bowels and mesentery need to be untwisted with utmost care. In case of malrotation, the 'Ladd Procedure' is applied. Subsequently, after the proximal and distal ends are located and the atretic portion is excised, the catheter is advanced through the distal segment, and warm saline is administered to investigate the presence of multiple atresia. The type of surgery to be performed is determined depending on the type and localization of atresia as well as the diameter difference between the proximal and distal ends. For a safe anastomosis, the diameter difference should not exceed a ratio of 4:1 (Puri, 2011). To minimize the diameter difference, the distal portion is cut at a 45-degree angle and the proximal part at a 90-degree angle (Figure 5). The distal bowel can be incised from the antimesenteric surface, and a fish-mouth anastomosis can be performed. In the presence of a greater diameter difference, the dilated part can be resected depending on the length of the bowel. If the remaining bowel length is less than 80 cm, the proximal bowel can be narrowed from the antimesenteric surface by the tapering method. Tapering can be performed safely up to 35 cm (Ramanujan, 1984). Afterwards, a single-row end-to-end anastomosis is performed between the proximal and distal ends. A mesenteric defect may be present, and it needs to be repaired. In the presence of multiple atresia, care should be taken to spare the least amount of bowel and perform the fewest number of anastomoses.

When intestinal atresia is accompanied by meconium ileus, it is safer to perform an ostomy rather than a primary anastomosis. In cases of atresia accompanied by anterior abdominal wall defects, primary anastomosis can be performed, or atresia repair can be postponed for a few weeks if there is no circulatory disorder. In the presence of necrotic bowel, performing an ostomy is preferable.

Nasogastric drainage is maintained in the postoperative period. Broad-spectrum antibiotic treatment is required. Fluid-electrolyte balance should be maintained. Total parenteral nutrition (TPN) support is essential since long-term enteral feeding is not possible. The more proximal the atresia is, the slower the bowel will function. The following day, rectal irrigation is needed to expel meconium, expand the distal portion of the bowel, and stimulate peristalsis. Enteral feeding can be restarted when it is determined that bowel functions have improved based on the following findings: gastric drainage decreases and lightens in color, the infant passes meconium, and abdominal distension decreases. Contrast-enhanced upper GI X-rays should be taken in patients in whom enteral feeding cannot be restarted on the 14th postoperative day. It has been shown that transanastomotic tube placement has no effect on early enteral nutrition and is not recommended since it increases the risk of tube-related complications.

The most common complications include stricture and anastomotic leakage (15%) (Nixon & Tawes, 1971). The type of atresia, presence of multiple atresia, presence of additional abnormalities, prematurity, and the remaining bowel length determine morbidity and mortality. In recent reports, mortality has been shown to decrease to less than 10% (Touloukian, 1993).

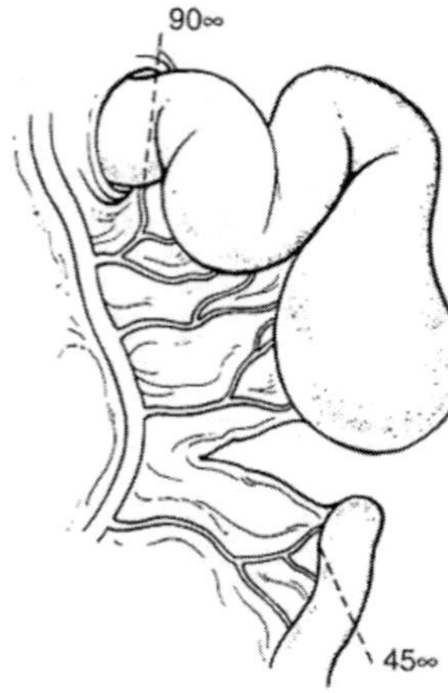

Figure 5. The proximal atretic segment is resected at a 90-degree angle and the distal segment at a 45-degree angle (Coran, 2012).

Colonic Atresia

It accounts for 10% of intestinal atresia (Benson et al., 1968). Its prevalence is 1 in 40,000 live births (Coran, 2012). Vascular events and maternal substance use are blamed in its embryopathogenesis. It is seen in the ascending colon in 28%, in the hepatic flexure in 3%, in the transverse colon in 23%, in the splenic flexure in 25%, and in the descending colon and sigmoid colon in 20% of the cases (Coran, 2012). It mostly presents as a single lesion. It may manifest with small bowel and duodenal atresia in 20% of the cases (Coran, 2012). It may accompany Hirschsprung's disease in 2% of the cases (Coran, 2012). It may be seen together with anterior abdominal wall defects and skeletal limb abnormalities (Arca et al., 1986).

There are three types of colonic atresia (Figure 6).

Type I: It presents with no mesenteric defect. Windsock deformity may accompany it.

Type II: There is a fibrous band between both atretic ends. There is a mesenteric defect.

Type III: It is the most common type (60%) (Etensel et al., 2005). There is no band between the atretic ends. There is a V-shaped mesenteric defect.

Common clinical signs and symptoms include distal obstruction findings. Bilious vomiting and abdominal distension are observed. The infant may pass meconium. Multiple different air-fluid levels are seen on the abdominal radiograph (Figure 7). The dilated bowel segment can be confused with pneumoperitoneum. Perforation risk is greater than in jejunoileal atresia. Mainstay treatment, as in other types of intestinal atresia, involves surgery after nasogastric decompression and regulation of electrolyte imbalance.

Surgical treatment is planned according to the level of atresia, additional abnormalities, and the presence of small bowel atresia. Primary anastomosis can be performed in atresia proximal to the splenic flexure, while in distal atresia, a colostomy is recommended as the initial method because the colon is blocked with solid mucus. Rectal biopsy is also recommended since it can be accompanied by Hirschsprung's disease (Kim et al., 2000; Lauwers et al., 2006).

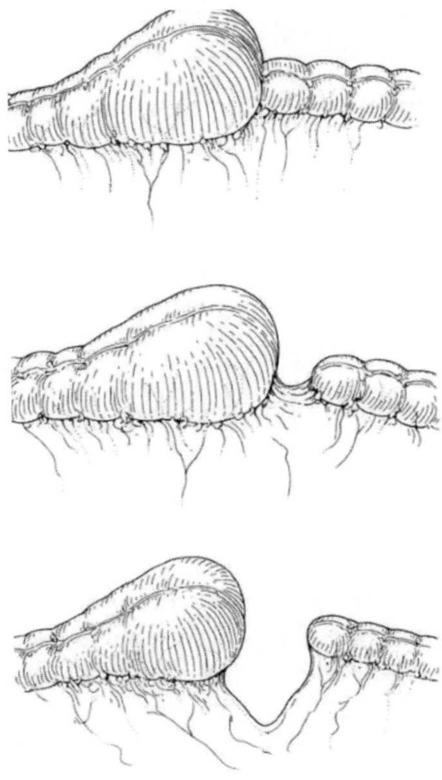

Figure 6. Types of colonic atresia (Puri, 2011).

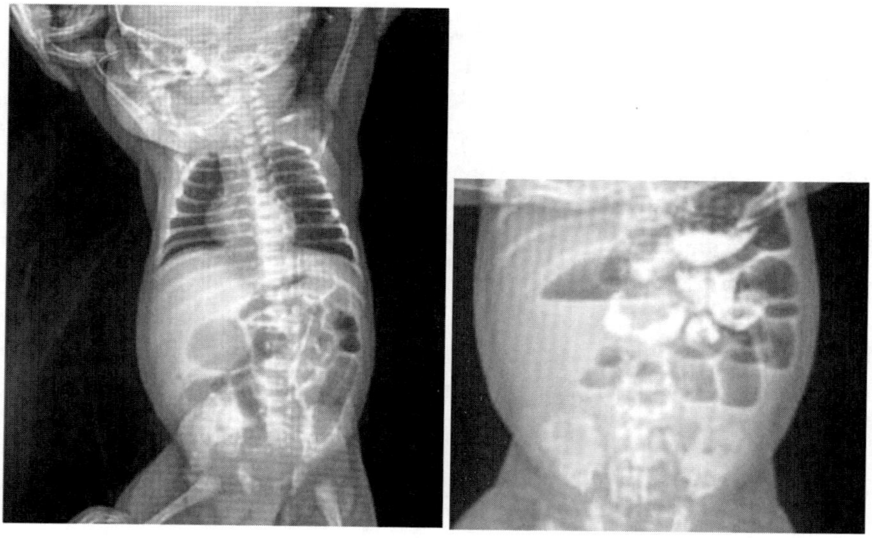

Figure 7. Multiple air-fluid levels are seen on the abdominal radiograph.

The atresia can be located by entering the abdomen with a transverse incision above the umbilicus. The presence of another atresia is investigated by administering warm saline through the distal end. Subsequently, primary anastomosis or colostomy is performed. The colostomy is closed after an average period of eight weeks (Puri, 2011). Postoperative complications are similar to those of small bowel atresia. If diagnosed early, survival rates are close to 100%.

Rectal Atresia

It is highly rare. Some scholars classify it as a colonic atresia, while others categorize it as an anorectal malformation. It constitutes less than 1% of all anorectal malformations (Puri, 2011). It is mostly located 1-3 cm above the anal canal. The anal canal, sacrum, and sphincter are usually normal. The incidence of additional abnormalities is low. It can be a component of multiple intestinal atresia. It results in distal atresia symptoms such as abdominal distension and failure to pass meconium.

There are five types of rectal atresia (Upadhyaya, 1996):

Type I: The bowel wall is intact. Continuity with the membrane is interrupted.

Type II: The gap between the blind ends is shorter than 2 cm.

Type III: It is the most common type. The gap between the ends is longer than 2 cm.

Type IV: It manifests with rectal stenosis.

Type V: It is accompanied by urinary fistula.

Diagnosis is made with multiple abdominal radiographies and lower GI tract radiography. A colostomy is performed in the neonatal period and enlarged until the infant is approximately eight weeks old. For definitive surgery, techniques such as abdominoperineal and sacroperineal Pull-Through, posterior sagittal anorectoplasty (PSARP), and transanal, end-to-end, rectorectal anastomosis (TERA) can be preferred. Mortality is around 35% (Puri, 2011). The most common complication is 'soiling.'

Conclusion

In newborns, intestinal obstruction is the most common congenital malformation requiring urgent surgical intervention. Proximal atresia, in particular, leads to polyhydramnios. Diagnosis is usually made with antenatal USG. Common symptoms include vomiting, abdominal distension, and failure to pass meconium. Normally, air reaches the stomach five minutes after birth, the small bowel 30 minutes later, the cecum two hours later, and the colon at the 4th hour after birth. It takes 18 hours to reach the sigmoid colon and rectum. Depending on the location of the atretic segment, the absence of gas in the distal part of the bowel and the dilation of the proximal portion on SDAR suggest intestinal atresia. In case of delayed diagnosis, perforation and peritonitis develop, causing mortality. Surgery is the mainstay treatment. Recently, mortality and morbidity rates have decreased remarkably due to the advancements in intensive care conditions and parenteral nutrition techniques.

References

Arca, M. J., & Oldham, K. T. (2012). Atresia, stenosis, and other obstructions of the colon. In A. G. Coran (Ed.), *Pediatric surgery* (7th ed., pp. 1247–1253). Mosby. https://doi.org/10.1016/B978-0-323-07255-7.00099-4.

Banieghbal, B., & Beale, P. G. (2007). Minimal access approach to jejunal atresia. *Journal of Pediatric Surgery, 42*(8), 1362–1364. https://doi.org/10.1016/j.jpedsurg.2007.03.034.

Başaklar, C. (2006). *Bebek ve çocukların cerrahi ve ürolojik hastalıkları* (pp. 465–489). Palme Yayınevi.

Benson, C. D., Lotfi, M. W., & Brogh, A. J. (1968). Congenital atresia and stenosis of the colon. *Journal of Pediatric Surgery, 3*(2), 253–257. https://doi.org/10.1016/0022-3468(68)90008-0.

Cloutier, R. (1975). Intestinal smooth muscle response to chronic obstruction: Possible applications in jejunoileal atresia. *Journal of Pediatric Surgery, 10*(1), 3–8. https://doi.org/10.1016/s0022-3468(75)80002-9.

Coran, A. G., Adzick, N. S., Krummel, T. M., Laberge, J.-M., Shamberger, R., & Caldamone, A. (2012). *Pediatric surgery* (7th ed.). Elsevier.

Dalla Vecchia, L. K., Grosfeld, J. L., West, K. W., Rescorla, F. J., Scherer, L. R., & Engum, S. A. (1998). Intestinal atresia and stenosis: A 25-year experience with 277 cases. *Archives of Surgery, 133*(5), 490–497. https://doi.org/10.1001/archsurg.133.5.490.

Etensel, B., Temir, G., Karkiner, A., Melek, M., Edirne, Y., Karaca, I., & Mir, E. (2005). Atresia of the colon. *Journal of Pediatric Surgery, 40*(8), 1258–1268. https://doi.org/10.1016/j.jpedsurg.2005.05.008.

Grosfeld, J. L. (1986). Jejunoileal atresia and stenosis. In M. M. Ravitch et al., (Eds.), *Pediatric surgery* (p. 838). Year Book Medical Publishers.

Grosfeld, J. L. (1986). Jejunoileal atresia and stenosis. In M. M. Ravitch et al., (Eds.), *Pediatric surgery* (pp. 1145–1158). Year Book Medical Publishers.

Grosfeld, J. L., Ballantine, T. V., & Shoemaker, R. (1979). Operative management of intestinal atresia and stenosis based on pathologic findings. *Journal of Pediatric Surgery, 14*(3), 368–375. https://doi.org/10.1016/s0022-3468(79)80502-3.

Holcomb, G. W., Murphy, J. D., & Ostlie, D. J. (2019). Ashcraft's pediatric surgery (6th edn). *Annals of the Royal College of Surgeons of England, 101*(8), 414–430. https://doi.org/10.1308/003588415x14181254788962.

Kim, S., Yedlin, S., & Idowu, O. (2000). Colonic atresia in monozygotic twins. *American Journal of Medical Genetics, 91*(3), 204–206.

Kumaran, N., Shankar, K. R., Lloyd, D. A., & Losty, P. D. (2002). Trends in the management and outcome of jejuno-ileal atresia. *European Journal of Pediatric Surgery, 12*(3), 163–167. https://doi.org/10.1055/s-2002-32726.

Lauwers, P., Moens, E., Wustenberghs, K., Deprettere, A., Ruppert, M., Balliu, L., Hubens, G., & Vaneerdeweg, W. (2006). Association of colonic atresia and Hirschsprung's disease in the newborn: Report of a new case and review of the literature. *Pediatric Surgery International, 22*(3), 277–281. https://doi.org/10.1007/s00383-005-1456-z.

Nixon, H. H., & Tawes, R. (1971). Etiology and treatment of small intestinal atresia: Analysis of a series of 127 jejunoileal atresias and comparison with 62 duodenal atresias. *Surgery, 69*(1), 41–51.

Puri, P. (2011). *Newborn surgery* (3rd ed., pp. 494–551). CRC Press. https://doi.org/10.1201/b13478.

Raffensperger, J. G. (1990). Intestinal obstruction in the neonate. In *Swenson's pediatric surgery* (5th ed., pp. 503–507).

Ramanujan, T. M. (1984). Functional capability of blind small bowel loops after intestinal remodelling techniques. *The Australian and New Zealand Journal of Surgery, 54*(2), 145–150. https://doi.org/10.1111/j.1445-2197.1984.tb06706.x.

Sweeney, B., Surana, R., & Puri, P. (2001). Jejunoileal atresia and associated malformations: Correlation with the timing of in utero insult. *Journal of Pediatric Surgery, 36*(5), 774–776. https://doi.org/10.1053/jpsu.2001.22958.

Touloukian, R. J. (1978). Antenatal intestinal adaptation with experimental jejunoileal atresia. *Journal of Pediatric Surgery, 13*(6), 468–474. https://doi.org/10.1016/s0022-3468(78)80307-8.

Touloukian, R. J. (1993). Diagnosis and treatment of jejunoileal atresia. *World Journal of Surgery, 17*(3), 310–317. https://doi.org/10.1007/BF01658697.

Upadhyaya, P. (1990). Rectal atresia: Transanal, end-to-end, rectorectal anastomosis - A simplified, rational approach to management. *Journal of Pediatric Surgery, 25*(5), 535–537. https://doi.org/10.1016/0022-3468(90)90567-S.

Chapter 8

Anterior Abdominal Wall Defects

Serap Samut Bülbül*, **MD**
Department of Pediatric Surgery, Faculty of Medicine, Samsun University, Samsun, Turkey

Abstract

The abdominal wall, consisting of skin, fascia, and muscle, is the body part that connects the abdomen, rib cage, and pelvis. Its most important function is to surround the abdominal cavity and vital internal organs. Abdominal wall defects may occur congenitally or later. Abdominal wall defects are also called ventral wall defects. In the newborn, abdominal wall defects can cause abdominal organs to protrude outside the body (Flynn & Vickerton, 2023). In addition, congenital anomalies and accompanying syndromes that develop in addition to abdominal wall defects may result in more complicated clinical presentations. Studies conducted to determine the prevalence of anterior abdominal wall defects in society report that these cases may have a frequency of approximately 1 in every 2,500 to 1 in 5,000 live births in the world. However, when abdominal wall defects are not treated surgically in the early period, in the presence of additional anomalies and in complicated cases, they pose a serious morbidity and mortality problem. In this chapter, frequently observed clinical conditions specific to anterior abdominal wall defects will be discussed.

Keywords: abdominal wall, congenital defect, gastroschisis, omphalocele

---

* Corresponding Author's Email: ssamutdr@hotmail.com

In: Current Approaches to Newborn Emergencies
Editors: Zuhal Keskin Sarılar and Serap Samut Bülbül
ISBN: 979-8-89530-999-5

Introduction

The anterior abdominal wall is divided into four quadrants - right, left, lower, and upper - by imaginary lines drawn vertically and horizontally from the umbilicus for better identification of pathological conditions. In addition, it can be divided into a total of 9 regions by two vertical lines drawn from the midline of each clavicle. Congenital defects are frequently seen in the anterior section surgically (Kostov et al., 2023).

The most common congenital abdominal wall defects that can be diagnosed by fetal ultrasonography in the pediatric age group are reported to be gastroschisis and omphalocele (Christison-Lagay et al., 2011). These defects are diagnosed before birth and are in the group of surgically treatable diseases. In gastroschisis, where the patient's prognosis is related to the amount and function of the intestine, there is no sac, and the defect is to the right of the belly button. It is common to have a sac in omphalocele. In addition, gastrointestinal anomalies such as intestinal atresia may accompany the disease in omphalocele, and the defect is located in the umbilicus. During the treatment phase, the approach to these defects and the prognosis of the patients may also differ. The aim of treatment in patients is to reduce intra-abdominal pressure and close the abdominal wall defect, but the presence of additional anomalies may be decisive in the patient's prognosis. Direct internal organ trauma due to a defect in the abdominal wall may also occur in these patient groups. One of the complications that may develop in the case of gastroschisis is intestinal dysfunction, which can cause morbidity and mortality in patients with abdominal wall defects. While trying to reduce the increased intra-abdominal pressure that often exists during surgical intervention, it is indirectly aimed to preserve vital internal organs (Christison-Lagay et al., 2011; Slater & Pimpalwar, 2020). Additionally, the size of the defect is also important in omphalocele cases. While small omphalocele defects are closed first, in the case of large defects, topical treatment may be preferred to allow initial skin coverage before closure. The embryological and epidemiological characteristics of the patients, existing additional anomalies, and the course of the cases during pregnancy are of surgical importance in these two groups of patients (Ledbetter, 2012).

Anatomy and Embryology

Abdominal wall defects can be broadly categorized as gastroschisis (intact umbilical cord, evisceration of intestines through a defect in the abdominal wall, usually to the right of the cord, without being covered by membrane), omphalocele (herniation of intestine, liver, and other organs into the intact umbilical cord, covered by membranes unless ruptured), and the rarer midline defects (Cantrell's pentalogy). These defects may also include exposed viscera in the lower or upper abdomen. Although researchers have attempted to find a common embryological origin to explain the existence of the various defects, most researchers suggest that they are distinct defects with similar appearances based on anatomy, incidence, presence of associated anomalies or chromosomal abnormalities, and their consequences (Weber et al., 2002). Recent work has clarified the normal development of the abdominal wall and umbilicus, and has proposed a convincing theory that these defects result from an imbalance between cell proliferation and apoptotic cell death (Robinson & Abuhamad, 2000). The embryonic folding process that transforms the developing embryo from a disc to a cylinder results from the rapid growth of the neuroectoderm and mesoderm. Apoptotic cell death in the umbilical ring region causes relative growth retardation in that area. Rapid development of the foregut also results in herniation of the intestine through the umbilical stalk. Inadequate mesoderm formation or migration results in failure of attachment of the umbilical ring to the yolk sac and stalk due to amniotic band or vascular disruption. In gastroschisis, the wall of the fold is dysplastic, probably related to decreased cell accumulation or vascular abnormality, resulting in a thinned area of abdominal wall to the right of the umbilicus that ruptures due to increased intra-abdominal pressure (Weber et al., 2002).

Gastroschisis

Gastroschisis is a paraumbilical, full-thickness abdominal wall defect. In gastroschisis, which rarely has a genetic basis, there is loss of the membrane covering the intestine exposed in the uterus. In some cases, this section may be matted, enlarged, and covered with a fibrous inflammatory crust (Rentea & Gupta, 2023). One of the pieces of evidence that gastroschisis is not related to omphalocele in etiology is the absence of chromosomal abnormalities and the lack of association with syndromes. It is suggested that factors such as young age, smoking, and alcohol use during pregnancy in mothers of babies with gastroschisis, and teratogens may cause at least some cases of this abdominal wall defect. It is also suggested that the use of paracetamol, aspirin, and pseudoephedrine during pregnancy increases the risk of developing gastroschisis (Weber et al., 2002). Intrauterine growth restriction is a common clinical picture in gastroschisis. In pregnant women, intestinal loops floating freely in the uterine cavity can be observed during ultrasound monitoring. In addition, laboratory tests of these pregnant women show high maternal serum alpha-fetoprotein (AFP) levels. The incidence of additional anomalies is seen at lower rates compared to omphalocele patients. Treatment begins at birth. The first intervention to be made in postpartum care should be to protect the herniated intestines and internal organs from heat loss and to prevent contact with the external environment with sterile wet sponges and dressings or stretch film or plastic bags. In addition, the patient should be laid on the right side to prevent vascular damage. Primary or staged intervention should be performed to close the defect. The monitoring of patients in intensive care conditions, temperature regulation, hydration, and the protection of the intestines are of great importance in stabilizing them. In addition to protecting the intestines from trauma, patients can be prepared for surgery by placing an orogastric tube for intestinal decompression. The preferred first treatment for gastroschisis is the placement of the bowel and internal organs, which have herniated outside the abdominal cavity, back into the abdomen, followed by the repair of the abdominal wall defect. If the patient's clinical condition is unstable and the reduction of the bowel into the abdomen could lead to compartment syndrome, staged repairs may be preferred. Until the defect can be repaired, a plastic silo is applied around the bowel, and the bowel is gradually pushed back into the abdomen. These interventions delay the transition to enteral feeding, while emergency repairs also lead to respiratory complications (Diyaolu et al., 2021; Prefumo & Izzi, 2014). Survival in babies with gastroschisis is more than 90%. However, intestinal atresia, volvulus, and intestinal loss are complications that may be encountered in these patients, and in these cases, morbidity and mortality rates are affected in patients (Christison-Lagay et al., 2011; Rentea & Gupta, 2023).

Without early intervention and surgical repair in patients with gastroschisis, it may cause short bowel syndrome in infancy and childhood. In addition, in children experiencing intestinal loss, total parenteral nutrition requirements may result in major socioeconomic losses (Moore et al., 1999). Cesarean delivery protocol and primary closure are preferred more frequently with a high survival rate (Jaczyńska et al., 2023).

Omphalocele

Omphalocele is a congenital abdominal wall defect that occurs due to disruption of organogenesis during the embryonic period. Omphalocele (also called exomphalos) is a translucent sac composed of amnion, Wharton jelly, and peritoneum, with an umbilical cord attached and containing herniated small intestine, liver, spleen, colon, and occasionally gonads. The intestines and organs are functionally and morphologically normal. Omphalocele can be seen alone or often with additional anomalies and syndromes (Lausten-Thomsen et al., 2024). All babies with an omphalocele should be delivered in a well-equipped center with neonatologists and surgical specialists. This allows for early diagnosis and management of associated anomalies, as well as evaluation and appropriate surgical treatment of the abdominal wall defect. Diseases seen in addition to omphalocele are Beckwith-Wiedemann syndrome (an overgrowth syndrome characterized by macrosomia, enlarged tongue, neonatal hypoglycemia, ear creases and pits, hemihypertrophy, visceromegaly, umbilical hernia, embryonal tumors, omphalocele, nephrocalcinosis, medullary sponge kidney disease, cardiomegaly, and nephromegaly), gastrointestinal anomalies, trisomy 13 (Patau syndrome: small eyes, cleft lip and palate, microcephaly, cryptorchidism, polydactyly, hypertelorism, micrognathia, cutis aplasia, and external ears anomalies), trisomy 18 (Edwards syndrome: dolichocephaly, external ear anomalies, micrognathia, short palpebral fissures, small face, clenched fist with overriding fingers, hypotonia, and rocker bottom feet), and others such as trisomy 21 (Down syndrome: hypotonia, upslanting palpebral fissures, brachycephaly, low-set ears, single palmar crease, flat nasal bridge, Brushfield spots around the iris, in-curved fifth digits, and a gap between the first and second toes) can be considered as congenital anomalies. Patients with Beckwith-Wiedemann syndrome are often accompanied by embryonal tumors (neuroblastoma, hepatoblastoma, and Wilms tumor) (Borjas Mendoza et al., 2024; Zahouani & Mendez, 2023). Pentalogy of Cantrell (omphalocele, Morgagni diaphragmatic hernia, sternal defect, pericardial defect, and intrinsic congenital heart disease), Shprintzen-Goldberg syndrome, CHARGE syndrome, cloacal exstrophy syndrome, Carpenter syndrome, Marshall-Smith syndrome, and Meckel-Gruber syndrome are other syndromic diseases that may accompany this picture. Intestinal obstructions and volvulus may occur as complications in cases (Cullis et al., 2024). In babies born with omphalocele, just like gastroschisis, the sac should not be infected, and the baby's heat loss should be prevented. If the sac ruptures, heat and fluid loss are as important as gastroschisis. Chest X-rays and echocardiography should be performed for heart anomalies. A nasogastric tube should be inserted to provide intestinal decompression fluid resuscitation, a careful physical examination looking for associated anomalies, and the sac should be covered with wet sterile gauze, and the baby should be taken to intensive care. Some babies with a large or ruptured omphalocele have significant respiratory distress at birth, requiring emergency intubation and ventilation. In treatment, the surgical stage is started when the baby's general condition becomes stable. Surgical closure is considered a good choice in omphalocele cases, especially in the first 72 hours of life. In large defects, the use of silos and patches may be necessary during the intervention. Especially after major surgical repairs, liquid nutrition monitoring and prophylactic antibiotic treatments when necessary can be considered as other options until patients are stabilized (Zahouani & Mendez, 2023; Roux et al., 2019). Babies who have undergone larger defect repairs usually require postoperative mechanical ventilation for days, depending on their lung condition. In this case, signs such as oliguria, intestinal ischemia, and liver dysfunction should be carefully observed for increased intra-abdominal pressure.

It has been reported that infections are common in patients with congenital abdominal wall defects. Approximately 1/3 of patients are infected with one or more types of bacteria or fungi. In cases where infection is observed, the most common infections are Enterobacteriaceae, Pseudomonas aeruginosa, and Acinetobacter spp.; Staphylococcus spp., Enterococcus spp., and Candida spp. are to be identified (Ţarcă et al., 2023).

Different Causes of Anterior Abdominal Wall Defect: Prune Belly Syndrome

Patients with Prune Belly syndrome have an abdominal wall defect due to inadequate abdominal wall skeletal muscle. In these cases, the abdominal wall has a loose, plum-like appearance and is named because of this appearance. In patients with Prune Belly syndrome, in addition to the abdominal wall defect, dysfunctional smooth muscle formation is observed in the patients, resulting in urinary system diseases (such as megalourethra, megacystis, hydroureteronephrosis, and renal dysplasia) and intra-abdominal testicles (Lopes et al., 2021).

Gastrointestinal, orthopedic, and cardiopulmonary comorbidities frequently accompany patients with Prune Belly syndrome. Although the pathogenesis of the disease is not fully known, it is suggested that the defect occurs due to a mesenchymal developmental disruption (Granberg et al., 2012; Arlen et al., 2019). Surgical abdominal wall reconstruction is required in patients with Prune Belly syndrome. In the abdominoplasty to be performed in the treatment of these patients, the aim is to support the inadequately formed parts of the abdominal wall. For this purpose, one of the main purposes of surgical intervention is to advance the peripheral abdominal wall (Arlen et al., 2019).

Conclusion

Omphalocele and gastroschisis are the most common congenital anomalies in anterior abdominal wall defects.

With these general features, anterior abdominal wall defects are conditions that can be treated surgically. However, in addition to early reparative surgical treatment for anterior abdominal wall defects, in complicated cases, complex surgical reconstructive techniques can also be used.

In addition, early diagnosis of congenital diseases in the fetal period and preoperative and postoperative follow-up and treatment of patients are of great importance. Therefore, follow-up and treatment should be carried out in equipped centers with a multidisciplinary approach by a team consisting of obstetricians, neonatologists, and pediatric surgeons with parental counseling.

References

Arlen, A. M., Nawaf, C., & Kirsch, A. J. (2019). Prune belly syndrome: Current perspectives. *Pediatric Health, Medicine and Therapeutics, 10*, 75–81. https://doi.org/10.2147/PHMT.S188014.

Borjas Mendoza, P. A., Daley, S. F., & Mendez, M. D. (2024). Beckwith-Wiedemann syndrome. In *StatPearls*. StatPearls Publishing.

Christison-Lagay, E. R., Kelleher, C. M., & Langer, J. C. (2011). Neonatal abdominal wall defects. *Seminars in Fetal & Neonatal Medicine, 16*(3), 164–172. https://doi.org/10.1016/j.siny.2011.02.003.

Cullis, P. S., Fouad, D., Goldstein, A. M., Wong, K. K. Y., Boonthai, A., Lobos, P., Pakarinen, M. P., & Losty, P. D. (2024). Major surgical conditions of childhood and their lifelong implications: Comprehensive review. *BJS Open, 8*(3), zrae028. https://doi.org/10.1093/bjsopen/zrae028.

Diyaolu, M., Wood, L. S., & Bruzoni, M. (2021). Sutureless closure for the management of gastroschisis. *Translational Gastroenterology and Hepatology, 6*, 31. https://doi.org/10.21037/tgh-20-185.

Flynn, W., & Vickerton, P. (2023). Anatomy, abdomen and pelvis: Abdominal wall. In *StatPearls*. StatPearls Publishing.

Granberg, C. F., Harrison, S. M., Dajusta, D., Zhang, S., Hajarnis, S., Igarashi, P., & Baker, L. A. (2012). Genetic basis of prune belly syndrome: Screening for HNF1β gene. *The Journal of Urology, 187*(1), 272–278. https://doi.org/10.1016/j.juro.2011.09.036.

Jaczyńska, R., Mydlak, D., Mikulska, B., Nimer, A., Maciejewski, T., & Sawicka, E. (2023). Perinatal outcomes of neonates with complex and simple gastroschisis after planned preterm delivery: A single-centre retrospective cohort study. *Diagnostics (Basel), 13*(13), 2225. https://doi.org/10.3390/diagnostics13132225.

Kostov, S., Dineva, S., Kornovski, Y., Slavchev, S., Ivanova, Y., & Yordanov, A. (2023). Vascular anatomy and variations of the anterior abdominal wall: Significance in abdominal surgery. *Prague Medical Report, 124*(2), 108–142. https://doi.org/10.14712/23362936.2023.9.

Lausten-Thomsen, U., Hedley, P. L., Conway, K. M., Løfberg, K. M., Johansen, L. S., Romitti, P. A., & Christiansen, M. (2024). Omphalocele prevalence and co-occurring malformations: A nationwide register-based study of Danish live births in 1997–2021. *Pediatric Surgery International, 41*(1), 1. https://doi.org/10.1007/s00383-024-05897-5.

Ledbetter, D. J. (2012). Congenital abdominal wall defects and reconstruction in pediatric surgery: Gastroschisis and omphalocele. *The Surgical Clinics of North America, 92*(3), 713–x. https://doi.org/10.1016/j.suc.2012.03.010.

Lopes, R. I., Baker, L. A., & Dénes, F. T. (2021). Modern management of and update on prune belly syndrome. *Journal of Pediatric Urology, 17*(4), 548–554. https://doi.org/10.1016/j.jpurol.2021.04.010.

Moore, T. C., Collins, D. L., Catanzarite, V., & Hatch, E. I., Jr. (1999). Pre-term and particularly pre-labor cesarean section to avoid complications of gastroschisis. *Pediatric Surgery International, 15*(2), 97–104. https://doi.org/10.1007/s003830050525.

Prefumo, F., & Izzi, C. (2014). Fetal abdominal wall defects. *Best Practice & Research. Clinical Obstetrics & Gynaecology, 28*(3), 391–402. https://doi.org/10.1016/j.bpobgyn.2013.10.003.

Rentea, R. M., & Gupta, V. (2023). Gastroschisis. In *StatPearls*. StatPearls Publishing.

Robinson, J. N., & Abuhamad, A. Z. (2000). Abdominal wall and umbilical cord anomalies. *Clinics in Perinatology, 27*(4), 947–ix. https://doi.org/10.1016/s0095-5108(05)70059-2.

Roux, N., Grangé, G., Salomon, L. J., Rousseau, V., Khen-Dunlop, N., & Beaudoin, S. (2019). Omphalocèle au premier trimestre: Valeur pronostique du contenu extériorisé pour le risque d'anomalie associée [Early diagnosis of omphalocele: Prognostic value of the herniated viscera for associated anomalies]. *Gynecologie, Obstetrique, Fertilite & Senologie, 47*(9), 637–642. https://doi.org/10.1016/j.gofs.2019.06.013.

Slater, B. J., & Pimpalwar, A. (2020). Abdominal wall defects. *NeoReviews, 21*(6), e383–e391. https://doi.org/10.1542/neo.21-6-e383.

Ţarcă, E., Cojocaru, E., Trandafir, L. M., Melinte Popescu, M. G., Luca, A. C., Butnariu, L. I., Hanganu, E., Moscalu, M., Ţarcă, V., Stătescu, L., Radu, I., & Melinte Popescu, A. S. (2023). Nosocomial infections affecting newborns with abdominal wall defects. *Healthcare (Basel), 11*(8), 1131. https://doi.org/10.3390/healthcare11081131.

Weber, T. R., Au-Fliegner, M., Downard, C. D., & Fishman, S. J. (2002). Abdominal wall defects. *Current Opinion in Pediatrics, 14*(4), 491–497. https://doi.org/10.1097/00008480-200208000-00023.

Zahouani, T., & Mendez, M. D. (2023). Omphalocele. In *StatPearls*. StatPearls Publishing.

Chapter 9

Malrotation and Volvulus

Mustafa Akçalı*, MD
Neonatology Clinic, Mersin City Training and Research Hospital, Mersin, Turkey

Abstract

Malrotation is a problem caused by abnormal positioning of the intestinal mesentery in the intrauterine period. This occurs intrauterinally but may not show any symptoms or signs until later in childhood. The abnormally positioned intestine can cause the mesentery to rotate and become obstructed. This is called volvulus. In volvulus, blood flow in the intestines decreases, segmental necrosis may occur at the involved site, and shock may occur in the following period. Malrotation or volvulus may not show any symptoms and may cause chronic gastrointestinal (GI) complaints in the long term. Sometimes the picture may progress very rapidly and lead to death. It is important to recognize and manage the problem early in these patients. Pediatric surgery should be contacted quickly. A preoperative and postoperative care plan should be made for hemodynamic management of the patient and prevention of deterioration of the intestinal structure.

Keywords: neonate, malrotation, volvulus

---

* Corresponding Author's Email: akcali_mustafa@hotmail.com

In: Current Approaches to Newborn Emergencies
Editors: Zuhal Keskin Sarılar and Serap Samut Bülbül
ISBN: 979-8-89530-999-5

Introduction

Rotational anomalies occur when the embryonic intestine fails to maintain its normal rotation during the intrauterine period. Since this condition may be asymptomatic, the actual incidence may not be known (Stockmann et al., 2005). The majority of life-threatening cases of malrotation-related volvulus occur in neonates and young children. The incidence of volvulus associated with malrotations decreases with increasing age (McCollough & Sharieff, 2003). The incidence of malrotation in newborns is 1 in 6000 live births (Aboagye et al., 2014). More than half of infants with malrotated bowel may be accompanied by other anomalies of the bowel, such as diaphragmatic hernia and congenital heart disease (Nehra & Goldstein, 2011; Filston & Kirks, 1981). Volvulus occurs as a result of the rotation of the small intestine around the superior mesenteric artery. Subsequently, ischemia of the small intestine occurs in a large part of the small intestine corresponding to the middle intestine. If we do not correct this situation quickly, there may be no return from the ischemia and necrosis that may develop in the intestine. Vomiting is the most common symptom of malrotation. Vomiting with or without bile occurs in 90% of cases with volvulus (Nehra & Goldstein, 2011). Necrosis of the intestines increases third-space fluid losses and sepsis. This contributes to the rapid progression of cardiovascular problems. Immediate intervention and restoring fluid balance is the most basic approach. In older children and adults with malrotation, 22% and 12%, respectively, present to the emergency department with volvulus (Nehra & Goldstein, 2011). Initial symptoms of volvulus are usually acute and noisy, but some children may have chronic episodic abdominal pain and vomiting suggestive of volvulus lasting for years (Nehra & Goldstein, 2011; Millar et al., 2003). In this article, an overview of the importance, diagnosis, and treatment of malrotation, which is one of the most important emergencies of the neonatal period and childhood, and volvulus, which sometimes accompanies this condition, will be presented.

Malrotation

Malrotation is a condition of improper rotation of the embryonic intestine in the intrauterine period due to the cessation of the rotational movement (Figure 1). Since it may be asymptomatic, the actual frequency of rotation anomalies is not clear (Stockmann et al., 2005). Symptomatic malrotation occurs in newborns once in 6000 births. Malrotation is rare after one year of age. It is usually diagnosed in 30% of patients before one month of postnatal age and 75% before 5 years of age (Nehra & Goldstein, 2011). The so-called middle intestine starts after the third part of the duodenum, continues with the ascending part of the colon, and ends by including the proximal 2/3 of the transverse colon. Mid-bowel volvulus occurs when the mesenteric root rotates around the superior mesenteric artery (SMA) and is rare. Midgut volvulus with classic malrotation is common in healthy newborns, and 75% of patients present to the hospital in the first postnatal month and 15% in the first year (Gross, 1953). The diagnosis can be both symptomatic and incidental.

Embryology and Pathogenesis

During intrauterine embryonic development at 4-8 weeks gestation, the embryonic cytosome cannot keep up with the rate of expansion of the gastrointestinal tract (GIT). As a result, the primitive intestinal stalk bends towards the yolk stalk (the thin tube connecting the embryo's midgut and yolk sac), and this stalk is directed towards the developing SMA. The primitive intestinal anus diverges outward from the abdomen, simultaneously bending 90° counterclockwise to begin the normal rotation of the intestine. During this initial rotation, the proximal part of the intestine grows faster than the distal part, and the liver is directed to grow faster (Stockmann et al., 2005). The primitive anus grows and returns to the abdomen at 8-10 weeks gestation (GA). During the return to the abdomen, it makes an additional 180° counterclockwise turn. The main expected movement is the 270° counterclockwise rotation of the intestine from the level of the primitive anus. After this last turn, the intestine is fixed to the posterior abdominal wall. In early pregnancy, the proximal part of the intestine is attached to the retroperitoneum, but the fixation of the distal part of the colon usually occurs closer to delivery and is gradual (Fonkalsrud, 2003).

Normal Intestinal Development

The proper rotation of the intrauterine intestine and its attachment to the retroperitoneum begins at the ligament of Treitz on the upper left and then extends to the ileocecal valve on the lower right, culminating in the formation of a large mesentery. When most rotation anomalies occur, the mesentery base becomes very narrow. In the 4th week of the primitive intestinal tract, the middle intestine is formed as a result of the exchange of the anterior, middle, and posterior intestine (Kluth et al., 2003). Almost all digestive organs and the alimentary tract are formed by this primitive tube, and the developmental pattern of the middle intestine is considered to include the stages of herniation, rotation, retraction, and fixation. The mesentery of the midgut has a broad base but hangs on a narrow vascular pedicle. This increases the risk of volvulus (bowel torsion).

Abnormal Intestinal Development

The most common rotation abnormalities are malrotation (incomplete rotation) or nonrotation (no rotation). Nonrotation occurs when the extension of the primitive intestinal anus on either side returns to the abdomen without rotation. The small intestine lies to the right of the abdomen, and the large intestine lies to the left of the abdomen. It is not easy to diagnose nonrotation radiologically. If the patient has symptoms, laparoscopy or open exploration may be required to confirm the diagnosis (Diaz et al., 2009). In the case of malrotation, the duodenojejunal appendage remains nonrotated, and the cecocolic appendage rotates 90° rather than 180°. The placement of the cecum is not normal; it moves towards the middle and upper abdomen, then forms peritoneal bands and attaches to the right lateral aspect of the abdomen. These bands of peritoneum are called Ladd bands. These bands pass over the duodenum, may compress it externally, and cause obstruction. Occasionally, a transverse column to the right of the SMA, dorsal to the artery, and an inverted rotation of the small intestine mesentery through the retroduodenal tunnel may also be seen (Ford et al., 1992).

Symptoms and Signs

In malrotation, vomiting with bile (green or bright yellow) is typical. Bilious vomiting occurs for three reasons: compression of the duodenum by Ladd's bands, additional duodenal atresia or web, and finally volvulus of the middle intestine (Langer, 2017). Malrotation, volvulus, and neonatal intestinal obstruction should be considered in this type of vomiting until proven otherwise. Some patients may also have vomiting without bile. Abdominal pain is very severe and fixed to a point (Lipsett & Bachur, 2021). The prominent findings in young children are abdominal distension and tenderness. At first, there is distension between the scaphoid and the abdomen (upper abdomen). Distension increases with increasing obstruction, vascular compression in the intestine increases when complete obstruction occurs, and peritonitis (wooden abdomen) occurs if perforation develops (Maxson et al., 1995). Ischemia and necrosis of the intestine occur several hours after the appearance of blood in the stool. The patient may develop septic shock, fluid loss, and hemodynamic status deterioration (Gross, 1953). If signs of intestinal ischemia develop, investigations should be performed for emergency operation (Maxson et al., 1995). In the newborn, vomiting with bile is usually the first finding. If vomiting with bile is present in patients under one year of age, it should be considered that malrotation may be accompanied by a volvulus. Patients may present to the hospital with three different clinical presentations, and the diagnosis and treatment of patients with all three clinical conditions should be urgent:

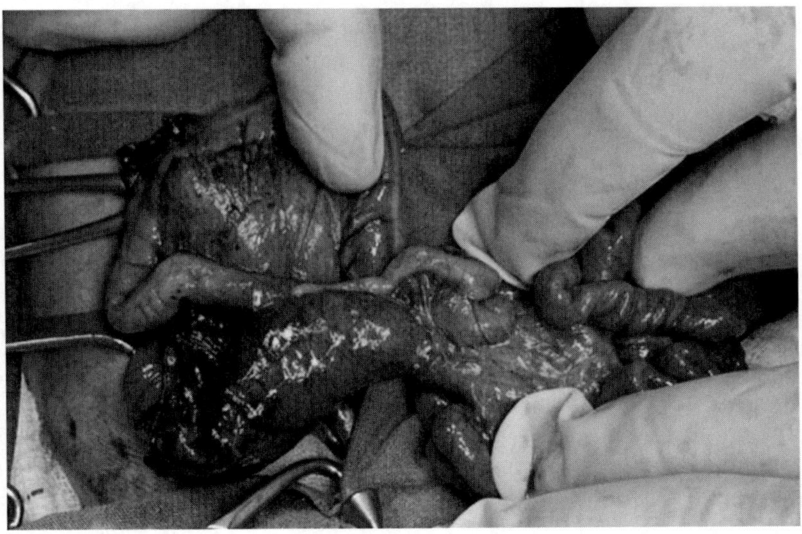

Figure 1. Demonstration of malrotation of the duodenum and small intestine during surgery (Retrieved from Mersin City Training and Research Hospital Pediatric Surgery Clinic archive).

1. An unexpected abdominal pain accompanied by vomiting with bile in a patient with no previous GI complaints. It is considered the most dangerous.
2. Sudden obstruction findings in a patient with feeding intolerance and intermittent bilious vomiting.
3. Developmental retardation in a child who cannot feed and has no desire to feed (Lipsett & Bachur, 2021).

In older children, the clinic may be silent (Pickhardt & Bhalla, 2002). The most common symptom in these infants is abdominal pain, which may or may not be accompanied by vomiting (Ford et al., 1992). In the long term, early feelings of satiety, inability to tolerate solid foods, inadequate weight gain, growth retardation, and malabsorption may also be observed. Prolonged diarrhea, protein-losing enteropathy, biliary obstruction, intestinal dysmobility, pancreatitis, and rarely ascites may develop. As children grow older, they may have long-term diagnoses such as allergy, gastroesophageal reflux, functional abdominal pain, irritable colon, and periodic vomiting (Maxson et al., 1995; Kirby et al., 2000). Malrotation may be a cause of duodenal obstruction in infants. Vomiting with bile may also be present even in the absence of abdominal distension (Zhang et al., 2017).

Volvulus

The narrow base of the mesentery leads to abnormal movement of the small intestine, followed by curvature of the mesentery. Volvulus occurs when the small intestine twists around the SMA, resulting in damage to the vascular structures in the midgut (Figure 2). This must be corrected very quickly; otherwise, ischemia and necrosis of the intestine are the inevitable outcomes (Figure 3). In infancy, vomiting (with or without bile) is the most common symptom in the presence of malrotation and associated volvulus, occurring in more than 90% of newborns with volvulus. Fluid passage to necrosis in the intestine occurs through the third space, and sepsis and heart failure can occur rapidly. Dehydration prevention and other emergency interventions must be done very quickly. Approximately 33% of children with malrotation present to the hospital with life-threatening complications related to volvulus in the first month of life (Fonkalsrud, 2003). Volvulus associated with malrotation occurs in 22% of older children (Nehra & Goldstein, 2011). Symptoms usually have an acute onset, but some children may present to the hospital with intermittent vomiting and abdominal pain that may last for years (Millar et al., 2003).

Types of association of malrotation and volvulus (Stewart et al., 1976):

1. No rotation
2. Malrotation not accompanied by volvulus
3. Malrotation with volvulus
4. Malrotation with partial or intermittent volvulus.

Sigmoid volvulus is rarely seen and causes constipation, irregular colonic bowel movements, and dilatation of the sigmoid colon. Although it is silent, it may cause sudden symptoms by obstruction. Sigmoid volvulus can be suspected if there are conditions such as colonic motility disorder, vomiting, abdominal distension, and very high abdominal pain (Lipsett & Bachur, 2021).

Congenital Conditions Associated with Malrotation

Approximately two-thirds of children with malrotation of the bowel have an anomaly associated with the condition (Table 1) (Ford et al., 1992).

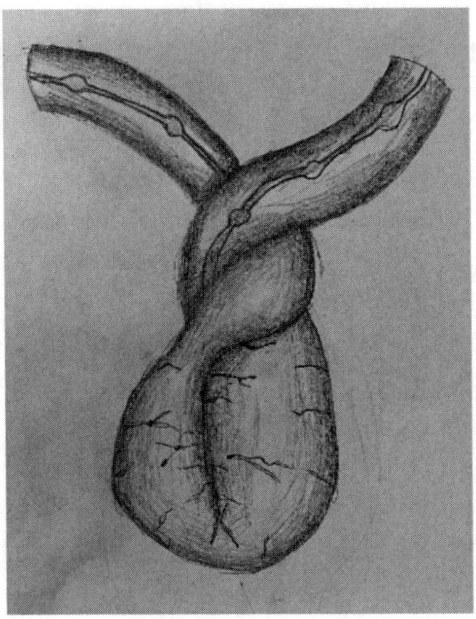

Figure 2. Image of small intestine volvulus (Image of intestinal volvulus by Ahmet Veli Akçalı illustrated).

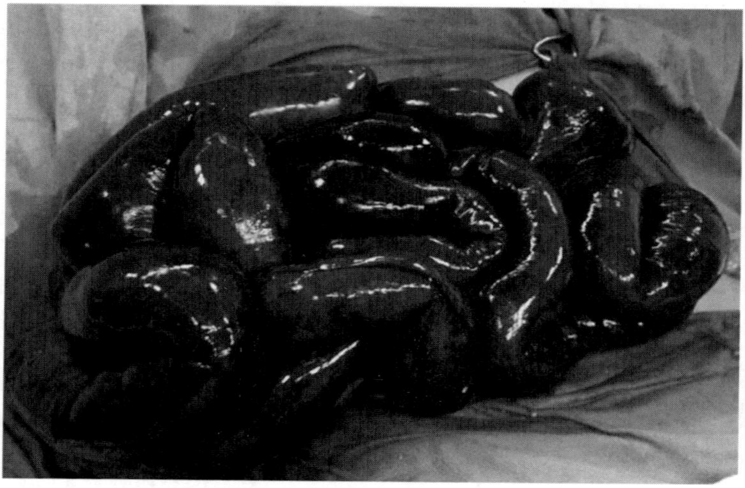

Figure 3. Appearance of necrosed small intestine after volvulus (Retrieved from Mersin City Training and Research Hospital Pediatric Surgery Clinic archive).

Diagnosis

Rotation-related anomalies may be asymptomatic or may give signs of obstruction and include a wide spectrum that may cause venous and lymphatic congestion and may be misdiagnosed as appendicitis (Langer, 2017). Malrotation should be considered in an infant admitted to the hospital with a tender abdomen, vomiting with or without bile, and urgent signs of duodenal obstruction. The hemodynamics of the patients may rapidly deteriorate, and a shock picture may develop (Shalaby et al., 2013). If this condition persists for more than two hours, necrosis may develop in the relevant intestinal segment (Lipsett & Bachur, 2021). If volvulus develops in the midgut, the entire small intestine and ascending colon may be lost. When we look at older children and adults, the most common symptom is abdominal pain. Abdominal pain may be of sudden onset or may be seen as chronic intermittent pain for many years. Other symptoms include chronic diarrhea, intermittent vomiting, malabsorption, and growth retardation (Nehra & Goldstein, 2011). In the differential diagnosis, obstruction, vomiting, and other causes should be considered in addition to the patient's age (Kiesewetter & Smith, 1958). Differentiation from necrotizing enterocolitis (NEC) may be difficult in premature patients, but the differential diagnosis becomes easier with imaging findings. In the presence of intussusception in children, abdominal distension, vomiting with bile, and blood in the stool may be seen. As children grow older, vomiting or abdominal pain includes a wide list of differential diagnoses. If volvulus has occurred, conditions that may cause peritonitis, such as appendicitis and perforation, should be excluded (Ford et al., 1992). Radiology plays an important role in the diagnosis of malrotation (Langer, 2017).

Imaging

Direct Graphics

Direct radiography is important to exclude perforation. In fact, it may not be very helpful in recognizing malrotation and the volvulus that may accompany this condition. When volvulus develops, the radiograph may be normal, or there may be mild dilatation of the bowel or, typically, no gas in the abdomen. Overlapping of the small bowel anus on the liver shadow may suggest malrotation. A “double-bubble” sign on direct radiography and abnormal positioning of the orogastric or nasogastric tube extending into the duodenum may be associated with malrotation. In the case of complete volvulus, an air-fluid level accompanied by a small number of dilated intestinal anuses may be seen. There may be little or no gas in the distal part of the volvulus (Lipsett & Bachur, 2021).

Table 1. Anomalies associated with malrotation

Congenital diaphragmatic hernia (100%)
Congenital heart disease (heterotaxy syndromes) (40-90%)
Gastroschisis, omphalocele (31-45%)
Prune-Belly syndrome
Esophageal atresia, tracheoesophageal fistula
Duodenal, jejunal, and ileal atresia
Biliary atresia
Meckel’s diverticulum
Anorectal malformations (isolated or associated with VACTERL anomalies)
Cornelia de Lange syndrome

VACTERL: vertebral, anal, cardiac, tracheoesophageal, renal, extremity (Aslanabadi et al., 2007).

Ultrasonography (USG)

USG is frequently used for diagnosis and screening purposes. In fact, although USG helps us more in the diagnosis of volvulus, it can be diagnostic for malrotation without volvulus (Zhang et al., 2017). If the USG image is compatible with volvulus, the patient should be operated on urgently. Findings suggestive of malrotation on USG are as follows (Orzech et al., 2006):

- The third part of the duodenum is not in its normal location in the retroperitoneal space (normally, the duodenum is located between the SMA and the aorta)
- Superior mesenteric vein not in its normal location (to the left of the SMA, in front of it, etc.)
- Presence of vortex sign seen in volvulus (caused by vessels surrounding the base of the pedicle to which the mesentery is attached)
- Dilated duodenum (shows duodenal obstruction through Ladd bands)
- Duodenal obstruction in the presence of distal air.

Normal USG findings do not exclude malrotation. Malrotation has been diagnosed in 2-3% of children with normal USG results as a result of detailed examinations performed in the upper digestive tract (Orzech et al., 2006). For this reason, differential diagnostic studies should be performed in the upper digestive tract if malrotation is suspected, even if USG findings are normal. In patients with acute volvulus, dilatation in the duodenum can be demonstrated by color Doppler USG in addition to SMA and vortex sign (Shimanuki et al., 1996).

Upper Digestive System Study (Sizemore et al., 2008)

- The duodenum is not in its normal location: it is misplaced and on the right side of the abdomen (Langer, 2017).
- Duodenum in "Corkscrew" view
- Duodenal obstruction with an appearance similar to duodenal atresia, 'beak sign' appearance in case of volvulus.

If obstruction in the distal intestine is considered, small bowel contrast imaging may be performed. If symptoms do not improve, the procedure may be repeated, or barium rectal enema and colon evaluation may be important for differential diagnosis (Long et al., 1996).

Barium Enema Radiography

Barium enema radiography is not preferred to reveal malrotation. The colon continues to settle until the end of pregnancy, which may mimic malrotation and may result in false positive results. In approximately 1/5 of cases with malrotation, the cecum is located in the right lower quadrant (Morrison, 1997). Volvulus findings may be as follows (Langer, 2017):

- 'Beak sign' in the segment with barium due to complete obstruction in the transverse colon
- The entire column is located on the left side.

Computed Tomography (CT)

It is the best test for confirmation of malrotation. CT with intravenous contrast is appropriate. The findings are as follows: (Taylor, 2011).

- The third part of the duodenum does not pass between the aorta and SMA.
- The proximal part of the intestine is on the right.
- The "vortex sign" seen in volvulus (caused by vessels surrounding the pedicle to which the mesentery is attached) is seen. (Figure 4)
- The superior mesenteric vein is not in its normal location (to the left or in front of the SMA).

Magnetic Resonance Imaging (MRI)

If there is a contraindication to radiation or contrast material, it may help to identify malrotation. MRI is difficult to access, which reduces its use (Taylor, 2011).

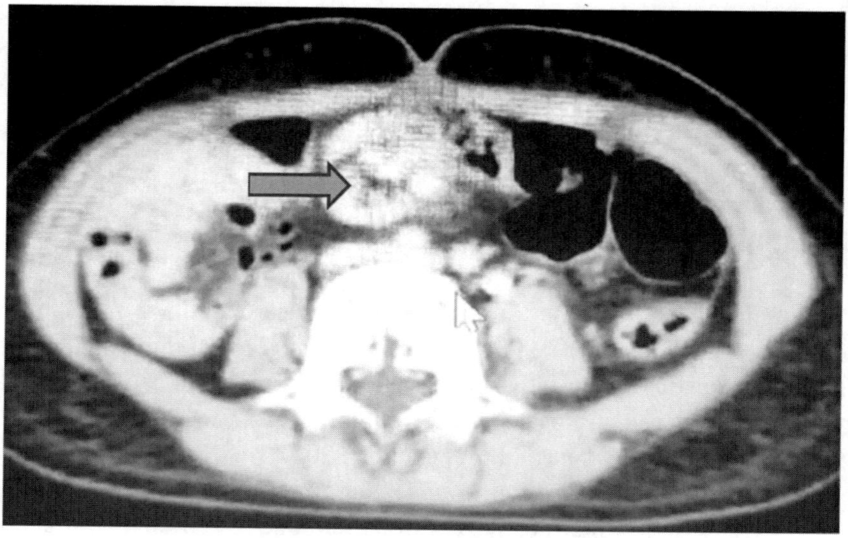

Figure 4. *"Vortex sign" seen in volvulus on CT* (Taken from the archive of the Radiology Clinic of Mersin City Training and Research Hospital).

Treatment

There is no clear answer as to the best therapeutic approach to incidentally detected malrotation in asymptomatic cases. If the risk of postoperative morbidity and mortality is low, elective surgery is recommended under appropriate conditions. The situation is complicated when malrotation is accompanied by volvulus or perforation, which requires urgent diagnosis and treatment. If the patient has signs of systemic decompensation such as hematochezia, hematemesis, abdominal distension, peritonitis, and shock, fluid replacement should be administered rapidly, and emergency explorative surgery should be performed. If the patient's hemodynamics are stable and there are no pathologic signs in the intestine, the diagnosis should be confirmed by radiologic examinations (Mazziotti et al., 1997).

Preoperative gastric contents are emptied, fluid replacement is performed if there is a fluid deficit, and appropriate antibiotherapy that may also affect the intestinal flora is started. If volvulus is detected during surgical intervention, it is rotated counterclockwise. Ladd surgery is preferred in malrotation surgery. The aim here is to minimize the risk of volvulus by expanding the mesentery rather than returning the bowel to an anatomically normal configuration. This method can be performed laparoscopically in older children without bowel ischemia, but the risk of recurrence is higher than open surgery if volvulus is present (Draus et al., 2007). Patients should undergo laparotomy if malrotation accompanied by symptoms and volvulus is suspected.

Considerations involving Ladd surgery (Lessin & Luks, 1998):

1. Separation of Ladd's bands.
2. Separation of adhesions between the duodenum and cecum, making the mesenteric floor wider.
3. If there are duodenal obstructions in newborns, a tube is advanced through the duodenum to detect them.
4. Restoring the bowel to its normal position (if we are unsure of the intactness of the bowel, the abdomen is closed and reopened and reassessed after 24-36 hours; any necrotic areas are cleaned, and stomas are created).

In fact, appendectomy was not part of the original Ladd operation but is commonly performed in patients operated on for malrotation (Newhall et al., 2017).

Complications

Surgical complications are not expected in malrotation and volvulus in the absence of ischemia. If necrotic areas are high and extensive bowel resection is required, short bowel syndrome may occur. Correct management of the diagnosis and treatment of mid-bowel volvulus is very important in this respect (Seashore et al., 1994). Small bowel obstruction may occur due to adhesions that develop after laparotomy. This complication may occur in 15% of patients. In malrotation surgery, widening the mesenteric floor reduces the recurrence of volvulus. However, recurrence is still possible because the underlying problem cannot be corrected. The risk of recurrence is 2-8% (Dilley et al., 2000). It has also been reported that 3.1% of patients develop postoperative intussusception after an open Ladd procedure (Kidd et al., 2000).

Survival

Symptoms return to normal in up to 89% of patients after surgery (Nehra & Goldstein, 2011). It has been found that 3-9% of malrotation cases die after surgery. Mortality is high in patients with volvulus, prematurity, development of intestinal necrosis and other anomalies, and close to zero in healthy children in the absence of intestinal ischemia (Messineo et al., 1992).

Conclusion

Malrotation and volvulus, a congenital problem of the intestine, are among the important surgical emergencies of newborns. Although the course is usually symptomatic in newborns and young children, it may be clinically silent in children as they grow older. The clinical course may be asymptomatic, or sepsis and rapid deterioration in hemodynamics may be observed, especially in the case of obstruction due to volvulus. In terms of the treatment plan, rapid differential diagnosis of other causes of acute abdomen and urgent treatment are extremely important. In addition to fluid replacement, fighting against sepsis, and stabilization of hemodynamics, the Ladd operation as a surgical procedure comes to the forefront in treatment. If urgent, rapid, and effective intervention is performed, complete resolution of symptoms in the presence of a non-necrotic intestinal anus is very high, and the mortality rate is very low.

Acknowledgments

I would like to thank Dr. Arman Api from Mersin Şehir Training and Research Hospital Pediatric Surgery Clinic for the surgical photos and my son Ahmet Veli Akçalı, the painter of our house, who successfully illustrated the volvulus picture.

References

Aboagye, J., Goldstein, S. D., Salazar, J. H., Papandria, D., Okoye, M. T., Al-Omar, K., Stewart, D., Lukish, J., & Abdullah, F. (2014). Age at presentation of common pediatric surgical conditions: Reexamining dogma. *Journal of Pediatric Surgery, 49*(6), 995–999. https://doi.org/10.1016/j.jpedsurg.2014.01.039.

Aslanabadi, S., Ghalehgolab-Behbahan, A., Jamshidi, M., Veisi, P., & Zarrintan, S. (2007). Intestinal malrotations: A review and report of thirty cases. *Folia Morphologica (Warsz), 66*(4), 277–282. https://pubmed.ncbi.nlm.nih.gov/18058748/.

Diaz, M. C., Reichard, K., & Taylor, A. A. (2009). Intestinal nonrotation in an adolescent. *Pediatric Emergency Care, 25*(4), 249–251. https://doi.org/10.1097/PEC.0b013e31819e36aa.

Dilley, A. V., Pereira, J., Shi, E. C., Adams, S., Kern, I. B., Currie, B., & Henry, G. M. (2000). The radiologist says malrotation: Does the surgeon operate? *Pediatric Surgery International, 16*(1–2), 45–49. https://doi.org/10.1007/s003830050012.

Draus, J. M. Jr., Foley, D. S., & Bond, S. J. (2007). Laparoscopic Ladd procedure: A minimally invasive approach to malrotation without midgut volvulus. *American Surgeon, 73*(7), 693–696. https://pubmed.ncbi.nlm.nih.gov/17674943/.

Filston, H. C., & Kirks, D. R. (1981). Malrotation: A common anomaly. *Journal of Pediatric Surgery, 16*(4), 614–620. https://doi.org/10.1016/0022-3468(81)90015-4.

Fonkalsrud, E. (2003). Rotational anomalies and volvulus. In J. A. O'Neill (Ed.), *Principles of Pediatric Surgery* (2nd ed., pp. 477). Mosby.

Ford, E. G., Senac, M. O. Jr., Srikanth, M. S., & Weitzman, J. J. (1992). Malrotation of the intestine in children. *Annals of Surgery, 215*(2), 172–178. https://doi.org/10.1097/00000658-199202000-00013.

Gross, R. E. (1953). Malrotation of the intestine and colon. In R. E. Gross (Ed.), *The Surgery of Infancy and Childhood* (pp. 192–203). W. B. Saunders.

Kidd, J., Jackson, R., Wagner, C. W., & Smith, S. D. (2000). Intussusception following the Ladd procedure. *Archives of Surgery, 135*(6), 713–715. https://doi.org/10.1001/archsurg.135.6.713.

Kiesewetter, W. B., & Smith, J. W. (1958). Malrotation of the midgut in infancy and childhood. *AMA Archives of Surgery, 77*(4), 483–491. https://doi.org/10.1001/archsurg.1958.04370010015002.

Kirby, C. P., Freeman, J. K., Ford, W. D., Davidson, G. P., & Furness, M. E. (2000). Malrotation with recurrent volvulus presenting with cholestasis, pruritus, and pancreatitis. *Pediatric Surgery International, 16*(1–2), 130–131. https://doi.org/10.1007/s003830050040.

Kluth, D., Jaeschke-Melli, S., & Fiegel, H. (2003). The embryology of gut rotation. *Seminars in Pediatric Surgery, 12*(4), 275–279. https://doi.org/10.1053/j.sempedsurg.2003.08.009.

Langer, J. C. (2017). Intestinal rotation abnormalities and midgut volvulus. *Surgical Clinics of North America, 97*(1), 147–159. https://doi.org/10.1016/j.suc.2016.08.011.

Lessin, M. S., & Luks, F. (1998). Laparoscopic appendectomy and duodenocolonic dissociation (Ladd) procedure for malrotation. *Pediatric Surgery International, 13*(2–3), 184–185. https://doi.org/10.1007/s003830050284.

Lipsett, S. C., & Bachur, R. G. (2021). Abdominal emergencies. In K. N. Shaw & R. G. Bachur (Eds.), *Fleisher & Ludwig's Textbook of Pediatric Emergency Medicine* (8th ed., pp. 5657–5665). Wolters Kluwer.

Long, F. R., Kramer, S. S., Markowitz, R. I., & Taylor, G. E., Liacouras, C. A. (1996). Intestinal malrotation in children: Tutorial on radiographic diagnosis in difficult cases. *Radiology, 198*(3), 775–780. https://doi.org/10.1148/radiology.198.3.8628870.

Maxson, R. T., Franklin, P. A., & Wagner, C. W. (1995). Malrotation in the older child: Surgical management, treatment, and outcome. *American Surgeon, 61*(2), 135–138. https://pubmed.ncbi.nlm.nih.gov/7856973/.

Mazziotti, M. V., Strasberg, S. M., & Langer, J. C. (1997). Intestinal rotation abnormalities without volvulus: The role of laparoscopy. *Journal of the American College of Surgeons, 185*(2), 172–176. https://doi.org/10.1016/s1072-7515(97)00058-6.

McCollough, M., & Sharieff, G. Q. (2003). Abdominal surgical emergencies in infants and young children. *Emergency Medicine Clinics of North America, 21*(4), 909–935. https://doi.org/10.1016/s0733-8627(03)00090-7.

Messineo, A., MacMillan, J. H., Palder, S. B., & Filler, R. M. (1992). Clinical factors affecting mortality in children with malrotation of the intestine. *Journal of Pediatric Surgery, 27*(10), 1343–1345. https://doi.org/10.1016/0022-3468(92)90293-G.

Millar, A. J., Rode, H., & Cywes, S. (2003). Malrotation and volvulus in infancy and childhood. *Seminars in Pediatric Surgery, 12*(4), 229–236. https://doi.org/10.1053/j.sempedsurg.2003.08.003.

Morrison, S. C. (1997). Controversies in abdominal imaging. *Pediatric Clinics of North America, 44*(3), 555–574. https://doi.org/10.1016/s0031-3955(05)70493-4.

Nehra, D., & Goldstein, A. M. (2011). Intestinal malrotation: Varied clinical presentation from infancy through adulthood. *Surgery, 149*(3), 386–393. https://doi.org/10.1016/j.surg.2010.07.004.

Newhall, K., Albright, B., Tosteson, A., Ozanne, E., Trus, T., & Goodney, P. P. (2017). Cost-effectiveness of prophylactic appendectomy: A Markov model. *Surgical Endoscopy, 31*(9), 3596–3604. https://doi.org/10.1007/s00464-016-5391-y.

Orzech, N., Navarro, O. M., & Langer, J. C. (2006). Is ultrasonography a good screening test for intestinal malrotation? *Journal of Pediatric Surgery, 41*(5), 1005–1009. https://doi.org/10.1016/j.jpedsurg.2005.12.070.

Pickhardt, P. J., & Bhalla, S. (2002). Intestinal malrotation in adolescents and adults: Spectrum of clinical and imaging features. *AJR American Journal of Roentgenology, 179*(6), 1429–1435. https://doi.org/10.2214/ajr.179.6.1791429.

Seashore, J. H., & Touloukian, R. J. (1994). Midgut volvulus: An ever-present threat. *Archives of Pediatrics & Adolescent Medicine, 148*(1), 43–46. https://doi.org/10.1001/archpedi.1994.02170010045009.

Shalaby, M. S., Kuti, K., & Walker, G. (2013). Intestinal malrotation and volvulus in infants and children. *BMJ, 347*, f6949. https://doi.org/10.1136/bmj.f6949.

Shimanuki, Y., Aihara, T., Takano, H., Moritani, T., Oguma, E., Kuroki, H., Shibata, A., Nozawa, K., Ohkawara, K., Hirata, A., & Imaizumi, S. (1996). Clockwise whirlpool sign at color Doppler US: An objective and definite sign of midgut volvulus. *Radiology, 199*(1), 261–264. https://doi.org/10.1148/radiology.199.1.8633156.

Sizemore, A. W., Rabbani, K. Z., Ladd, A., & Applegate, K. E. (2008). Diagnostic performance of the upper gastrointestinal series in the evaluation of children with clinically suspected malrotation. *Pediatric Radiology, 38*(5), 518–528. https://doi.org/10.1007/s00247-008-0762-8.

Stewart, D. R., Colodny, A. L., & Daggett, W. C. (1976). Malrotation of the bowel in infants and children: A 15-year review. *Surgery, 79*(6), 716–720. https://pubmed.ncbi.nlm.nih.gov/1273757/.

Stockmann, P. T. (2005). Malrotation. In K. T. Oldham, P. M. Colombani, R. P. Foglia, & M. A. Skinner (Eds.), *Principles and Practice of Pediatric Surgery* (2nd ed., Vol. 2, p. 1283). Lippincott Williams & Wilkins.

Taylor, G. A. (2011). CT appearance of the duodenum and mesenteric vessels in children with normal and abnormal bowel rotation. *Pediatric Radiology, 41*(11), 1378–1383. https://doi.org/10.1007/s00247-011-2118-z.

Zhang, W., Sun, H., & Luo, F. (2017). The efficiency of sonography in diagnosing volvulus in neonates with suspected intestinal malrotation. *Medicine (Baltimore), 96*(42), e8287. https://doi.org/10.1097/MD.0000000000008287.

Chapter 10

Necrotizing Enterocolitis (NEC)

Şerife Tutar[1,*], PhD, and Hande Özgörü[2], PhD

[1]Department of Pediatric Nursing, Süleyman Demirel University, Isparta, Turkey
[2]Department of Medical Services and Techniques, Süleyman Demirel University, Isparta, Turkey

Abstract

Necrotizing enterocolitis (NEC) is a life-threatening disease particularly seen in premature and low-birth-weight infants. The incidence of NEC worldwide varies between 0.3 and 2.4 per 1,000 live births, with approximately 70% of cases occurring in premature infants born before the 36th gestational week. It affects 2-4% of premature infants and is responsible for about 8% of all neonatal intensive care admissions. Many factors contribute to the development of this disease, whose etiology and pathophysiology are not fully understood. The lack of a clear definition and specific findings related to the disease complicates the diagnostic process. Clinical, laboratory, and radiological findings are utilized during this process. NEC treatment includes supportive medical care and, in some cases, surgical intervention. Considering that the incidence of NEC cases has not declined, it continues to be one of the significant gastrointestinal problems in neonatal intensive care units, associated with high morbidity and mortality, a lack of specific findings for diagnosis, and many unclear factors regarding diagnosis, treatment, prevention, and care. Therefore, this section will discuss the risk factors, diagnosis, treatment, and prevention methods related to NEC in light of the literature.

* Corresponding Author's Email: serifeguven@sdu.edu.tr

In: Current Approaches to Newborn Emergencies
Editors: Zuhal Keskin Sarılar and Serap Samut Bülbül
ISBN: 979-8-89530-999-5

Keywords: necrotizing enterocolitis, preterm newborn, newborn emergencies

Introduction

Necrotizing enterocolitis (NEC) is an emergency condition primarily affecting premature and very low birth weight infants, characterized by inflammation and necrosis of the small intestine and colon, with potential consequences including sepsis, peritonitis, perforation, and death (Roberts et al., 2024). NEC is characterized by necrosis of the mucosa of the small and large intestines, most commonly in the distal ileum and proximal colon. The necrosis may be very superficial and only detectable microscopically, or it may extend through the bowel wall. Mild disease may be completely reversible, but neonates with extensive involvement may not survive (Potts & Mandleco, 2012). Technological advancements in neonatal intensive care have increased survival rates among preterm and very low birth weight infants, but the incidence of NEC has also risen (Patole, 2013). The prevention, treatment, and nursing care of NEC, which is a significant cause of mortality and morbidity in preterm infants, is thus seen as crucial (Ginglen & Butki, 2023). Therefore, this section will focus on the risk factors, diagnosis, treatment, and preventive methods related to NEC in light of the literature.

Incidence and Etiology

NEC commonly occurs in preterm, low birthweight neonates and is rarely seen in term infants (Potts & Mandleco, 2012). Worldwide, the incidence of NEC, which varies between 0.3 and 2.4 per 1,000 live births, is observed in approximately 70% of premature infants born before 36 weeks of gestation. It affects 2-4% of premature infants and is responsible for about 8% of all neonatal intensive care admissions (Ginglen & Butki, 2023). It affects both sexes equally (Potts & Mandleco, 2012).

The exact etiology of NEC is unclear; however, several factors are associated with its development. Perinatal asphyxia, respiratory distress syndrome, exchange transfusions, and umbilical artery catheters may all contribute to ischemia of the bowel (Potts & Mandleco, 2012; Neu, 2014). In addition, it has been noted that genetic factors, erythrocyte transfusions, H2 receptor antagonists, unnecessary prolonged antibiotic treatments, and enteral feeding with hypertonic solutions - which are commonly used in clinical practice - are also associated with NEC (Patole, 2013; Roberts et al., 2024).

Pathophysiology

Although the pathophysiology of NEC, which is frequently encountered in preterm infants, is not fully understood, it is associated with many different etiological factors and largely with the immaturity of the gastrointestinal system (Neu, 2014). However, prematurity continues to be accepted as the single most important risk factor for the illness (Patole, 2013). Immature motility, digestion, absorption, and vascular circulation in the gastrointestinal system increase the risk of intestinal damage in preterm infants. In addition, immunologic host defense is significantly impaired in these patients due to disruption of the physical barrier in the gastrointestinal tract. Accordingly, many biochemical factors such as lactoferrin, epidermal growth factor (EGF), heparin-binding (HB)-EGF, transforming growth factor, insulin-like growth factor, oligosaccharides, and polyunsaturated fatty acids (PUFA) are deficient or absent (Choi, 2014).

In NEC, damage to the mucosal cells that line the intestinal wall disrupts blood circulation to these cells and leads to cell death. In this process, the secretion of protective, lubricating mucus ceases, and the thin and unprotected intestinal wall is attacked by proteolytic enzymes. Protective IgM cannot be synthesized, and the mucosa becomes permeable to macromolecules (e.g., exotoxins), further complicating intestinal defense. Gas-producing bacteria invade the damaged areas, creating intestinal pneumatosis and generating gas on the submucosal or subserosal surfaces of the intestine (Potts & Mandleco, 2012; Fraser, 2015).

Diagnosis

Diagnosis is made using clinical, laboratory, and radiological findings. The clinical condition that is most challenging to differentiate in NEC cases is feeding intolerance. Feeding intolerance can be a symptom of NEC, but it can also occur independently before the onset of NEC, with vomiting and abdominal distension being the primary clinical conditions that come to mind.

Evidence that routine gastric residual volume monitoring prevents the development of NEC is insufficient (Özgörü et al., 2023).

However, due to non-specific clinical findings such as vomiting, apnea, lethargy, and bradycardia, gastric residual volume can be assessed at the physician's discretion. If residue is checked, a residue of more than 5 ml/kg or more than 50% of the feeding volume in newborns is suggestive of feeding intolerance. If the newborn with abdominal distension and residue has normal laboratory tests and no other clinical symptoms or radiologic findings, the diagnosis of feeding intolerance for the newborn is focused (Yee et al., 2012).

Clinical, Radiological, and Laboratory Findings

Necrotizing enterocolitis can present a variable clinical course, ranging from nonspecific findings such as lethargy, episodes of apnea, thermoregulation irregularities, and perfusion abnormalities to rapidly progressing shock, peritonitis, and severe outcomes leading to mortality. The earliest signs in the gastrointestinal system are feeding intolerance, vomiting, and abdominal distension, while erythema of the abdominal skin and palpable mass are late gastrointestinal findings. In 20-30% of cases, NEC is associated with bacteremia, and the clinical signs of bacteremia accompany the condition. The disease can have an early or late onset related to the pathogenesis in preterm neonates (Yee et al., 2012; Cuna et al., 2018; Ginglen & Butki, 2023; Roberts et al., 2024).

Currently, the lack of a clear definition of NEC and disease-specific findings complicates diagnosis. Imaging methods such as abdominal x-ray or abdominal ultrasonography evaluate the status of bowel perforation, bowel wall thickness and dilation, pneumatosis, and motility conditions. Nonspecific findings used to support diagnosis include gas distension, dilated intestinal loops, and edema in the intestinal wall in the early period. The definitive radiological finding for NEC is pneumatosis intestinalis, characterized by gas produced in the bowel wall by bacteria. Additional radiological findings include the appearance of gas in the portal vein, ascites, and pneumoperitoneum. When pneumoperitoneum is suspected, a left lateral decubitus X-ray can be helpful (Kim, 2019; Christian et al., 2018). Additionally, the appearance of intestinal bubbles in radiological evaluations can be confused with feces. Therefore, a follow-up film after 6 hours is suggested to make this distinction. While the detection of crescent-shaped gas is not a specific finding for NEC, it may also arise from another pathology, such as bowel perforation or cardiogenic ischemic bowel necrosis. Thus, there is no gold standard finding that can be considered definitive for NEC. Furthermore, NEC can be confused with congenital bowel anomalies such as Hirschsprung's disease, volvulus, and meconium ileus due to cystic fibrosis (Neu, 2020). Another clinical condition that can be confused with NEC is sepsis. Findings that differentiate NEC from sepsis include the presence of pneumatosis intestinalis and/or portal venous gas or direct visualization of necrotic bowel during surgery (Robinson et al., 2017; Christian et al., 2018; Hong et al., 2018).

Table 1. Modified bell criteria

Kriterler	Possible NEC suspicion	Definitive NEC	Advanced Level NEC
Abdominal Findings	-Distention, vomiting, occult blood in stool, rectal hemorrhage	-Distention, absence of bowel sounds, abdominal tenderness, palpable bowel loops -Abdominal cellulitis or palpable mass in the right lower quadrant	-Distention, absence of bowel sounds, abdominal tenderness, abdominal cellulitis, or palpable mass in the right lower quadrant -Generalized peritonitis
Systemic Findings	-Apnea, lethargy, thermoregulation imbalances	-Apnea, lethargy, thermoregulation imbalances -Moderate metabolic acidosis -Thrombocytopenia	-Severe apnea, drop in blood pressure, acidosis, coagulopathy, neutropenia
Radiological Findings	-Absence of gas in the intestines or moderate intestinal distension	-Intestinal distension, pneumatosis intestinalis, gas in the portal vein, ascites	-Intestinal distension, pneumatosis intestinalis, gas in the portal vein, significant ascites -Significant ascites, pneumoperitoneum

When NEC is suspected, common laboratory tests include blood tests such as complete blood count (C-reactive protein (CRP)), biochemical tests (liver and kidney function tests, serum electrolytes), arterial blood gas assessment, and coagulation tests, while blood cultures and acute phase markers are used for sepsis monitoring. Although not routinely recommended, peritoneal culture assessment for identifying the causative microorganism can be utilized but is not common. The sensitivity, specificity, and positive predictive value of these tests for NEC diagnosis are low, indicating a need for better biomarkers (Goldstein & Sylvester, 2019).

Clinical Staging

NEC was initially staged by Bell and colleagues. Later, Walsh and Kliegman reorganized the Bell criteria by considering clinical, radiological, and laboratory findings (Bell et al., 1978; Walsh & Kliegman, 1986).

Risk Factors

Below are the commonly accepted risk factors for NEC (Gephart et al., 2014; Naberhuis et al., 2016):

- Low gestational age
- Intrauterine growth restriction or low birth weight
- Newborns fed with formula
- Postnatal factors (blood transfusion, prolonged antibiotic treatment, congenital heart diseases, polycythemia, prolonged mechanical ventilation support, asphyxia, etc.)
- Perinatal maternal factors (smoking during pregnancy, substance use, premature rupture of membranes, placental abruption, lack of antenatal corticosteroid use, etc.).

Treatment

NEC is one of the gastrointestinal problems that is a source of serious morbidity and mortality, especially in preterm neonates. In addition to high costs, its long-term complications include intestinal obstruction and adhesions, cholestasis, short bowel syndrome, and neurodevelopmental delay (Neu, 2020). For this reason, early diagnosis and treatment approaches are likely to increase the effectiveness before the clinical picture progresses. Moreover, one of the most challenging aspects of NEC treatment is distinguishing it from clinical conditions such as feeding intolerance and making an accurate diagnosis. This is because the treatment approach for each clinical issue is often different, and sometimes neonates may be subjected to unnecessary treatment practices, such as the use of antibiotics, even when they do not have NEC. NEC treatment includes supportive medical therapy and, in some cases, surgical treatment (Mashriq et al., 2019; Hong et al., 2018). Evidence regarding when surgical treatment should be performed, apart from neonates with intestinal perforation, is unclear. Most clinical experts still continue to use the modified Bell staging to determine the severity of cases. However, this staging has not been validated in terms of clinical management and guidance (Hackam et al., 2019). Generally, supportive medical treatment is preferred for neonates classified as Bell Criteria stages 1 and 2, while surgical treatment is considered for those with stage 3 or accompanying bowel perforation. It is important that the healthcare facility where surgical intervention is planned also has the capacity to provide postoperative care services (Robinson et al., 2017). Supportive care should be initiated for all patients suspected of having NEC, regardless of the stage of the disease (Hong et al., 2018; Neu, 2020).

Components of Supportive Care Include

- Cessation of enteral feeding (48-72 hours for Stage I NEC, 7 days for Stage II NEC, 10-14 days for Stage III NEC)
- Gastric decompression (until enteral feeding is initiated)
- Total parenteral nutrition
- Fluid and electrolyte support
- Cardiovascular and respiratory support
- Other supportive treatments (multi-organ failure).

Medical Treatment

NEC suspicion should prompt the initiation of medical treatment. Supportive care and medical treatment are critically important for the clinic's progress (Hong et al., 2018). Broad-spectrum antibiotics covering Gram (-) and anaerobic bacteria (ampicillin, gentamicin (amikacin), and metronidazole) are appropriate for treatment, while for CNS (coagulase-negative staphylococci) and MRSA (methicillin-resistant Staphylococcus aureus) or ampicillin-resistant enterococci (+), vancomycin may be started as an alternative to ampicillin. If cultures from blood or other sterile sites are positive, treatment can be narrowed or expanded if necessary. For Stage 1 NEC, early discontinuation of antibiotics and the resumption of enteral feeding may be considered after 48-72 hours, depending on the patient's course. For Stage ≥2 NEC, a 10-14 day course of antibiotics is recommended even if culture results are negative (Robinson et al., 2017). The fluid-electrolyte support provided to an infant whose enteral feeding has been halted should be calculated while considering both the maintenance fluid volume and the replacement of fluids coming from gastric aspiration. In cases of NEC, lactic acidosis may occur due to inadequate perfusion of intestinal tissue and accompanying necrosis, negatively affecting vascular tone and cardiac output. Cardiovascular and respiratory problems may arise due to this condition, and inotropic support may be added to the infants' treatment. As a result, necessary measures should be taken to correct acidosis, and one of the primary goals should be to stop tissue damage and necrosis (Christian et al., 2018).

Surgical Treatment

Surgical treatment is determined based on the width of the affected intestinal segment. The surgical techniques used in babies diagnosed with NEC are laparotomy (resection of the intestinal regions, proximal enterostomy [colostomy, ileostomy], and placement of a distal mucosal fistula) or primary peritoneal drainage (PPD). Although the standard approach for babies with perforation is laparotomy, PPD can be used as a salvage procedure or, in some cases, as a definitive method. Enterostomy formation followed by intestinal resection can be applied after laparotomy, while primary intestinal anastomosis can be performed in limited NEC cases (Robinson et al., 2017; Thakkar & Lakhoo, 2016).

The evaluation of treatment response is quite important for shaping the intervention plan and early identification of adverse situations. Therefore, monitoring the effectiveness of supportive care and antibiotic treatment (medical treatment) should be conducted through serial physical examinations, follow-up of physiological parameters, monitoring of laboratory values, and abdominal imaging (Hong et al., 2018). In infants diagnosed with NEC but not undergoing surgical treatment, strictures (narrowing) in the intestines can be observed in 3-36% of cases, while in infants requiring surgical intervention, this rate increases to 24-65%. In cases of stricture development, the treatment approach involves surgical resection followed by end-to-end anastomosis or creation of an ostomy. Additionally, surgical treatment may result in anatomical short bowel syndrome and intestinal failure. In severe cases of intestinal failure, intestinal transplantation may be the only solution. Parenteral nutrition, ultimately, increases the risk of growth failure, central catheter-associated sepsis, and liver disease associated with total parenteral nutrition. Infants who have received medical treatment have a high likelihood of achieving normal intestinal function and feeding tolerances (Wertheimer et al., 2019).

Serial physical examination: In cases of NEC, the clinical course can change very quickly, making serial physical examination an important aspect of disease management and monitoring. Detecting changes in physiological parameters and abdominal examination will help determine the severity and progression of the disease. This allows for earlier surgical evaluation. Differences in abdominal examination, such as erythema or bruising indicating possible intestinal perforation, along with increased abdominal distension and tenderness, are critical signals that the condition is worsening. The frequency of physical examinations is related to the onset speed of symptoms and can be performed every few hours. In short, serial physical examination involves more frequent monitoring of newborns diagnosed with NEC (Robinson et al., 2017).

There are unclear areas in the treatment or prevention, and current research is still needed in this field (Neu, 2020). Provided that premature newborns are hemodynamically stable and have no gastrointestinal problems, it is important to initiate enteral feeding with breast milk without delay for the development of their immature gastrointestinal system. Accelerating the transition to full enteral feeding can reduce complications of parenteral nutrition. Additionally, assessing the amount and color of gastric residual volume before enteral feeding can guide decisions regarding the course of enteral feeding (Özgörü et al., 2023). This is because biliary gastric residual and/or retrieving more than half of the feeding amount may indicate NEC. Moreover, the risk of NEC increases in preterm newborns who are not fed breast milk or who are started on enteral feeding very rapidly after a prolonged period of parenteral nutrition. Although evidence in the literature is not conclusive, situations such as withholding feeding during blood transfusions or administering medications like ibuprofen or other vasoactive drugs may influence the development of NEC. Monitoring gastric residual volume is critical for the early diagnosis of necrotizing enterocolitis (NEC), which affects 7-14% of premature infants, and is often used as a criterion for evaluating feeding tolerance. However, there is very little scientific evidence for gastric residual volume. There are studies suggesting that there is no relationship between the gastric residual volume and its color with feeding intolerance (Özgörü et al., 2023; Rysavy et al., 2020; Thomas et al., 2018). In the study by Rysavy et al., (2020), one group of two preterm newborn groups underwent gastric residual volume monitoring, while the other group did not. The study found that enteral feeding progressed more rapidly in the group without gastric residual volume monitoring (Rysavy et al., 2020). In the study by Thomas et al., (2018), the measurement of abdominal circumference before feeding and the monitoring of gastric residual volume were compared during the process of preterm newborns reaching full enteral feeding. It was determined that the group measured only for abdominal circumference transitioned to full enteral feeding more quickly (Thomas et al., 2018). In the study by Torrazza et al., (2015), 61 low birth weight preterm newborns were randomized into two groups, one with gastric residual volume measurements and the other without. It was observed that preterm newborns without gastric residual volume monitoring began full enteral feeding six days earlier than those with monitoring (Torrazza et al., 2015). There are significant differences in the results of studies examining the gastric residual volume technique. Although routine gastric residual volume assessment has been discontinued in some neonatal intensive care units, there is insufficient evidence to support the discontinuation or continuation of this practice (Li et al., 2014; Özgörü et al., 2023).

Postoperative Care and Rehabilitation

After surgical treatment in NEC, cardiovascular, hemodynamic, and respiratory support is required in postoperative care. During the postoperative period, fluid-electrolyte resuscitation, bowel rest, broad-spectrum antibiotics, and total parenteral nutrition support should be maintained. In neonates, hypergastrinemia may develop after extensive resection of the small intestine. Therefore, acid suppression with a proton pump inhibitor or H2-blocker may be beneficial. Ensuring enteral feeding requires a multidisciplinary approach, and the timing of initiating enteral feeding post-surgery depends on the neonate's clinical stability, other comorbidities, stool/ostomy output, and bowel anatomy. At the same time, potential postoperative complications such as sepsis, intestinal strictures, wound infections, obstructive adhesions, delayed anastomotic strictures, anastomotic ulcers, short bowel syndrome, and issues related to stomas must be recognized early, and appropriate treatments should be provided (Hong et al., 2018).

Short bowel syndrome is the most common cause of intestinal failure in infants who have experienced severe NEC. Advances in parenteral nutrition, infection prevention strategies, surgical treatment, and intestinal transplantation have significantly improved survival in patients with short bowel syndrome. With an appropriate and individualized management plan and a multidisciplinary approach, most newborns with short bowel syndrome can transition to enteral feeding and achieve normal growth and development (Christian et al., 2018; Neu, 2020). Enteral feeding will be restarted after the postoperative recovery period (at least 7 days). Total parenteral nutrition should be continued until the enteral feeding goal is reached. In cases of severe NEC, especially when intestinal resection is required, some newborns may take weeks to recover. Additionally, infants who cannot tolerate full enteral feeding for several months may require total parenteral nutrition for more than 21 days (Christian et al., 2018). Breast milk is the preferred form of nutrition during the recovery process for infants with NEC. However, formula may be preferred due to maternal medical conditions or parental preferences. Another factor to consider is cow's milk protein allergy. In such cases, specialized formulas like extensively hydrolyzed formula or elemental formula may be preferred (Wertheimer et al., 2019; Lapillonne et al., 2016). Additionally, non-nutritive sucking (using a pacifier) may support the transition to full enteral feeding by increasing mesenteric blood flow (Christian et al., 2018).

The Prevention of NEC

Approaches to prevent NEC development in newborns are listed below (He et al., 2018; Huang et al., 2018; Patel et al., 2017; Gupta et al., 2013):

- Antenatal corticosteroid administration (Evidence level A)
- Feeding with breast milk (Evidence level A)
- Feeding with donor milk in the absence of breast milk (Evidence level A)
- Maintaining postnatal oxygen saturation between 91-95% (Evidence level A)
- Administration of ibuprofen (paracetamol) for the treatment of patent ductus arteriosus (Evidence level A)
- Standard feeding protocol (Evidence level B)
- Withholding feeding during erythrocyte transfusion (Evidence level B)
- Limiting initial empirical antibiotic treatment to ≤ 5 days (if culture negative) (Evidence level C)
- Limiting the use of H2 blockers (Evidence level C)
- Use of probiotics (Evidence level C)
- Use of lactoferrin (Evidence level C).

Current Approaches in Diagnosis and Treatment

The management of newborn nutrition is critically important, especially for the most vulnerable group, preterm newborns (Evsyukova et al., 2020). Enteral nutrition is ideal for the development of the gastrointestinal system in premature newborns due to its ability to reduce the risk of nosocomial infections, enhance intestinal motility, stimulate the release of gastrointestinal hormones through trophic effects, and improve nutritional tolerance. However, preterm newborns are at risk for gastrointestinal complications such as feeding intolerance and NEC (Özkan et al., 2021). Currently, the suspicion of NEC is based on clinical findings, and abdominal X-rays are used for diagnosis. However, since clinical signs are not specific to the diagnosis, they may be confused with other pathological conditions like sepsis and feeding intolerance. For this reason, NIRS (Near Infra-Red Spektroskopisi), which has the potential to differentiate other diseases at an early stage, can be used to prevent unnecessary treatment in suspected cases (Van Der Heide et al., 2021).

Regional (cerebral, abdominal) tissue oxygen saturation measured by NIRS has become an increasingly used parameter for monitoring cerebral hemodynamics in newborns and for diagnosing and treating gastrointestinal complications such as feeding intolerance and necrotizing enterocolitis

(Özkan et al., 2021). It has also been noted that enteral feeding in stable preterm newborns increases abdominal oxygenation, that splanchnic oxygenation does not change in breastfed preterms, and that there is a temporary decrease in those fed enriched breast milk, while a continuous decrease is observed in formula-fed infants (Yücel et al., 2024). It is stated that the frequency of blood transfusions increases the likelihood of NEC development, that abdominal oxygenation increases during the procedure compared to afterward, but studies on the effects of feeding during the procedure on splanchnic tissue oxygenation have shown variable results (Pavlek et al., 2021). Özkan and colleagues (2021) indicated that the decrease in mesenteric tissue oxygenation during continuous monitoring of the first enteral feeding could be used to predict NEC development during follow-up (Özkan et al., 2021). It has also been shown that there can be a decrease in mesenteric perfusion in the presence of hemodynamic ductus arteriosus. Therefore, the limited number of abdominal NIRS studies and the variable results highlight the need for increased research in this area (Van Der Heide et al., 2021).

Systematic reviews of randomized controlled studies have shown that the prophylactic use of enteral probiotics significantly reduces mortality, length of hospital stay, and time to full enteral feeding in very low birth weight preterm newborns at risk of ≥Stage II necrotizing enterocolitis (AlFaleh & Anabrees, 2014; Deshpande et al., 2015). Many developed countries, including Australia, Canada, Finland, Denmark, and Germany, use probiotics as a standard practice to prevent necrotizing enterocolitis in preterm newborns (Deshpande et al., 2015). Additionally, stem cell therapy (such as mesenchymal stem cells and enteric-oral stem cells) is among the promising treatment approaches for NEC. Research is being planned based on the idea that the direct application of stem cells or particles to the damaged intestine may contribute to the healing process and reduce the risk of this complication in infants with short bowel syndrome in the long term. Research in this area is ongoing (Drucker et al., 2018; McCulloh et al., 2018).

Conclusion

The fact that the incidence of NEC cases has not decreased in recent times, that it is associated with high morbidity and mortality, that there are no specific findings for diagnosis, and that there are many factors that lack clarity in diagnosis, treatment, prevention, and care indicates that it continues to be one of the significant gastrointestinal problems in neonatal intensive care units. Due to the limited options available after the disease develops, preventing the disease in cases and raising awareness among healthcare professionals is critically important. Providing sufficient evidence through current studies related to diagnosis, treatment, and prevention is essential. In particular, emphasis should be placed on raising awareness of NEC alongside other preventive approaches, such as breastfeeding, which has proven effective in preventing NEC.

References

Afzal, B., Elberson, V., McLaughlin, C., & Kumar, V. H. (2017). Early onset necrctizing enterocolitis (NEC) in premature twins. *Journal of Neonatal-Perinatal Medicine, 10*(1), 109–112. https://doi.org/10.3233/NPM-1616.

AlFaleh, K., & Anabrees, J. (2014). Probiotics for prevention of necrotizing enterocolitis in preterm infants. *Evidence-Based Child Health: A Cochrane Review Journal, 9*(3), 584–671.

Bell, M. J., Ternberg, J. L., Feigin, R. D., Keating, J. P., Marshall, R., Barton, L., & Brotherton, T. (1978). Neonatal necrotizing enterocolitis: Therapeutic decisions based upon clinical staging. *Annals of Surgery, 187*(1), 1–7.

Caplan, M. S. (2010). Neonatal necrotizing enterocolitis: Clinical observations, pathophysiology, and prevention. In R. J. Martin, A. A. Fanaroff, & M. C. Walsh (Eds.), *Fanaroff & Martin's Neonatal-Perinatal Medicine* (9th ed., pp. 1431–1442). Elsevier Mosby.

Choi, Y. Y. (2014). Necrotizing enterocolitis in newborns: Update in pathophysiology and newly emerging therapeutic strategies. *Korean Journal of Pediatrics, 57*(12), 505–513. https://doi.org/10.3345/kjp.2014.57.12.505.

Christian, V. J., Polzin, E., & Welak, S. (2018). Nutrition management of necrotizing enterocolitis. *Nutrition in Clinical Practice, 33*(4), 476–482.

Cuna, A., George, L., & Sampath, V. (2018). Genetic predisposition to necrotizing enterocolitis in premature infants: Current knowledge, challenges, and future directions. *Seminars in Fetal & Neonatal Medicine, 23*(6), 387–393. https://doi.org/10.1016/j.siny.2018.08.006.

Deshpande, G., Rao, S., & Patole, S. (2015). Probiotics in neonatal intensive care: Back to the future. *Australian and New Zealand Journal of Obstetrics and Gynaecology, 55*(3), 210–217.

Drucker, N. A., McCulloh, C. J., Li, B., Pierro, A., Besner, G. E., & Markel, T. A. (2018). Stem cell therapy in necrotizing enterocolitis: Current state and future directions. *Seminars in Pediatric Surgery, 27*(1), 57–64.

Evsyukova, I. I., Zvereva, N. A., Gurieva, N. G., & Velichko, T. A. (2020). The feature of brain oxygenation in the sleep cycle of healthy newborn babies. *Pediatrician (St. Petersburg), 10*(6), 5–11.

Fraser, D. (2015). The high risk newborn and family. In M. J. Hockenberry & D. Wilson (Eds.), *Wong's Nursing Care of Infants and Children* (10th ed., pp. 386–387). Elsevier Mosby.

Gephart, S. M., Spitzer, A. R., Effken, J. A., Dodd, E., Halpern, M., & McGrath, J. M. (2014). Discrimination of Gut Check NEC: A clinical risk index for necrotizing enterocolitis. *Journal of Perinatology, 34*(6), 468–475.

Ginglen, J. G., & Butki, N. (2023). Necrotizing enterocolitis. In *StatPearls* [Internet]. StatPearls Publishing. https://www.ncbi.nlm.nih.gov/books/NBK513357/.

Goldstein, G. P., & Sylvester, K. G. (2019). Biomarker discovery and utility in necrotizing enterocolitis. *Clinics in Perinatology, 46*(1), 1–17.

Hackam, D. J., Sodhi, C. P., & Good, M. (2019). New insights into necrotizing enterocolitis: From laboratory observation to personalized prevention and treatment. *Journal of Pediatric Surgery, 54*(3), 398–404.

He, Y., Cao, L., & Yu, J. (2018). Prophylactic lactoferrin for preventing late-onset sepsis and necrotizing enterocolitis in preterm infants: A PRISMA-compliant systematic review and meta-analysis. *Medicine, 97*(35), e11976.

Hong, C. R., Han, S. M., & Jaksic, T. (2018). Surgical considerations for neonates with necrotizing enterocolitis. *Seminars in Fetal & Neonatal Medicine, 23*(6), 420–425.

Huang, X., Wang, F., & Wang, K. (2018). Paracetamol versus ibuprofen for the treatment of patent ductus arteriosus in preterm neonates: A meta-analysis of randomized controlled trials. *Journal of Maternal-Fetal & Neonatal Medicine, 31*(16), 2216–2222.

Kim, J. H. (2019). Role of abdominal US in diagnosis of NEC. *Clinics in Perinatology, 46*(1), 119–127.

Lapillonne, A., Matar, M., Adleff, A., Chbihi, M., Kermorvant-Duchemin, E., & Campeotto, F. (2016). Use of extensively hydrolysed formula for refeeding neonates post-necrotising enterocolitis: A nationwide survey-based, cross-sectional study. *BMJ Open, 6*(7), e008613.

Li, Y. F., Lin, H. C., Torrazza, R. M., Parker, L., Talaga, E., & Neu, J. (2014). Gastric residual evaluation in preterm neonates: A useful monitoring technique or a hindrance? *Pediatrics & Neonatology, 55*(5), 335–340.

Mashriq, A., Lee, C., Edoardo, B., Li, B., & Agostino, P. (2019). Recent advances in understanding necrotizing enterocolitis. *F1000Research, 8.*

McCulloh, C. J., Olson, J. K., Wang, Y., Zhou, Y., Tengberg, N. H., Deshpande, S., & Besner, G. E. (2018). Treatment of experimental necrotizing enterocolitis with stem cell-derived exosomes. *Journal of Pediatric Surgery, 53*(6), 1215–1220.

Naberhuis, J., Wetzel, C., & Tappenden, K. A. (2016). A novel neonatal feeding intolerance and necrotizing enterocolitis risk–scoring tool is easy to use and valued by nursing staff. *Advances in Neonatal Care, 16*(3), 239–244.

Neu, J. (2014). Necrotizing enterocolitis: The mystery goes on. *Neonatology, 106*(4), 289–295.

Neu, J. (2020). Necrotizing enterocolitis: The future. *Neonatology, 117*(2), 240–244.

Özgörü, H., Mutlu, B., & Erkut, Z. (2023). Effect of lying position on gastric residual volume in premature infants: A systematic review. *Nutrition in Clinical Practice, 39*(2), 295–310.

Özkan, H., Çetinkaya, M., Dorum, B. A., & Köksal, N. (2021). Mesenteric tissue oxygenation status on the development of necrotizing enterocolitis. *The Turkish Journal of Pediatrics, 63*(5), 811–817.

Patel, A. L., Panagos, P. G., & Silvestri, J. M. (2017). Reducing incidence of necrotizing enterocolitis. *Clinics in Perinatology, 44*(3), 683–700.

Patole, S. (2013). Prevention and treatment of necrotising enterocolitis in preterm neonates. In S. Patole (Ed.), *Nutrition for the Preterm Neonate* (pp. 71–96). Springer. https://doi.org/10.1007/978-94-007-6812-3.

Pavlek, L. R., Mueller, C., Jebbia, M. R., Kielt, M. J., & Fathi, O. (2021). Near-infrared spectroscopy in extremely preterm infants. *Frontiers in Pediatrics, 8,* 624113.

Potts, N. L., & Mandleco, B. L. (2012). *Pediatric Nursing: Caring for Children and Their Families* (3rd ed., pp. 769–771). Delmar, Cengage Learning.

Roberts, A. G., Younge, N., & Greenberg, R. G. (2024). Neonatal necrotizing enterocolitis: An update on pathophysiology, treatment, and prevention. *Paediatric Drugs, 26*(3), 259–275. https://doi.org/10.1007/s40272-024-00626-w.

Robinson, J. R., Rellinger, E. J., Hatch, L. D., Weitkamp, J. H., Speck, K. E., Danko, M., & Blakely, M. L. (2017). Surgical necrotizing enterocolitis. *Seminars in Perinatology, 41*(1), 70–79.

Rysavy, M. A., Watkins, P. L., Colaizy, T. T., & Das, A. (2020). Is routine evaluation of gastric residuals for premature infants safe or effective? *Journal of Perinatology, 40*(3), 540–543.

Thakkar, H. S., & Lakhoo, K. (2016). The surgical management of necrotising enterocolitis (NEC). *Early Human Development, 97,* 25–28.

Thomas, S., Nesargi, S., Roshan, P., Raju, R., Mathew, S., Sheeja, P., & Rao, S. (2018). Gastric residual volumes versus abdominal girth measurement in assessment of feed tolerance in preterm neonates: A randomized controlled trial. *Advances in Neonatal Care, 18*(4), E13–E19.

Thompson, A. M., & Bizzarro, M. J. (2008). Necrotizing enterocolitis in newborns: Pathogenesis, prevention and management. *Drugs, 68,* 1227–1238.

Van Der Heide, M., Hulscher, J. B. F., Bos, A. F., & Kooi, E. M. W. (2021). Near-infrared spectroscopy as a diagnostic tool for necrotizing enterocolitis in preterm infants. *Pediatric Research, 90*(1), 148–155.

Walsh, M. C., & Kliegman, R. M. (1986). Necrotizing enterocolitis: Treatment based on staging criteria. *Pediatric Clinics of North America, 33*(1), 179–201.

Wertheimer, F., Arcinue, R., & Niklas, V. (2019). Necrotizing enterocolitis: Enhancing awareness for the general practitioner. *Pediatrics in Review, 40*(10), 517–527

Yee, W. H., Soraisham, A. S., Shah, V. S., Aziz, K., Yoon, W., Lee, S. K., & Canadian Neonatal Network. (2012). Incidence and timing of presentation of necrotizing enterocolitis in preterm infants. *Pediatrics, 129*(2), e298–e304.

Yücel, A., Küçükoğlu, S., & Soylu, H. (2024). The effect of breast milk odor on feeding cues, transition time to oral feeding, and abdominal perfusion in premature newborns: A randomised controlled trial. *Biological Research for Nursing, 26*(1), 160–175.

Chapter 11

Meconium Ileus

Gül Doğan*, MD
Department of Pediatric Surgery, Hitit University, Çorum, Turkey

Abstract

Meconium is the first stool produced by the fetal gastrointestinal system, typically accumulating in the large intestine towards the end of pregnancy. This initial stool, which constitutes the newborn's first bowel movement, is thick and sticky in consistency and dark brown or green in color. It is expected to pass through the infant's system within the first 24 to 48 hours after birth. Meconium ileus is a condition commonly observed in newborns that leads to intestinal obstruction. This obstruction occurs due to the failure of meconium accumulated in the large intestine during fetal development to be expelled normally. Meconium ileus is frequently associated with genetic disorders such as cystic fibrosis, but it can also occur due to other causes. Conditions such as intestinal anomalies, metabolic disorders, and intrauterine urinary tract obstruction can also lead to meconium ileus.

The symptoms of meconium ileus typically manifest within the first few days after birth. Normally, stool passage is expected in the initial days post-delivery. In newborns with meconium ileus, stool output is often reduced or absent. Associated symptoms include vomiting, abdominal distention, and feeding intolerance. The diagnosis of meconium ileus is primarily based on clinical findings and radiological examinations. During physical examination, abdominal distention and tenderness may be observed. Radiological assessments, especially abdominal ultrasound and X-ray, are utilized to evaluate the condition of the intestines. Radiographs may reveal gas and meconium accumulation in the bowel.

---

* Corresponding Author's Email: guldemirdag_982@hotmail.com

In: Current Approaches to Newborn Emergencies
Editors: Zuhal Keskin Sarılar and Serap Samut Bülbül
ISBN: 979-8-89530-999-5

The treatment of meconium ileus varies depending on the severity and underlying causes. One of the most frequently employed methods involves the mechanical removal of meconium from the intestine, which can be performed using a rectal tube or other instruments. If mechanical removal is unsuccessful or if there is significant bowel damage, surgical intervention may be required. During the treatment process, the newborn is often provided with intravenous fluid support for nutrition. If meconium ileus is associated with cystic fibrosis, appropriate cystic fibrosis management should also be initiated. In such cases, thinning of mucus and clearing the airways may also be necessary.
Meconium ileus can represent a significant health concern in newborns, requiring timely diagnosis and intervention. Early management reduces the risk of complications. The presence of underlying conditions, such as cystic fibrosis, plays a critical role in the management of meconium ileus. Therefore, careful evaluation of such cases and the development of appropriate treatment plans are essential.

Keywords: newborn, meconium, ileus, cystic fibrosis

Introduction

Meconium ileus is a congenital condition characterized by intestinal obstruction in newborns (Boczar et al., 2015). This condition arises when meconium, the first stool produced in the fetal intestines, accumulates and obstructs normal bowel function. Meconium is a green-black, sticky substance typically expelled within the first few days after birth (Carlyle et al., 2012). Meconium ileus usually results from an anatomical or physiological problem that impairs the normal movement of meconium. One of the most common causes is genetic disorders such as cystic fibrosis (CF), which affects mucus production in the intestines, increasing the viscosity of meconium and leading to obstruction (Boczar et al., 2015). Clinically, meconium ileus presents with symptoms such as abdominal distension, vomiting, and feeding difficulties in newborns. Prompt recognition and management of this condition are crucial to prevent complications. While surgical intervention is often required for treatment, conservative approaches may be considered in certain cases (Hill et al., 1964).

In conclusion, meconium ileus is a serious medical condition in newborns that necessitates timely intervention for optimal outcomes.

Main Body

Meconium begins to form around the 16th week of fetal life, gradually moving downward throughout the remainder of pregnancy and remaining in the upper rectum until birth. Meconium consists of bile, mucus secretions from the intestines, swallowed amniotic fluid, stratified squamous epithelium, and desquamated intestinal epithelial cells. Meconium ileus occurs when meconium becomes impacted in the distal ileum and colon, leading to intraluminal obstruction (Burge & Drewett, 2004). Although meconium ileus was first described by Landsteiner in 1905, Anderson provided a more detailed characterization of its clinical features. It is most commonly observed in patients with CF and is often the earliest clinical manifestation of this condition. However, it can also be seen in cases of ileal atresia and terminal ileum aganglionosis, which cause lower gastrointestinal obstructions (Serban et al., 2002).

In neonates with CF, meconium ileus results from the accumulation of thickened meconium, which adheres tightly to the intestinal wall, leading to mechanical obstruction. As a consequence, there is widespread proximal small bowel distension due to the obstruction caused by the meconium filling the intestinal lumen (Rescorla & Grosfeld, 1993). CF is an autosomal recessive disorder with an incidence of approximately 1 in 2500 live births. It is the most common fatal genetic disease in the Caucasian population. The frequency of CFTR (cystic fibrosis transmembrane conductance regulator) gene mutation is 1 in 2500 in the United States and 1 in 17,000 in Africa, while the exact prevalence in Turkey remains unknown; however, it is higher in societies with a high rate of consanguineous marriages. The average life expectancy for individuals with CF is approximately 40 years (Ziegler et al., 2012).

Meconium ileus is an early clinical manifestation of CF, observed in approximately 10-20% of newborns with the disease. Under normal conditions, meconium is soft and is propelled forward by the infant's bowel movements, passing through the small intestine, colon, and anus. However, in CF, meconium becomes thickened and loses its fluidity, leading to intestinal obstruction, particularly at the level of the terminal ileum. The thickening of meconium is primarily attributed to CF, which affects mucus-secreting organs and systems, including the lungs, pancreas, gastrointestinal tract, and sweat glands (Ziegler et al., 2012). This dysfunction results in the production of thick, viscous mucus that disrupts normal physiological processes. The adhesive and hyperviscous nature of meconium in meconium ileus results from abnormal mucus secretion. In CF, exocrine glands are primarily affected, and the disease occurs due to mutations in the CFTR gene. The CFTR gene is located on chromosome 7q22-31 and encodes the CFTR protein, consisting of 1480 amino acids (van der Doef et al., 2011).

The CFTR protein plays a key role in regulating ion transport across the epithelial cells of various exocrine tissues, including the airway epithelium, submucosal glands, pancreas, liver, sweat glands, and reproductive organs. It forms a channel that facilitates the passive movement of electrolytes, such as sodium (Na^+) and chloride (Cl^-), across the cell membrane. In CF, mutations affecting CFTR protein function lead to impaired sodium, chloride, and water transport. The inability to secrete these components results in epithelial surface dehydration and mucus stasis.

As a consequence of dehydrated mucus accumulation, hyperviscous mucoid secretions form, which can obstruct the intestinal lumen, particularly at the terminal ileum, leading to the clinical presentation of meconium ileus (van der Doef et al., 2011; Chaudry et al., 2006).

Clinical Findings

Patients present with abdominal distension and vomiting starting from birth. The infant has not passed meconium within the first 24-48 hours; evacuation of distal colonic secretions with enemas may be mistakenly perceived as defecation. Two types of meconium ileus have been defined: simple and complicated. The simple type typically manifests with postnatal abdominal distension, bilious vomiting, and failure to pass meconium within 24-48 hours. In the complicated type, unlike the simple form, abdominal distension frequently occurs within the first 24 hours after birth (Maurica et al., 2020). Meconium ileus presents with a picture of terminal ileal obstruction. In the newborn, typical signs of small bowel obstruction such as bilious vomiting, feeding intolerance, abdominal distension, and inability to pass stool are present. In advanced stages, abdominal distension increases, and pneumoperitoneum, peritonitis, and inflammation of the abdominal wall may develop. This type is often accompanied by signs of hypovolemia and sepsis (Borowitz & Gelfond, 2013).

Diagnosis

The diagnosis is typically established based on clinical findings, physical examination, and imaging methods. Imaging techniques such as X-ray or ultrasound support the diagnosis by demonstrating meconium accumulation and bowel obstruction.

Prenatal ultrasound can aid in diagnosing meconium ileus. Findings include significantly distended bowel loops, increased echogenicity, and an increase in abdominal circumference measurements compared to the gestational age. Although these findings can also be observed in meconium ileus cases unrelated to CF, they should prompt evaluation for CF in the neonatal period. Postnatal upright abdominal X-rays are helpful for diagnosis, though findings can vary. In CF-related cases, there is dilation of the small bowel; however, the typical air-fluid levels observed in obstructions are absent. This is due to the thick, non-fluid meconium obstructing the air passage. Air bubbles trapped within thick meconium create a soap-bubble appearance or a ground-glass pattern. Intra-abdominal calcifications should raise suspicion for complicated meconium ileus presenting as meconium peritonitis due to prenatal perforation. The presence of ascites and pneumoperitoneum suggests postnatal perforation. Nevertheless, abdominal X-rays can appear normal in approximately 35% of cases.

Contrast imaging can be both diagnostic and therapeutic. High-osmolar contrast material draws fluid from the bowel wall into the lumen, inducing osmotic diarrhea, which helps expel thickened meconium through the anus, thus providing simultaneous treatment. Water-soluble contrast imaging may reveal a characteristic “pearl grains” appearance in the terminal ileum caused by meconium, which is diagnostic (Houwen et al., 2010; Borowitz & Gelfond, 2013).

Laboratory

In all cases of meconium ileus, a sweat test and CF genetic testing should be performed to confirm the diagnosis of CF. Newborn CF screening tests have been implemented in our country since 2016. In suspected cases, sweat tests and genetic tests should be conducted. However, in some cases of meconium ileus, although clinical findings are consistent with intestinal involvement typical of CF, the sweat test or genetic test may occasionally yield negative results. Furthermore, clinical symptoms can be significant and require treatment even in heterozygous-positive cases (Johnson et al., 2010; Serban et al., 2002).

Differential Diagnosis

CF can be confused with meconium plug syndrome. In cases without CF, transient obstruction may occur due to colonic motility disorders and viscous meconium, leading to meconium plugs. It is most commonly mistaken for meconium ileus. Meconium plugs are located in the distal colon and can be differentiated from meconium ileus by their black-green color. Meconium plug syndrome typically resolves with evacuating enemas, and surgical intervention is rarely required. However, Hirschsprung disease, which can rarely accompany these cases, should be kept in mind, and a sweat test for CF must be performed.

Hirschsprung disease, total colonic aganglionosis, and meconium ileus can present with similar clinical findings. Hirschsprung disease is observed in approximately 5% of meconium ileus cases. Additionally, neuronal intestinal dysplasia can also present with a clinical picture resembling meconium ileus. Therefore, in cases of suspicion, a definitive diagnosis requires a rectal biopsy (Burge & Drewett, 2004; Serban et al., 2002).

Treatment

The treatment of meconium ileus generally requires surgical intervention. The process begins with stabilizing the infant's overall condition. Intravenous fluids are administered to maintain fluid balance, and feeding is discontinued. Imaging methods are then used to determine the level and cause of the obstruction. Initially, rectal enemas containing *N-acetylcysteine* are administered to soften and evacuate the meconium. If this approach is unsuccessful, surgical treatment becomes necessary. The goal of surgery is to mechanically clear the thick meconium obstructing the intestines, particularly the terminal ileum. The contrast agent used for imaging or intraoperative irrigation also has therapeutic effects. Before the procedure, patients must be well-hydrated and protected with broad-spectrum antibiotics (O'Neill et al., 1970; Evans et al., 2001). When medical management fails or in complicated cases of meconium ileus with intestinal obstruction, surgical intervention is often required. During surgical exploration, sticky meconium is removed, and based on the condition of the bowel, surgical options such as primary resection-anastomosis or stoma creation (ileostomy) are performed. In patients with a stoma, bowel irrigation with *N-acetylcysteine* solution is initiated in the early postoperative period, which is generally successful. However, in complicated cases of meconium ileus, such as intestinal volvulus, atresia, perforation, or gangrene, bowel resections or ileostomy may be necessary. When oral feeding is resumed, pancreatic enzyme preparations must be administered. In these patients, respiratory physiotherapy and pulmonary care are also essential (Evans et al., 2001; Perman et al., 1975).

Prognosis

Regardless of whether a stoma is created, ileus episodes may occur from time to time. Patients who do not receive an appropriate dose of pancreatic enzyme replacement therapy often present with ileus attacks. These patients are typically lost in their 30s, not due to gastrointestinal complications, but rather as a result of pulmonary issues stemming from the enzymatic defects observed in CF (Houwen et al., 2010).

Conclusion

Meconium ileus is a form of intestinal obstruction observed in newborn infants, typically becoming evident within the first days after birth. This condition occurs due to the accumulation of meconium in the intestines, leading to obstruction. While meconium ileus is commonly associated with genetic disorders such as CF, in some cases, the underlying cause may remain unknown. Diagnosis is established through clinical findings and imaging methods, and treatment often requires surgical intervention. With early diagnosis and appropriate treatment, the chances of recovery are high. Raising awareness about meconium ileus plays a critical role in the effective management of neonatal health.

References

Boczar, M., Sawicka, E., & Zybert, K. (2015). Meconium ileus in newborns with cystic fibrosis: Results of treatment in the group of patients operated on in the years 2000–

2014. *Developmental Period Medicine, 19*(1), 32–40. https://doi.org/10.1055/s-0037-1609027.

Borowitz, D., & Gelfond, D. (2013). Intestinal complications of cystic fibrosis. *Current Opinion in Pulmonary Medicine, 19*(6), 676–680. https://doi.org/10.1097/MCP.0b013e3283659ef2.

Burge, D., & Drewett, M. (2004). Meconium plug obstruction. *Pediatric Surgery International, 20*(2), 108–110. https://doi.org/10.1007/s00383-003-1098-y.

Carlyle, B. E., Borowitz, D. S., & Glick, P. L. (2012). A review of pathophysiology and management of fetuses and neonates with meconium ileus for the pediatric surgeon. *Journal of Pediatric Surgery, 47*(4), 772–781. https://doi.org/10.1016/j.jpedsurg.2012.02.019.

Chaudry, G., Navarro, O. M., Levine, D. S., & Oudjhane, K. (2006). Abdominal manifestations of cystic fibrosis in children. *Pediatric Radiology, 36*(3), 233–240. https://doi.org/10.1007/s00247-005-0049-2.

Evans, A. K., Fitzgerald, D. A., & McKay, K. O. (2001). The impact of meconium ileus on the clinical course of children with cystic fibrosis. *European Respiratory Journal, 18*, 784–789. https://doi.org/10.1183/09031936.01.00053701.

Hill, J. T., Snyder, W. H., Jr., & Pollock, W. F. (1964). Management of complicated meconium ileus. *American Journal of Surgery, 108*(2), 233–238. https://doi.org/10.1016/0002-9610(64)90014-5.

Houwen, R. H., van der Doef, H. P., Sermet, I., Munck, A., Hauser, B., Navarro, J., ... & Colombo, C. (2010). Defining DIOS and constipation in cystic fibrosis with a multicentre study on the incidence, characteristics, and treatment of DIOS. *Journal of Pediatric Gastroenterology and Nutrition, 50*(1), 38–42. https://doi.org/10.1097/MPG.0b013e3181a6e01d.

Johnson, J. A., Bush, A., & Buchdahl, R. (2010). Does presenting with meconium ileus affect the prognosis of children with cystic fibrosis? *Pediatric Pulmonology, 45*(10), 951–958. https://doi.org/10.1002/ppul.21271.

Maurica, A., Escobar, J. R., & Caty, M. G. (2020). Meconium disease. In G. W. Holcomb, J. P. Murphy, & S. D. St. Peter (Eds.), *Holcomb and Ashcraft's pediatric surgery* (7th ed., pp. 517–535). Saunders/Elsevier. https://doi.org/10.1016/B978-1-4160-6127-4.00033-1.

O'Neill, J. A., Jr., Grosfeld, J. L., Boles, E. T., Jr., & Clatworthy, H. W., Jr. (1970). Surgical treatment of meconium ileus. *American Journal of Surgery, 119*(1), 99–105. https://doi.org/10.1016/0002-9610(70)90019-X.

Perman, J., Breslow, L., & Ingal, D. (1975). Nonoperative treatment of meconium ileus equivalent. *American Journal of Diseases of Children, 129*(10), 1210–1211. https://doi.org/10.1001/archpedi.1975.02120470056016.

Rescorla, F. J., & Grosfeld, J. L. (1993). Contemporary management of meconium ileus. *World Journal of Surgery, 17*(3), 318–325. https://doi.org/10.1007/BF01658698.

Serban, D. E., Florescu, P., & Miu, N. (2002). Fibrosing colonopathy revealing cystic fibrosis in a neonate before any pancreatic enzyme supplementation. *Journal of Pediatric Gastroenterology and Nutrition, 35*(3), 356–359. https://doi.org/10.1097/00005176-200209000-00022.

van der Doef, H. P., Kokke, F. T., van der Ent, C. K., & Houwen, R. H. (2011). Intestinal obstruction syndromes in cystic fibrosis: Meconium ileus, distal intestinal obstruction syndrome, and constipation. *Current Gastroenterology Reports, 13*(3), 265–270. https://doi.org/10.1007/s11894-011-0185-9.

Ziegler, M. M., Coran, A., Adzick, N. S., Krummel, T., Laberge, J. M., Shamberger, R., & Caldamone, A. (Eds.). (2012). Meconium ileus. In *Pediatric surgery* (7th ed., pp. 1073–1083). Saunders/Elsevier. https://doi.org/10.1016/0011-3840(94)90040-X.

Chapter 12

Anorectal Malformations

Mehtap Durukan*, MD
Department of Mersin Training and Research Hospital, Department of Pediatrics, Division of Neonatology, Mersin, Turkey

Abstract

Anorectal malformations (ARM) are the most common cause of neonatal surgery. It is a spectrum of structural congenital defects involving variable segments of the anorectal and urogenital systems in males and females. The prevalence in the population is 1/3000-5000. ARM is defined as a wide spectrum of diseases ranging from simple anatomic changes to severe atresia of the anogenital region. Abnormal septation of the hindgut with an abnormal cloacal membrane between 6 and 9 weeks of gestation forms the basis of a series of anomalies. Although it is often associated with syndromes, 1/3 of cases are isolated. Careful perineal examination of the baby after birth leads to a clinical diagnosis. ARM is surgically corrected with different approaches for boys and girls. The quality of life of patients with ARM can be improved by knowing the long-term problems and managing them correctly. Continuous research is needed to determine antenatal diagnostic methods and ARM's preventability, explain genetic and epigenetic changes, and develop optimal surgical procedures.

Keywords: anorectal malformation, cloaca, imperforate anus, incontinence

---

* Corresponding Author's Email: mehtap.durukan@gmail.com

In: Current Approaches to Newborn Emergencies
Editors: Zuhal Keskin Sarılar and Serap Samut Bülbül
ISBN: 979-8-89530-999-5

Introduction

Anorectal malformations are the most common group of surgical diseases in neonates. The incidence is 1/3000-5000. It can affect both sexes but is more common in male neonates. The incidence of ARM may increase up to 1/100 in the presence of a sibling with ARM. Antenatal diagnosis of an isolated case of ARM is difficult. It can be diagnosed early with careful and detailed genital examination of the newborn after birth or in the absence of fecal output in the first 24 hours. Defects range from minor defects that can be easily treated with excellent results to complex defects with poor prognosis. Although anorectal malformations may present as an isolated finding, it is important to note that anorectal malformations are associated with VACTERL Syndrome (vertebral, anorectal, cardiac, tracheoesophageal fistula/esophageal atresia, renal, and limb), MURCS (Müllerian duct aplasia, renal aplasia, and cervicothoracic somite dysplasia), OEIS (omphalocele, exstrophy, imperforate anus, and spinal defects), Axial mesodermal dysplasia, and Klippel-Feil syndrome are frequently associated anomalies. Therefore, additional investigations are also required (Coran et al., 2012; de Blaauw et al., 2024; Mahmud et al., 2021).

History

Centuries ago, attempts were made to perforate the perineum of neonates born without an anus with cutting instruments similar to knives, and some of the mild forms of ARMs could be kept alive in the conditions of that day without antibiotics and parenteral fluids. Hippocrates was the first person to mention anorectal surgery. Aristotle stated that congenital malformations of the anorectal region occur more frequently in boys than in girls. The first record related to anal atresia is associated with the opening and dilatation of the anus with a cutting instrument in a patient with anal atresia by Paul Aegina (625-690 AD), who lived in the Aegean region in Turkey (3).

Etiology

The etiology of anorectal malformations has not been determined. Only one-third of ARMs are isolated. Congenital urogenital, cardiovascular, skeletal-muscular, and gastrointestinal anomalies are frequently associated. Therefore, the etiology is thought to be multifactorial. Autosomal dominant inheritance is thought to be possible due to the similarity and frequency of associated congenital anomalies. The incidence of ARM in other children is 1/100, and the presence of a neonate with ARM in the family supports this possibility. Chromosome 7q39 contains the SHH, EN2, and HLXB9 loci that play a role in the development of ARM. The most frequently associated syndromes are those with autosomal dominant modes of inheritance, such as Down syndrome, Townes-Brocks syndrome, Currarino syndrome, and Pallister-Hall syndrome. Experimental studies have shown that exposure to Adriamycin, etretinate, and vitamin A deficiency during pregnancy may cause ARM. Maternal fever in the first trimester of pregnancy, maternal diabetes, excessive weight gain, maternal exposure to tobacco smoke, caffeine, and asthma medications have been reported to be associated with ARM cases. It is known that there is a significant relationship between ARM and consanguinity, and the risk of recurrence is high in first-degree relatives (3-6).

Embryology and Anatomy

In typical embryonic development, the anorectum forms from the cloaca, and by the sixth week of gestation, the urorectal septum (URS) divides the embryonic cloaca into urogenital and anorectal sections, while the URS merges with the cloacal membrane (CM). During the sixth to eighth week of embryonic development, apoptotic cells concentrated in the CM and dorsal rectum cause localized detachment of the CM, allowing the URS to contact it. The dorsal cloaca, positioned near the tail of the embryo, gives rise to the anal orifice through the dorsal part of the cloacal membrane (CM). Secondary obstruction of the anorectal canal occurs when the walls adhere to each other and an epithelial cell plug forms at the level of the anal orifice due to a pause or defect in the separation process. Recanalization is observed with apoptotic cell death in the ninth week of pregnancy. Local muscle and nerve development in the region is disrupted due to abnormal anorectal and urogenital formations. Various ARMs occur according to the time and degree of pause and separation. It is common to classify ARMs as low, medium, or high localization. The rectal pouch is named according to its position relative to the levator ani muscule (LA) or pelvic floor. In low-type ARMs with mild developmental defects of the cloacal membrane (CM), the rectal pouch lies beneath the pelvic floor. In contrast, in high-type ARMs with severe CM defects, the rectal pouch is positioned above the pelvic floor, resulting in the longitudinal axis (LA) being displaced anteriorly and upward, just behind the posterior urethra. In a typical anorectum, the anal canal is surrounded by the anal sphincter complex, which consists of longitudinal muscle fibers of the internal sphincter canal and transverse muscle fibers. In high-type ARMs, the terminal rectum does not pass from the pelvic floor to the perineal skin, so the fibers of the internal sphincter do not develop connections between the longitudinal smooth muscle fibers and transverse muscle fibers, and the LA is thinner, indicating that the LA is significantly thinner, asymmetric, and deviated from the midline in high-type ARMs compared to low-type ARMs. Highly located ARMs are more difficult to operate and have a worse prognosis and morbidity (Li et al., 2020; Miyake et al., 2022; Miyake et al., 2022).

Diagnosis

Antenatal Diagnosis

It is very difficult to diagnose in the antenatal period. 3D ultrasonography can detect the absence of perianal muscles, and 2D ultrasonography can show distal bowel dilatation and calcified meconium within the lumen, but these findings are generally not sufficient to diagnose ARM. However, a large cystic mass originating from the pelvis could point toward a presumptive diagnosis of cloaca (King & Levitt, 2022).

In the postnatal period, a detailed and careful perineal examination of a neonate is sufficient for clinical diagnosis. Atresia, or abnormal position of the anus, is diagnostic. In male infants, in addition to the absence of the anus, the anal pit should also be evaluated in detail for the presence of a fistula. In cases where the fistula diameter is narrow, it may be difficult to see the fistula, so it should be re-evaluated after 24 hours. In male infants, especially anocutaneous fistula, bucket handle, and pearl sign should be noted in terms of ARM. Diagnosis by physical examination is different in female infants compared to male infants; the diagnosis is made by the appearance of the perineum. In a healthy female newborn, three openings should be seen in the perineum, respectively, urethra, vagina, and anus in the posterior part. The first two of these openings are in the vestibule. The presence of the three openings in anatomically different locations or fewer in number supports the diagnosis of ARM (Gangopadhyay & Pandey, 2015).

Imaging Findings

Invertogram

It was first described in 1930. Inversion radiography was used to indicate the distance between the air in the terminal colon and the skin of the perineum. By placing a radio-opaque marker on the skin, the location of the atresia is determined by direct measurement between the gas-filled bowel and the skin of the anus.

Cross-Table Lateral View

The neonate is held in the genu pectoral position for 3 minutes with the hips flexed, torso in the prone position, and face down. Similar to an invertogram, lateral prone radiographs are obtained, and the location of the atresia is determined by gas distribution.

Ultrasonographic Evaluation

Ultrasonographic examination is used to measure the perineal distance from the atresia. It can be done transperineally or infracoccygeally. The infracoccygeal region can show the puborectalis directly as a hypoechoic U-shaped band. It has the advantage of being non-invasive, but its sensitivity and specificity are low due to its dependence on the evaluator.

Computed Tomography and Magnetic Resonance Imaging

Computed tomography (CT) and magnetic resonance imaging (MRI) can be performed to evaluate the sphincter muscles in detail. They provide important information for preoperative and postoperative evaluation of the sphincters, atresia, and blind bowel. The presence and location of the fistula and its relationship with the pelvic floor can be demonstrated by MRI or CT imaging and provide important information for ease of surgical approach. MRI is considered superior to CT because of its better soft tissue resolution, ability to obtain thin sections and multiple planar images, and non-invasiveness (Gangopadhyay & Pandey, 2015; Le Bayon et al., 2010).

Classification

In the Wing Spread classification made according to the relationship of the blunt end of the rectum with the levator muscles, anorectal malformations are divided into three basic groups: high type (supralevator), low type (infralevator), and intermediate type (intermediate), which does not fit high or low type (Table 1).

Considering the classifications and operations performed, a new classification, the PENA classification, has emerged in which gender, fistula type, treatment approach, and clinical outcomes are evaluated (Table 2).

When surgically treated cases and their morbidities were evaluated for many years, it was inevitable that the 'Krickenbeck classifications' emerged in 2005 (Table 3). With this classification, both surgical methods (Table 4) and evaluation of long-term morbidities (Table 5) have become easier and more effective.

Table 1. The Wingspread conference classification (1984)

Level of Anomaly	Male	Female
High type	Anorectal agenesis	Anorectal agenesis
	Rectovesical fistula	Rectovesical fistula
	Without fistula	Without fistula
	Rectal atresia	Rectal atresia
Intermediate type	Rectourethral fistula	Rectovestibular fistula
	Anal agenesis without fistula	Rectovaginal fistula
Low type	Anocutaneous fistula	Anal agenesis without fistula
	Anal stenosis-fistula	Anovestibular fistula
		Anocutaneous fistula
Miscellaneous		Anal stenosis
		Persistent cloacal anomaly
	Rare malformations	Rare malformations

Table 2. Pena classification (1995) (Gangopadhyay & Pandey, 2015; Levitt & Peña, 2007; Pena, 2005)

Male	**Female**
Perineal fistula	Perineal fistula
Rectourethral fistula	Vestibular fistula
Bulbar	*Persistent cloaca*
Prostati	
Retrovesical fistula	
	<3 cm common channel *>3 cm common channel*
Imperforate anus without fistula	Imperforate anus without fistula
Rectal atresia	**Rectal atresia**

Table 3. Krickenbeck classifications (2005)

Major clinical groups	*Rare/Regional variants*
Perineal (cutaneous) fistula	Pouch colon
Rectourethral fistula	Rectal atresia/stenosis
Rectovesical fistula	
Vestibular fistula	H-type fistula
No fistula	Others
Anal stenosis	

Table 4. Krickenbeck's classification of surgical procedures

Operative procedures
Perineal operation
Anterior sagittal approach
Sacroperineal approach
Posterior sagittal anorectoplasty
Abdominosacroperineal pull-through
Abdominoperineal pull-through
Laparoscopic-assisted pull-through

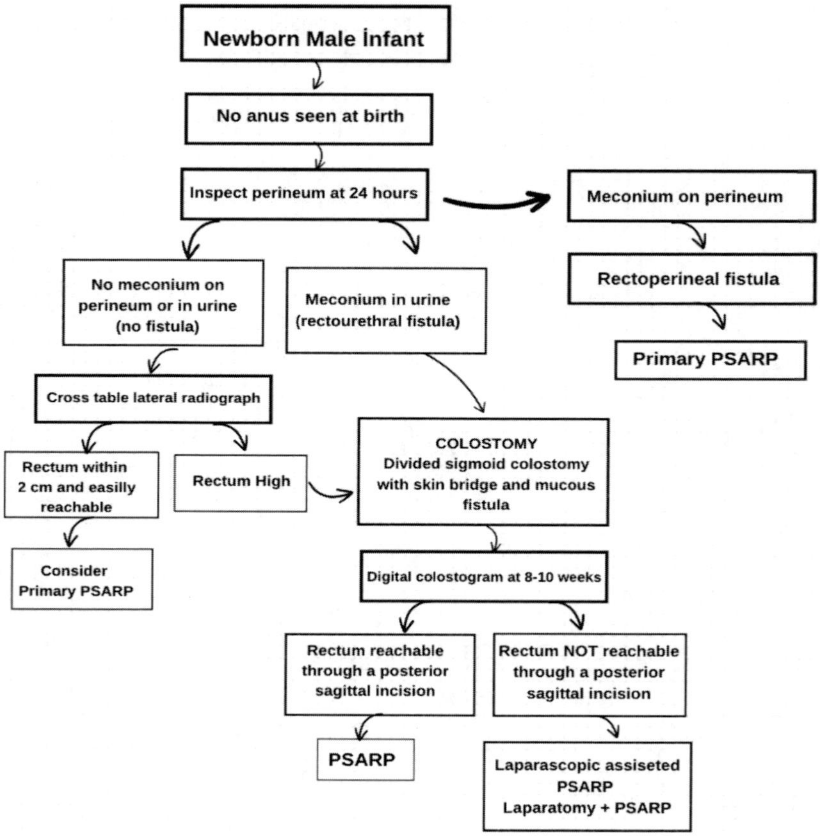

Figure 1. Management of male infant.

Male Infants

Colostomy is not necessary for male infants with a rectoperineal fistula. Posterior sagittal anoplasty, or PSARP, will be sufficient. Male infants who are thought to have a connection between the rectum and the urinary system should have colostomy and fecal diversion. Patients with rectobulbar and rectoprostatic fistulas may benefit from PSARP surgery. Cases with a fistula between the rectum and bladder neck require an abdominal approach to access the fistula. In cases of perforation, a protective colostomy is initially performed during the neonatal period to divert stool from the affected area. This is followed by colostomy closure and bowel reconstruction at 3 to 6 months of age, allowing time for the infant to grow stronger and for the affected area to heal. Before the operation, a pressurized distal colonogram and a micturition cystoureterogram should be performed to reveal the location of the rectourethral fistulas (Wood & Levitt, 2018) (Figure 1).

Female Infants

The general condition of the neonate and the number of openings in the vestibule are the primary determinants of the appropriate management strategy. A colostomy is indicated in the presence of abdominal distension or a single opening, which may be indicative of a permanent cloaca. The most prevalent anomaly in females is the rectovestibular type of ARM, which is characterized by the presence of a normal urethra and vagina, in addition to a rectal fistula in the vestibule. These cases can be treated with a colostomy and PSARP. In some instances, primary PSARP or primary anterior sagittal anorectoplasty may also be recommended. The definitive treatment for a permanent cloaca is achieved through PSARP. When the common duct exceeds 3 cm in length, mobilizing the vagina during PSARP becomes more difficult. In such instances, an abdominoperineal approach is necessary. In cases where the common canal is less than 3 cm, total urogenital mobilization is possible, whereby the vagina and urethra are mobilized as a unit without separation. If the distance between the vagina and perineum is long, the gap can be closed using a segment of bowel, preferably a colon segment. Alternatively, in cases of bicornuate uterus, vaginal passage can be performed. (Wood & Levitt, 2018) (Figure 2).

Table 5. Krickenbeck classification for postoperative results (Age >3 years, no therapy) (Sharma & Gupta, 2017)

Questions	Reply
Voluntary bowel movements	Yes/No
Soiling	Yes/No
Grade 1	Occasionally (once/twice per week)
Grade 2	Every day, no social problem
Grade 3	Constant, social problem
Constipation	Yes/No
Grade 1	Manageable by changes in diet
Grade 2	Requires laxatives
Grade 3	Resistance to laxatives and diet

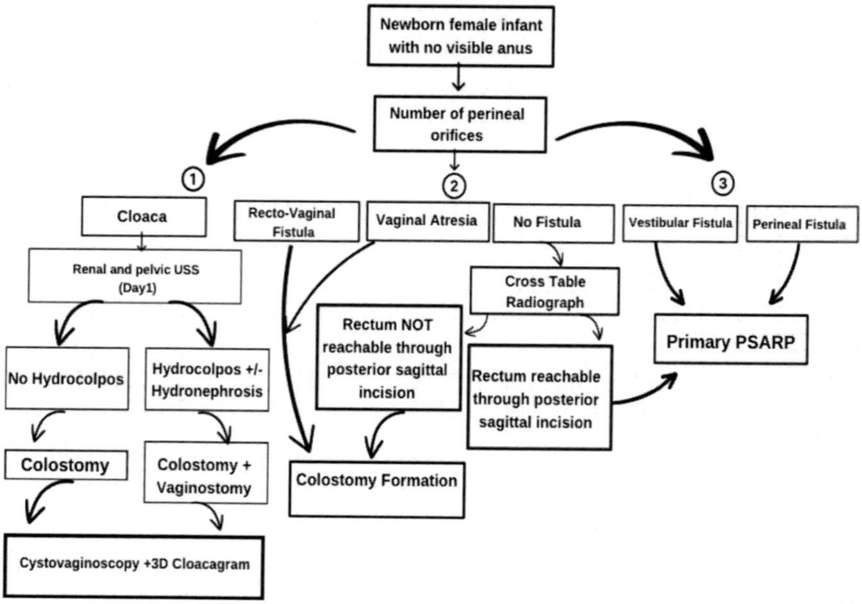

Figure 2. Management of female infant.

Surgical Management

The most commonly used surgical procedure to treat ARMs is posterior sagittal anorectoplasty (PSARP). Another approach, laparoscopic or laparotomic anorectoplasty (LAARP), is preferred in ARMs with an abnormal pelvic floor, especially in high-type ARMs with severe CM developmental disorders. PSARP requires midline excision of the pelvic floor muscles, so the PSARP method can be used in patients with a symmetrical pelvic floor. Regardless of the method used, high-type ARM cases tend to have more severe bowel dysfunction in the postoperative period than low-type ARM cases. A comprehensive evaluation of LA muscle mass and symmetry with MRI is recommended to improve functional outcomes and prevent damage to the LA, especially in patients with high-type ARM (Georgeson, 2007; Pena, 1986).

The location of the rectal pouch, resulting from defects in the development of the cloacal membrane, plays a crucial role in planning and performing the surgical procedure. During PSARP, if the distal rectal pouch is positioned below the coccyx, it can be easily located through direct downward dissection.

Anatomical variations may lead to issues such as inadequate defecation and postoperative complications following PSARP (Fujiwara et al., 2021; Yamataka et al., 2013).

Urinary retention, which often occurs after both PSARP and LAARP anorectoplasty, is considered to be caused by damage to the autonomic pelvic nerve plexus during fistula dissection. To prevent harm to the muscular cuff and peripheral nerve plexus, the fistula tract must be identified and sealed by approaching the rectal mucosa from the interior.

In early embryonic development, the rectal outlet is constricted, and in cases of ARMs, the rectum is obstructed before birth due to impaired development, leading to the prenatal expansion of the rectal pouch. It has been reported that the dilated terminal rectum is hypoganglionic; resection of the distal dilated rectal pouch may be beneficial to improve postoperative outcomes and prevent late morbidities (Li et al., 2020; Miyake et al., 2022).

Long-Term Morbidities

Anorectal malformations are the most common surgical disease group of the neonates. The main goal of surgery is to ensure a good quality of life at all stages of life. Since the presentation of the disease varies from a simple displacement to anomalies with severe procedures, it requires meticulous monitoring and care. Knowing, recognizing, and preventing long-term morbidities will contribute to the ease of life of individuals.

Bowel Dysfunction

Most infants with sphincter defects who undergo surgery for ARMs experience varying degrees of fecal incontinence, depending on the type and location of the defect and associated anomalies. Functional outcomes after surgical correction of ARMs are usually evaluated by manometric study, neural electrophysiologic studies, magnetic spinal stimulation, and fecal flowmetry. In cases with distally located ARMs, bowel function is usually better and does not severely affect the social life of the patient. Fecal incontinence may be seen in one-third of patients with high or moderate ARM. In treatment, incontinence can be prevented by keeping the rectum empty. Incontinence can be prevented with an enema, colon irrigation, or suppositories. In refractory cases, the Malone antegrade continence enema procedure offers a useful alternative. Patients with severe fecal incontinence may require secondary reconstruction. For many years, the gracilis muscle, or gluteus maximus muscle, has been used for transplantation to strengthen the anal sphincter (Bischoff et al., 2009; Gangopadhyay & Pandey, 2015).

Urinary Incontinence

Patients with anorectal malformations are often accompanied by urinary tract anomalies or sacral anomalies. Urinary incontinence is not a rare finding. Incontinence is seen in approximately 10% of patients undergoing surgery, especially with the PRSAP method (Harris & Wilcox, 2023).

Sexual Dysfunctions

Male infants with urogenital anomalies or sacral anomalies often have problems with erection and ejaculation at an older age. About 40% of adolescent boys with high and medium ARMs have sexual problems such as erection and ejaculation dysfunction. In females, high and intermediate ARMs usually do not cause serious problems, whereas sexual activity disorders are more common in those with low-lying ARMs. Other common problems in women are vaginal anomalies, agenesis, and uterine septation anomalies. In sexually active women, these anomalies often cause infertility and sexual problems (Harris & Wilcox, 2023).

Assessment of Growth and Development

Anorectal malformations are a group of surgical diseases affecting the gastrointestinal and urogenital systems, and growth and development are adversely affected, especially in the first two years of life in infants. Growth and developmental retardation are common due to prolonged hospitalization, surgical procedures, periods when feeding cannot be started, and repeated reconstruction surgeries. Children with ARM are at risk of gross motor function problems; therefore, close follow-up of patients who have undergone ARM surgery by a commission formed by pediatric surgery, social pediatrics, developmental pediatrics, pediatric surgery, pediatric urology, pediatric gastroenterology, child and adolescent psychiatry, and physiotherapists with multidisciplinary methods will reduce the problems of these infants in the future. The genetic characteristics of each infant, the degree of ARM, differences in associated malformations, nutritional deficiency, and bowel management should be individually optimized to prevent extensive physical and mental development, and social support for these children who start life 1-0 behind will make their lives easier (Divarci & Ergun, 2020).

Conclusion

Anorectal malformations are the most common group of neonatal diseases requiring surgery. Apart from post-operative complications, patients face various problems in the long term. Education of the parents of sick infants will help them to understand the long-term problems that the child will potentially face regarding continence. The diagnosis, follow-up, and treatment of these patients should be carried out by a multidisciplinary team who should work collaboratively to treat this population comprehensively and successfully and provide the lifelong management they need. Future research should be related to patient-centered outcomes, especially to improve the quality of life of these infants.

Acknowldegments

Thanks to Eda DURUKAN, MD, who contributed to the editing of the graphics and tables.

References

Bischoff, A., Levitt, M. A., Bauer, C., Jackson, L., Holder, M., & Peña, A. (2009). Treatment of fecal incontinence with a comprehensive bowel management program. *Journal of Pediatric Surgery*, *44*(6), 1278-1284. https://doi.org/10.1016/j.jpedsurg.2009.02.047.

Coran, A. G., Adzick, N. S., Krummel, T. M., Laberge, J.-M., Shamberger, R., & Caldamone, A. (2012). *Pediatric Surgery: Expert Consult-Online and Print* (Vol. 2). Elsevier Health Sciences.

de Blaauw, I., Stenström, P., Yamataka, A., Miyake, Y., Reutter, H., Midrio, P., Wood, R., Grano C., Pakarinen, M. (2024). Anorectal malformations. *Nature Reviews Disease Primers*, *10*(1), 88. https://doi.org/10.1038/s41572-024-00574-2.

Divarci, E., & Ergun, O. (2020). General complications after surgery for anorectal malformations. *Pediatric Surgery International*, *36*(4), 431-445. https://doi.org/10.1007/s00383-020-04629-9.

Fujiwara, K., Ochi, T., Koga, H., Miyano, G., Seo, S., Okazaki, T., Urao, M., Lane, G. J., Rintala, R. J., Yamataka, A. (2021). Lessons learned from lower urinary tract complications of anorectoplasty for imperforate anus with rectourethral/rectovesical fistula: Laparoscopy-assisted versus posterior sagittal approaches. *Journal of Pediatric Surgery*, *56*(7), 1136-1140.https://doi.org/10.1016/j.jpedsurg.2021.03.04.

Gangopadhyay, A. N., & Pandey, V. (2015). Anorectal malformations. *Journal of Indian Association of Pediatric Surgeons*, *20*(1), 10-15. https://doi.org/10.4103/0971-9261.145438.

Georgeson, K. (2007). Laparoscopic-assisted anorectal pull-through. Seminars in pediatric surgery, 16(4),266-9. https://doi.org/10.1053/j.sempedsurg.2007.06.009.

Harris, K. T., & Wilcox, D. T. (2023). Management of the urological tract in children with anorectal malformations–a contemporary review. *Therapeutic Advances in Urology*, *15*, 17562872231161468. https://doi.org/10.1177/17562872231161468.

King, S. K., & Levitt, M. A. (2022). Advances in the Management of the Neonate Born with an Anorectal Malformation. *Clinics in perinatology*, *49*(4), 965-979. https://doi.org/10.1016/j.clp.2022.08.002.

Le Bayon, A., Carpentier, E., Boscq, M., Lardy, H., & Sirinelli, D. (2010). Imaging of anorectal malformations in the neonatal period. *Journal de radiologie*, *91*(4), 475-483. https://doi.org/10.1016/s0221-0363(10)70062-7.

Levitt, M. A., & Peña, A. (2007). Anorectal malformations. *Orphanet journal of rare diseases*, *2*(1), 33. https://doi.org/10.1186/1750-1172-2-33.

Li, L., Ren, X., Xiao, H., Wang, C., Xu, H., Ming, A., Wang, X., Li, Z., Diao, M., Cheng, W. (2020). Normal anorectal musculatures and changes in anorectal malformation. *Pediatric Surgery International*, *36*, 103-111.https://doi.org/10.1007/s00383-019-04583-1.

Mahmud, A., Khan, N., Islam, M., Islam, S., Bari, M., Das, S., Uddin, M.B., Kamal, N., Banu, N., Akhtaruzzaman, M. (2021). Anorectal Malformations and Associated Anomalies in Children. *Mymensingh Medical Journal: MMJ*, *30*(1), 62-68.

Miyake, Y., Lane, G. J., & Yamataka, A. (2022). Embryology and anatomy of anorectal malformations. Seminars in Pediatric Surgery,31(6):151226. https://doi.org/10.1016/j.sempedsurg.2022.151226.

Miyake, Y., Ochi, T., Yamashiro, Y., Seo, S., Miyano, G., Koga, H., Lane, G. J., Kuwatsur, R., Yamataka, A. (2022). Levator ani asymmetry and deviation in high-type anorectal malformation evaluated by magnetic resonance imaging. *Pediatric Surgery International*, *38*(5), 749-753. https://doii.org/10.1007/s00383-022-05104-3.

Pena, A. (1986). Posterior sagittal approach for the correction of anorectal malformations. *Advances in surgery (Chicago)*, *19*, 69-100.

Pena, A. (2005). Anorectal Malformations: Operative Pediatric Surgery Edited by: Ziegler, Azizkhan. *Gauderer & Weber. Boston: Appleton & Lange*.

Sharma, S., & Gupta, D. K. (2017). Diversities of H-type anorectal malformation: a systematic review on a rare variant of the Krickenbeck classification. *Pediatric Surgery International*, *33*, 3-13. https://doi.org/10.1007/s00383-016-3982-2.

Wood, R. J., & Levitt, M. A. (2018). Anorectal malformations. *Clinics in colon and rectal surgery*, *31*(02), 061-070. https://doi.org/10.1055/s-0037-1609020.

Yamataka, A., Lane, G. J., & Koga, H. (2013). Laparoscopy-assisted surgery for male imperforate anus with rectourethral fistula. *Pediatric Surgery International*, *29*, 1007-1011. https://doi.org/10.1007/s00383-013-3391-8.

Chapter 13

Physical Assessment of the Newborn

Aylin Kul Türköz, MD
Department of Pediatrics, Samsun Training and Research Hospital, Samsun, Turkey

Abstract

The neonatal period refers to the first 28 days of life after birth. The first 7 days of this period are called the "early neonatal period." The period from the 7th to the 28th day is known as the "late neonatal period."

The normal pregnancy duration is 37-42 weeks, or 259-293 days, averaging 280 days, starting from the first day of the last menstrual period. Newborns born within this period are referred to as "term" or "full-term" newborns. Those born before completing the 37th week or 259 days intrauterinally are called "preterm" or "premature" newborns, while those born after the 42nd week or 293 days are called "postterm" or "postmature" newborns.

Every newborn's first systemic examination should be conducted within the first hour after birth, following the necessary interventions for adaptation to extrauterine life, at the resuscitation and intervention table designated for the baby in the delivery room. The second examination should be performed within 24-72 hours after birth. Besides these routine checkups, any newborn presenting with complaints should undergo an examination similar to the second checkup.

Keywords: neonatal examination, newborn assessment, congenital anomalies, vital signs, physical findings

In: Current Approaches to Newborn Emergencies
Editors: Zuhal Keskin Sarılar and Serap Samut Bülbül
ISBN: 979-8-89530-999-5

Introduction

The neonatal period, encompassing the first 28 days of life, represents a critical window for the detection and management of life-threatening conditions and congenital anomalies. A comprehensive and systematic physical examination is essential for early diagnosis and timely intervention. This chapter outlines a detailed framework for neonatal examination, beginning with vital signs and anthropometric measurements and extending through a region-specific inspection including the head, neck, thorax, abdomen, genitalia, and extremities. Special attention is paid to dermatological manifestations, cranial morphology, and neurological reflexes, all of which can provide important clues to underlying pathologies. By integrating current guidelines and evidence-based practices, this guide aims to support healthcare providers in ensuring optimal neonatal care during this vulnerable period.

Neonatal Examination Guidelines

Newborns should undergo a detailed examination within the first 24 hours after birth. The examination should start from the least disturbing area and proceed to the more invasive regions.

Vital Signs

- *Temperature:* Usually measured axillary; if abnormal, rectal measurement is performed.
- *Respiration:* Normal respiratory rate is 40-60 breaths per minute.
- *Blood Pressure:* Varies with gestational age, postnatal age, and birth weight.
- *Heart Rate:* Normal heart rate for newborns is 100-180 beats per minute. In healthy infants, the heart rate increases with stimulation.
- *Pulse Oximetry:* Effective for screening congenital cyanotic heart conditions. Measurements above 95% from any extremity and a difference of less than 3% between the right hand and any foot are considered normal.

Head Circumference, Length, Weight, Chest, and Abdominal Measurements

- *Head Circumference:* Measured from the forehead, above the eyebrows, and across the occipital area. The normal range for term infants is 32-37 cm.
- *Length and Percentiles:* The normal length is 48-52 cm.
- *Weight and Percentiles:* Assessed as part of growth and development.
- *Chest Circumference:* Measured at the level of the nipples while the infant is lying on their back. Normal range is 30-35 cm.
- *Abdominal Circumference:* Measured at the level of the umbilicus; important for identifying abdominal distension.
- *Gestational Age and Birth Weight Classification:* Classified based on Ballard scoring into preterm, late preterm, and term. Birth weight is categorized into very low, low, or appropriate weight for gestational age.

General Appearance

The newborn's activity level, skin color, and the presence of congenital anomalies are evaluated. The infant's overall smell is also assessed.

Skin Examination

- Color:
  1. *Plethora:* Observed in polycythemic infants or those exposed to excessive oxygen. Hematocrit levels should be checked.
  2. *Jaundice:* Appears if bilirubin levels exceed 5 mg/dL. Onset within the first 24 hours suggests conditions like Rh incompatibility, TORCH infections, or sepsis.
  3. *Pallor:* May indicate anemia, congenital asphyxia, or PDA.
  4. *Hyperpigmentation:* Common in the scrotum, ear folds, nail beds, or labia.
  5. *Cyanosis:* Requires >3-4 mg/dL of desaturated hemoglobin. Can be central, peripheral, acrocyanosis, or perioral.
  6. *Bruising and Petechiae.*

7. *Harlequin Sign:* Transient vascular condition caused by hypothalamic immaturity.
8. *Cutis Marmorata:* Temporary marbling of the skin, may persist in Down syndrome or hypothyroidism.
9. *Lanugo:* Fine, soft hair covering the body.
10. *Vernix Caseosa:* Covers the body up to 38 weeks of gestation, with moisturizing properties.
11. *Dry Skin:* Flaking and peeling may indicate post-term maturity.

- Rashes:
  1. *Milia:* Very small sebaceous retention cysts found on the chin, nose, and cheeks. They are completely benign.
  2. *Sebaceous Hyperplasia:* Appears more yellowish, is known as neonatal miniature puberty, and is benign.
  3. *Erythema Toxicum:* Small, red patches with central yellow or white papules.
  4. *Candidiasis Rash:* Sharp-bordered, erythematous plaques, often found near diaper areas.
  5. *Transient Neonatal Pustular Melanosis:* Rashes begin in utero and can be found all over the body.
  6. *Infantile Seborrheic Dermatitis:* Found on the scalp, face, neck, and diaper area.
  7. *Neonatal Acne:* Comedones and papules on the cheeks, chin, and forehead.
  8. *Herpes Simplex:* Vesicular or pustular lesions.
  9. *Sucking Blisters*: Fluid-filled blisters on the hands and forearms, caused by the baby's sucking.

- Birthmarks (Nevi):
  1. *Nevus Simplex:* Macular lesions commonly seen on the occipital area, eyelids, and glabella; often resolves within a year.
  2. *Port-Wine Stain:* Non-blanching lesion; if located on the forehead or upper lip, Sturge-Weber syndrome should be ruled out.
  3. *Mongolian Spots:* Blue-gray spots on the sacral region; usually disappear by age four.
  4. *Cavernous Hemangioma:* Large, red, cyst-like lesions.

Head Examination

The shape and condition of the head should be evaluated. Mild molding of the cranial bones is normal for all newborns.

- *Macrocephaly:* Head circumference above the 90th percentile.
- *Microcephaly:* Head circumference below the 10th percentile.
- *Fontanelles:*
  - Anterior: Average size is 2.5 cm.
  - Posterior: Average size is 0.5 cm.
  - Bulging fontanelles can indicate increased intracranial pressure, meningitis, or hydrocephalus.
  - Sunken fontanelles may indicate dehydration.
- *Cranial Molding:* Temporary asymmetry of the skull due to the birthing process; resolves within one week.
- *Caput Succedaneum:* Swelling of the scalp that crosses suture lines; resolves in a few days.
- *Cephalohematoma:* Subperiosteal bleeding that does not cross suture lines. It may grow after birth and resolve within 2-3 weeks.
- *Subgaleal Hematoma:* A large collection of blood between the scalp and skull; crosses suture lines.
- *Intracranial Pressure Increase:* Associated with hydrocephalus, hypoxic-ischemic encephalopathy, or intracranial hemorrhage.
- *Craniosynostosis:* Premature closure of one or more sutures, leading to skull asymmetry.
- *Cranial Softness (Cranial Tabes):* Congenitally thin cranial bones, often near sutures.
- *Plagiocephaly:* Flattened, asymmetrical skull shape, common in preterm infants or those lying in the same position.
- *Brachycephaly:* Short and broad head due to early fusion of coronal sutures.
- *Dolichocephaly:* Long and narrow skull due to premature sagittal suture closure.
- *Acrania/Anencephaly:* Congenital absence or malformation of the brain and skull.

Neck Examination

The neck is inspected by stimulating the rooting reflex, which allows better assessment.

- *Short Neck:* May indicate syndromes like Turner, Noonan, or Klippel-Feil.
- *Webbed Neck:* Found in Turner or Noonan syndromes.
- *Brachial Cleft Cyst:* Firm, small cyst located anterior to the sternocleidomastoid muscle.
- *Cystic Hygroma:* Most common neck cyst; fluctuant and located near the clavicle.
- *Thyroid Enlargement (Goiter):* Assessed for any abnormal growth.
- *Thyroglossal Duct Cyst:* A midline cyst moving with swallowing.
- *Torticollis:* Shortening of the sternocleidomastoid muscle causing the head to tilt; corrected with physical therapy.

Facial Examination

The face is inspected for distinct anomalies:

- *Coarse Facial Features:* May indicate lysosomal storage disorders.
- *Hypertelorism:* Wide spacing between the eyes.
- *Low-Set Ears:* Often associated with syndromes.
- *Micrognathia:* Small lower jaw.
- *Facial Nerve Damage:* Includes asymmetric facial movements, drooping, or impaired crying.

Ears

Examined for structural abnormalities:

- *Low-Set Ears:* Associated with genetic syndromes.
- *Skin Tags:* Small growths near the ear.
- *Hair Growth:* Excessive hair on the ear.
- *Anotia:* Absence of the ear.

- *Microtia/Macrotia:* Abnormally small or large ears.

Eyes

Key eye findings include:

- *Leukocoria:* Loss of red reflex; white pupil appearance.
- *Congenital Cataracts:* Requires urgent referral; associated with galactosemia and Zellweger syndrome.
- *Glaucoma:* Presents with corneal opacity.
- *Retinoblastoma:* Emergency referral needed.
- *Coloboma:* Congenital defect of the eye structure.
- *Brushfield Spots:* Whitish spots on the iris seen in Down syndrome.
- *Subconjunctival Hemorrhage:* Common and benign.
- *Epicanthal Folds:* Skin folds near the inner corner of the eye.
- *Nystagmus and Strabismus:* Involuntary eye movement or misalignment.
- *Ptosis:* Drooping eyelids.

Nose

Newborns are obligate nasal breathers.

- *Bilateral Choanal Atresia:* Causes cyanosis and difficulty breathing.
- *Nasal Flaring:* Indicates respiratory distress.
- *Nasal Discharge or Septum Deviation:* Should be assessed.

Mouth

- *Cleft Lip/Palate:* Assessed for structural abnormalities.
- *Bifid Uvula:* Split uvula.
- *Epstein Pearls:* Keratin cysts on the gums or palate.
- *Ranula:* Mucus-filled cyst under the tongue.
- *Macroglossia:* Enlarged tongue.

- *Ankyloglossia:* Tight frenulum restricting tongue movement.
- *Micrognathia:* Small jaw, often positional.
- *Natal Teeth:* Rarely present at birth.

Chest

- *Retractions:* May indicate respiratory distress.
- *Stridor or Hoarseness:* Associated with upper airway obstruction.
- *Weak Cry:* Can indicate neurological issues.
- *Clavicle Fractures:* Common birth injury.
- *Chest Deformities:*
  - *Pectus Excavatum:* Sunken chest.
  - *Pectus Carinatum:* Protruding chest.
  - *Barrel Chest*: Rounded chest shape.
- *Newborn Breasts:*
  - Breast enlargement or discharge is normal.
  - *Polymastia or Polytelia:* Extra breasts or nipples.

Heart

- *Murmurs:* May suggest congenital heart defects like ASD, VSD, TOF, or PDA.

Abdomen

- *Abdominal Wall Defects:* Includes omphalocele or gastroschisis.
- *Organomegaly:* Enlarged organs.
- *Linea Nigra:* Dark line on the abdomen.
- *Diastasis Recti:* Separation of the abdominal muscles.
- *Scaphoid Abdomen*: Sunken abdominal appearance.

Umbilicus

Normally, the umbilical cord contains two arteries and one vein.

- *Single Umbilical Artery:* May indicate congenital anomalies.
- *Patent Urachus:* Urine leakage from the umbilicus.
- *Wharton's Jelly Cyst:* Benign cyst in the umbilical cord.

Genital Examination

- *Male Genitalia:*
  - Scrotal discoloration may indicate testicular torsion.
  - Meatus location should be assessed for epispadias or hypospadias.
  - Penile length should be at least 2 cm.
  - Cryptorchidism, hydrocele, or inguinal hernias are evaluated.

- *Female Genitalia:*
  - Clitoral size, vaginal tags, or discharge are assessed.

Anus and Rectum

- *Imperforate Anus:* Ruled out by inserting a probe 1 cm into the anus.
- *Meconium Passage*: Should occur within 48 hours of birth in term infants.

Extremities

- *Syndactyly:* Webbed fingers or toes.
- *Polydactyly:* Extra digits.
- *Brachydactyly:* Shortened digits.
- *Clubfoot:* Abnormal foot positioning.
- *Hypoplasia or Aplasia:* Underdeveloped or absent extremities.

Spine

- *Sacral Dimple:* Simple or coccygeal dimples are evaluated for spinal abnormalities.
- *Meningomyelocele:* A neural tube defect.

Nervous System

- *Movement Disorders:* Jitteriness, seizures, or irritability are assessed.
- *Hypotonia or Hypertonia:* Indicates abnormal muscle tone.
- *Primitive Reflexes:* Includes rooting, Moro, Babkin, glabella, and grasp reflexes.
- *Cranial Nerve Assessment:* Evaluated for eye movement, nystagmus, and pupillary reactions.
- *Peripheral Nerve Injuries:*
  - *Erb-Duchenne Paralysis:* Injury to cervical nerves C5-C6.
  - *Klumpke Paralysis:* Injury to C7-C8.
  - *Facial Nerve Palsy:* Asymmetry in facial expressions.

Conclusion

A meticulous and standardized approach to the neonatal examination is vital for the early identification of congenital anomalies and physiological irregularities. Recognition of normal versus pathological findings across different organ systems allows healthcare professionals to initiate appropriate diagnostic and therapeutic actions. The examination must be performed systematically, ideally within the first 24 hours and repeated within 72 hours post-delivery, to capture any delayed-onset conditions. Ensuring accuracy in this critical phase contributes significantly to improving neonatal outcomes and long-term child health.

References

De-Wahl Granelli, A., Wennergren, M., Sandberg, K., Mellander, M., Bejlum, C., Inganäs, L., Eriksson, M., Segerdahl, N., Agren, A., Ekman-Joelsson, B. M., Sunnegårdh, J.,

Verdicchio, M., & Östman-Smith, I. (2009). Impact of pulse oximetry screening on the detection of duct dependant congenital heart disease: A Swedish prospective screening study in 39,821 newborns. *BMJ, 338*, a303. https://doi.org/10.1136/bmj.a303.

Green, K., & Oddie, S. (2008). The value of the postnatal examination in improving child health. *Archives of Disease in Childhood - Fetal and Neonatal Edition, 93*(5), F389–F393. https://doi.org/10.1136/adc.2007.134833.

Health & Wellbeing Division. (2016). *Evidence review for the child health model* (Version 3). Scottish Government. https://www.gov.scot/publications/evidence-review-child-health-programme-model/

Kemper, A. R., Mahle, W. T., Martin, G. R., Cooley, W. C., Kumar, P., Morrow, R. W., Kelm, K., Pearson, G. D., Glidewell, J., Grosse, S.D., & Howell, R. R. (2011). Strategies for implementing screening for critical congenital heart disease. *Pediatrics, 128*(5), e1259–e1267. https://doi.org/10.1542/peds.2011-1317.

Royal College of Physicians in Ireland. (2017). *The impact of early childhood on future health: Position paper of the Faculty of Public Health Medicine*. https://rcpi-live-cdn.s3.amazonaws.com/wp-content/uploads/2021/04/Faculty-of-Public-Health-Medicine_Position-Paper_The-Impact-of-Early-Childhood-on-Future-Health.pdf.

National Institute for Health and Care Excellence. (2016). *Jaundice in newborn babies under 28 days* (NICE Guideline CG98). National Institute for Health and Care Excellence.

National Institute for Health and Clinical Excellence. (2006). *Postnatal care up to 8 weeks after birth* (NICE Guideline CG37). National Institute for Health and Clinical Excellence.

Russell, H., McDougall, V., & Dutton, G. (2011). Congenital cataract. *BMJ, 342*, d3075. https://doi.org/10.1136/bmj.d3075.

Shorter, D., Hong, T., & Osborn, D. A. (2011). Screening programmes for developmental dysplasia of the hip in newborn infants. *Cochrane Database of Systematic Reviews, 2011*(9), CD004595. https://doi.org/10.1002/14651858.CD004595.pub2.

World Health Organization. (2006). *WHO child growth standards: Length/height-for-age, weight-for-age, weight-for-length, weight-for-height and body mass index-for-age: Methods and development*. World Health Organization. ISBN: 9789241546935.

Chapter 14

Neonatal Resuscitation

Emre Sanrı*, MD
Department of Pediatrics, Samsun University Faculty of Medicine, Samsun, Turkey

Abstract

Neonatal resuscitation is a critical set of interventions designed to support oxygenation and perfusion of vital organs in the immediate postnatal period. Globally, neonatal mortality remains a major public health concern, with marked disparities between resource-poor and resource-rich settings. This chapter examines the physiological transitions of the neonatal circulatory and respiratory systems, emphasizing the importance of understanding these mechanisms for effective resuscitation. High-risk deliveries, particularly those involving preterm infants, are highlighted as situations requiring advanced preparation and multidisciplinary intervention. This chapter aims to provide clinicians with a comprehensive framework for improving neonatal outcomes through the implementation of timely and effective resuscitation practices, supported by a thorough review of current evidence and international guidelines.

Keywords: neonatal resuscitation, high-risk deliveries, post-resuscitation care

---

* Corresponding Author's Email: emresanri@yahoo.com

In: Current Approaches to Newborn Emergencies
Editors: Zuhal Keskin Sarılar and Serap Samut Bülbül
ISBN: 979-8-89530-999-5

Introduction

Neonatal resuscitation is defined as the set of interventions performed with the objective of supporting the oxygenation and circulation of vital organs during the critical postpartum period. The neonatal period is one of the most vulnerable stages of life in terms of mortality and morbidity.

Globally, the annual rate of neonatal mortality is estimated to be 2.4 million. Approximately 47% of these deaths occur on the first day of life, with 75% occurring within the first week (Janet et al., 2018). The most common causes of these deaths are asphyxia at birth, infections, and complications of prematurity. Epidemiological data indicate that globally, approximately 23.4% of newborns do not initiate crying within the first minute after birth, and 17% of this group do not exhibit spontaneous respiration. Furthermore, it is estimated that 4.4% of these infants require advanced resuscitative interventions (Kc et al., 2021). In low- and middle-income countries, 98% of infant mortality is attributed to neonatal deaths. Conversely, in developed nations, the implementation of standard resuscitation protocols has resulted in a notable reduction in mortality rates (Shikuku et al., 2018).

Neonatal resuscitation confers dual benefits, namely the saving of lives and the preservation of the neurological and physical health of infants. The implementation of timely and appropriate interventions has been demonstrated to significantly reduce the risk of mortality while also contributing to the prevention of neurological injuries, such as hypoxic-ischemic encephalopathy (Fischer et al., 2019). Effective neonatal resuscitation is of paramount importance for improving long-term outcomes for these vulnerable infants, who are at an elevated risk of developmental delays, cognitive impairments, and other adverse health consequences if resuscitation is not provided promptly and correctly. Early and skilled resuscitation efforts can be a determining factor in whether an infant survives or dies, as well as in whether they have a healthy future or one marked by significant disabilities.

Study of the Circulatory and Respiratory Physiology of Neonates

The circulatory and respiratory systems of newborns undergo substantial physiological alterations during the transition from the intrauterine to the extrauterine environment. Following birth, the fetal blood circulation and gas exchange systems undergo a rapid reorganization. The transition of gas exchange from the fetal to the neonatal state is accompanied by a profound alteration in the circulatory and respiratory mechanisms, which require the simultaneous adaptation of the cardiovascular and respiratory systems (Hooper et al., 2018).

Cardiovascular Physiology

The fetal circulatory system depends on the placenta as the primary source of gas exchange and nutrient supply. Subsequently, following the birth process, the placental circulation is terminated, and the lungs become the primary site for gas exchange. The principal adaptations that occur during this transition are as follows:

1. *Closure of the ductus arteriosus:* The reduction in pulmonary vascular resistance and increase in oxygen levels that occur with the onset of birth serve as the impetus for the closure of the ductus arteriosus. This process allows for an increase in blood flow to the pulmonary circulation (Singh & Tissot, 2018).
2. *Closure of the foramen ovale:* After birth, the increased pressure in the left atrium exceeds that in the right atrium, resulting in the closure of the foramen ovale. This change facilitates the passage of oxygenated blood from the right ventricle to the lungs (Frugoni & Downey, 2018).
3. *Reduction in Pulmonary Vascular Resistance:* The high pulmonary vascular resistance present before birth rapidly decreases as the lungs expand and oxygen concentrations increase (Lakshminrusimha & Saugstad, 2016).

Respiratory Physiology

It is during the intrauterine period that the fetus lives with lungs filled with amniotic fluid and receives its oxygen requirements through the placenta. Subsequent to birth, it is essential that this fluid be removed and an air-filled lung environment be established.

1. *Ventilation of the lungs:* During birth, the removal of fetal lung fluid is achieved through the pressurized birth canal and the pulmonary lymphatic system. The first breath allows for lung ventilation (Hooper et al., 2018).
2. *Functional residual capacity:* Newborn babies have a low functional residual capacity in their lungs. This condition renders them vulnerable to rapid depletion of oxygen reserves and desaturation (Neumann & von Ungern-Sternberg, 2014).
3. *Respiratory mechanics:* Neonates have a highly compliant chest wall and low lung elasticity, a situation that requires the respiratory muscles to use more energy, and the risk of respiratory failure is particularly high in premature infants.

During the neonatal period, coordinated adaptation between the circulatory and respiratory systems is an essential imperative for survival. The increase in pulmonary circulation facilitates more efficient delivery of oxygenated blood to the body, while the remodeling of the cardiovascular system regulates systemic blood pressure and optimizes the distribution of oxygen to tissues (Vrancken et al., 2018).

High-Risk Deliveries and the Need for Resuscitation

Successful neonatal resuscitation is critically dependent on adequate preparation for the intervention. While the majority of newborns do not require any resuscitation during birth, approximately 10% need positive pressure ventilation, and 1% require advanced resuscitation (Kc et al., 2021).

Evaluations conducted prior to delivery are essential in determining the need for resuscitation. This approach facilitates the anticipation of potential complications that may arise during or immediately after birth. Specifically, it is imperative to address the following four key questions prior to delivery:

1. What is the gestational age?
2. What is the appearance of the amniotic fluid?
3. Are there any additional risk factors present?
4. Is there a plan for the timing of cord clamping?

Table 1. Equipment list required for neonatal resuscitation

Aspiration Equipment - Bulb syringe - Mechanical aspirator - Aspiration catheters (sizes 5F, 6F, 8F, 10F, 12F, or 14F) - 8F feeding tube and 20 mL syringe - Meconium aspiration device	Umbilical Venous Catheterization Equipment - Sterile gloves - Scissors or scalpel - Antiseptic solution (e.g., povidone-iodine) - Adhesive tape - Umbilical catheters (sizes 3.5F, 5F) - Three-way stopcock - Syringes (1 mL, 3 mL, 5 mL, 10 mL, 20 mL, 50 mL) - Needles (sizes 25G, 21G, 18G)
Bag-Mask Equipment - Masks for term and preterm neonates - Self-inflating or flow-inflating bag (250-270 mL) - Oxygen source - Gas source - Flowmeter - Oxygen-air blender and tubing - Pulse oximeter and probes - T-piece resuscitator	Medications - Epinephrine: 1:10,000 (0.1 mg/mL) in ampoules (1 mL, 0.5 mL, 0.25 mL diluted in sterile water) - Volume expanders: isotonic crystalloid (e.g., saline or Ringer's lactate, 100-250 mL) - Dextrose 10% (250 mL) - Normal saline for flushing - Sterile water
Intubation Equipment - Laryngoscope blades (size 0 for preterm, size 1 for term) - Spare bulbs and batteries for the laryngoscope - Endotracheal tubes (inner diameter 2.5 mm, 3.0 mm, 3.5 mm, 4.0 mm) - Stylet (optional) - Scissors - Adhesive tape or endotracheal tube holder - Alcohol swabs - CO_2 detector (if available) - Laryngeal mask - Orogastric tube (5F or 6F)	Other Equipment - Gloves, caps, and other personal protective equipment - Umbilical cord clamps - Radiant warmer - Firm, flat surface for resuscitation - Stopwatch (or chronometer) - Warm towels - Stethoscope (preferably neonatal-specific) - Adhesive tape - Cardiac monitor and electrodes (if available) - Intraosseous needles (optional)

Table 1. (Continued)

For Extremely Preterm Infants
- Large polyethylene plastic bag
- Nasal CPAP cannulas, ventilator set
- Transport incubator capable of maintaining the baby's body temperature (preferably with ventilator support)
- Laryngoscope blade size 00

Answering these questions helps to identify risk factors early and formulate an appropriate birth plan. High-risk pregnancies in particular benefit greatly from the establishment of a specialized perinatal team. This multidisciplinary team of pediatricians and obstetricians works together to develop and implement tailored intervention strategies that can significantly reduce neonatal morbidity and mortality.

Equally important is the availability of resuscitation equipment. All necessary equipment, as outlined in standardized checklists (Table 1), should be readily available and in optimal working condition. Regular routine checks are essential to confirm functionality and address any deficiencies prior to delivery (Oygür et al., 2018).

Premature Infants and Resuscitation Requirement

Premature infants have been shown to require resuscitation at a higher rate in the postnatal period when compared to term infants. They are also more prone to the development of complications. In particular, very low birth weight (VLBW) babies with a birth weight of less than 1000 grams carry serious health risks (Bajaj et al., 2018). In instances where premature birth is anticipated, perinatal transfer of the mother and delivery of the infant in a tertiary neonatal intensive care center has been demonstrated to result in a substantial reduction in both mortality and morbidity rates (Katheria et al., 2016).

Factors Increasing the Need for Resuscitation in Premature Babies

- *Risk of Hypothermia:* The absence of subcutaneous adipose tissue, thin skin structure, and a large surface-to-volume ratio in premature infants results in rapid heat loss after birth. Complications related to hypothermia have been shown to increase the mortality rate in premature infants (De Almeida et al., 2014). Therefore, it is recommended to maintain the delivery room temperature above 25°C, pre-activate radiant heaters, and apply protective methods such as polythene bags.

- *Ventilation Problems:* In premature infants, inadequate lung maturation, lack of surfactant, and weak respiratory muscles result in difficulties in providing adequate ventilation. Approaches such as nasal continuous positive airway pressure (CPAP) and exogenous surfactant therapy, when necessary, may improve the respiratory stability of these infants (Tana et al., 2023).
- *Susceptibility to Infections:* It is well established that premature babies are susceptible to infection during both the antenatal and postnatal periods, due to their underdeveloped immune systems. Maternal infections have been shown to be a contributing factor to preterm delivery, which in turn can result in an increased risk of infectious complications after birth (El-Naggar & McNamara, 2012).
- *Organ Damage and Complications:* Inadequate tissue and vascular maturation in premature infants have been demonstrated to result in the development of serious complications. These include, but are not limited to, intracranial hemorrhage, bronchopulmonary dysplasia (BPD), and retinopathy of prematurity (Lakshminrusimha et al., 2020).

Thermoregulation and Heat Management in Premature Infants

Temperature control of preterm infants should be optimized by measures in the delivery room:

- *Room temperature:* Should be set above 25°C.
- *Radiant heaters:* Switch on before birth to provide warmth.
- *Protective equipment:* Babies should be wrapped in polyethylene plastic covers, and hats should be placed on their heads.
- *Warming beds:* Can be used for babies <32 weeks. The baby's temperature can be maintained by activating the chemical gel (De Almeida et al., 2014).

Healthcare Team and Equipment in Resuscitation of Premature Infants

The resuscitation of premature infants requires a multidisciplinary approach. It is important to have the following equipment available:

- Positive Pressure Ventilation (PPV) equipment.
- Materials required for nasal CPAP and exogenous surfactant therapy.
- Heated transport incubators (Schilleman et al., 2012).

During labor, at least two certified health care professionals who can manage resuscitation procedures must be present. For premature babies born at less than 30 weeks' gestation, equipment should be fully prepared for the possibility of ventilation and surfactant therapy (Bajaj et al., 2018).

General Approach to Neonatal Resuscitation

Neonatal resuscitation is a process that is carried out in accordance with guidelines established by international organizations. These guidelines are published by entities such as the American Heart Association (AHA), the American Academy of Pediatrics (AAP), the International Liaison Committee on Resuscitation (ILCOR), and the European Resuscitation Council (ERC) (Figure 1) (Wyllie et al., 2015). The implementation of these guidelines is based on a standardized algorithm, ensuring a consistent and systematic approach to resuscitation procedures (Wyckoff et al., 2020). The clinical condition of the newborn is assessed in all these guidelines by answering the following three questions:

- Is the infant full-term?
- Does the infant exhibit a good tone?
- Does the infant exhibit either crying or breathing?

In the event that the response to all three questions is affirmative, it is assumed that resuscitation is not required. In such cases, the infant is not separated from the mother, is dried with a dry cloth, and routine neonatal care is applied by ensuring skin contact. The Apgar score is not used to determine the need for resuscitation; however, it may provide information about the general condition of the newborn and its response to resuscitation (Ramaswamy et al., 2021).

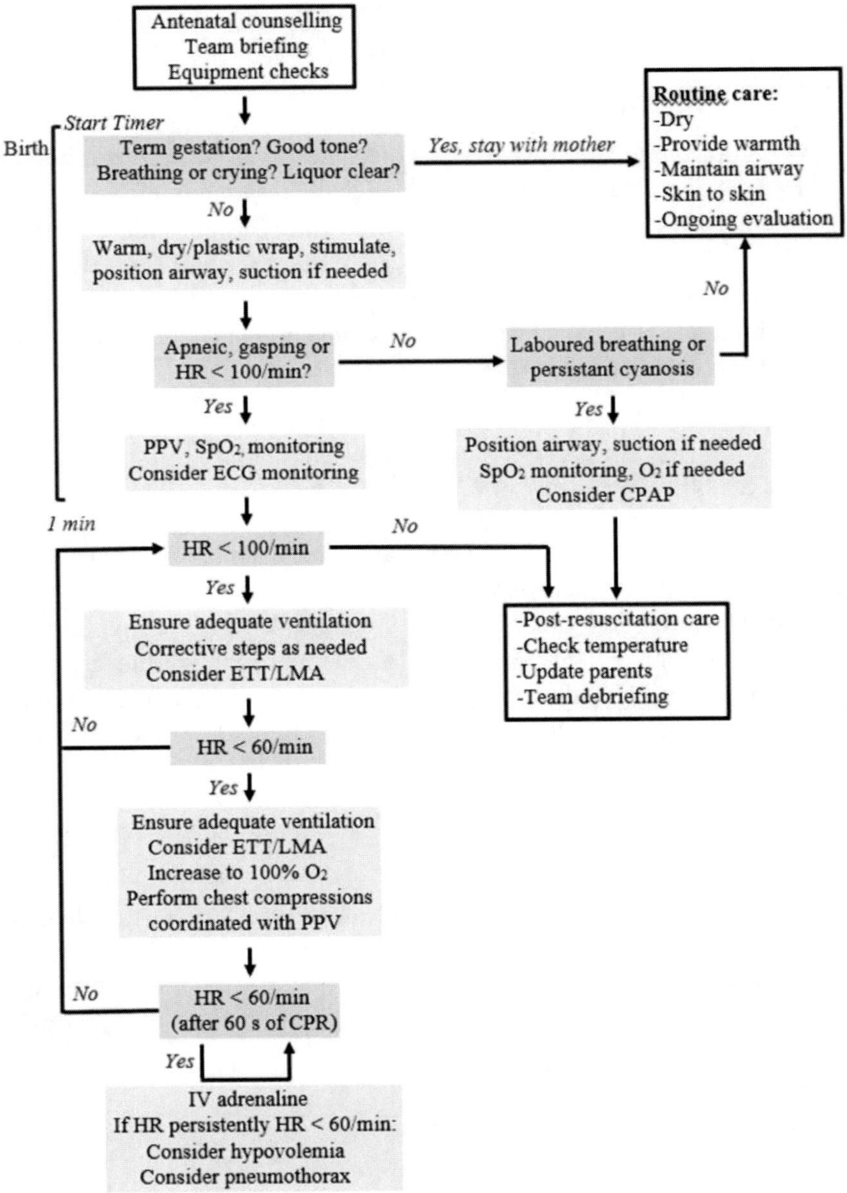

Figure 1. Flowchart depicting the steps of resuscitation.

Initial Steps and Evaluation

The initial steps in the assessment of a newborn's respiratory status include warming, drying, positioning, and clearing secretions. Subsequent to these preparatory measures, the respiratory effort and heart rate of the newborn are evaluated.

- *Respiration:* Chest movements are expected to be adequate, and the baby is expected to demonstrate effective respiratory effort.
- *Heart Rate (HR):* A heart rate above 100 beats per minute (bpm) is considered sufficient. HR should be measured by precordial auscultation or an electrocardiogram (ECG). Pulse oximetry can be used to assess oxygenation, but it is not sufficient alone to determine heart rate (Thakre, 2021).

Late Cord Clamping and Meconium Staining

According to the 2020 ILCOR and ERC guidelines, the recommendation for uncomplicated preterm and term deliveries is for late cord clamping (30-60 seconds). However, this procedure is contraindicated in cases of impaired placental circulation or depressed infants. Furthermore, intrapartum aspiration is not recommended in the presence of meconium-stained amniotic fluid. (Soraisham & Srivastava, 2021).

Tactile Stimulation

Tactile stimulation has been demonstrated to be an efficacious method for stimulating neonatal respiration. The stimulus should be applied for no longer than 30 seconds. It is preferable to gently flick the sole of the infant's foot or pat the back. Harsh interventions should be avoided (Weiner & Zaichkin, 2022).

Stabilization and Monitoring

Subsequent to the completion of the preliminary steps, infants exhibiting adequate tone and respiration may be reunited with their mothers. However, infants demonstrating inadequate respiratory effort or heart rate should undergo stabilization through the implementation of advanced resuscitation procedures. During the stabilization phase, the following measures are implemented:

- Maintenance of the infant's temperature
- Attainment of the desired respiratory and oxygenation targets
- Monitoring of cardiac activity (Wyckoff et al., 2020).

Respiratory Distress and Bradycardia (<100 bpm) in Neonates at Birth

Apnea, sigh-like breathing, and a heart rate (HR) below 100/min during labor are among the conditions requiring urgent intervention in neonatal resuscitation. The management of these conditions necessitates the prompt commencement of ventilation and circulatory support. Positive pressure ventilation (PPV) represents the primary intervention for respiratory support in newborns with these conditions (Wyckoff et al., 2020).

Positive-pressure ventilation should be administered at a rate of 40 to 60 breaths per minute. The newborn's heart rate and oxygen saturation levels should be continuously monitored using pulse oximetry. Electrocardiogram monitoring enables a more accurate and rapid assessment of heart rate (Berisha et al., 2021).

In the event that the rib cage does not rise, ventilation should be transitioned to a corrective approach, which involves the following steps:

- A thorough examination should be conducted to ascertain the proper fit of the mask to the face, ensuring the availability of appropriate-size masks for both term and preterm infants.
- The head of the newborn should be positioned in a neutral or slightly extended position.
- Mouth and nose aspiration should be performed to remove secretions.
- Airway patency should be facilitated by lifting the chin.

- The pressure can be gradually increased by continuing positive pressure breathing (5-10 cm H2O increments, up to a maximum of 40 cm H2O). Alternative airway methods (endotracheal intubation or laryngeal mask) should be considered (Wyckoff et al., 2020).

Devices and Techniques Used for Ventilation

The three main devices utilized in positive-pressure ventilation applications are

- *Self-Inflating Balloon:* This device does not rely on an external gas source and is suitable for straightforward ventilation needs. By adding a reservoir, it can deliver 100% oxygen concentration.
- *Anesthesia Balloon:* This device provides both positive inspiratory pressure and positive end-expiratory pressure.
- *T-piece Resuscitator:* This device allows for more precise pressure settings and is generally the preferred choice for infants requiring positive end-expiratory pressure or continuous positive airway pressure (Ersdal et al., 2012).

Pulse Oximetry and Target Oxygen Saturation Values

In the context of neonatal resuscitation, the pulse oximeter should be positioned in the following manner: preductally on the right wrist or medial palm. The recommended oxygen saturation targets are as follows:

- 1st minute: 60%-65%
- 2nd minute: 65%-70%
- 3rd minute: 70%-75%
- 4th minute: 75%-80%
- 5th minute: 80%-85%
- 10th minute: 85%-95% (Kapadia et al., 2020).

It is imperative to adjust oxygen concentration with the objective of averting hypoxemia and hyperoxia:

- ≥35 weeks gestation: Begin resuscitation with 21% oxygen
- <35 weeks gestation: Use 21-30% oxygen (Logan et al., 2014).

Evaluation and Management of Heart Rate

In the event that heart rate variability increases following ventilatory corrective measures, positive-pressure ventilation is to be continued, with heart rate monitoring occurring at 15-second intervals. At the conclusion of the 30-second interval, if the heart rate is ≥100 beats per minute and there is spontaneous effective respiration, positive-pressure ventilation is to be discontinued, and free breathing is to be initiated. Oxygen support is to be adjusted to the target oxygen saturation. In instances where the heart rate fails to attain the desired thresholds or exhibits persistent variability despite the implementation of corrective measures, further interventions must be executed to address the underlying issues and stabilize the newborn's condition.

- If the heart rate is <100 bpm, positive-pressure ventilation is continued, and the patient's chest is lifted or not. If there is no chest movement, ventilation correction steps are applied. If necessary, intubation or laryngeal mask application is initiated.
- If the heart rate is <60 bpm, vascular access is established, and intravenous adrenaline is administered. The possibility of hypovolemia and pneumothorax should also be considered (Wyckoff, 2010).

Patients exhibiting persistent respiratory distress or persistent cyanosis, along with a heart rate ≥100 beats per minute (bpm) in the initial postnatal minute, necessitate meticulous monitoring. The following protocol is recommended for such patients:

- Position the patient in a manner that maximizes airway patency.
- Implement pulse oximetry monitoring to ensure optimal oxygen saturation levels.
- Administer supplemental oxygen to achieve the targeted oxygen saturation level.
- Initiate continuous positive airway pressure (CPAP) ventilation to support the respiratory function (Nesterenko et al., 2023).

Alternative Airways: Endotracheal Tube and Laryngeal Mask

Endotracheal Intubation

Endotracheal intubation is a critical procedure in neonatal resuscitation, providing a safe and effective airway to ensure adequate ventilation and oxygenation in situations where non-invasive methods are inadequate. Endotracheal intubation is indicated in the following scenarios:

- Inadequate or protracted positive pressure ventilation (PPV): When adequate ventilation cannot be achieved with a mask.
- Need for chest compressions: During advanced neonatal resuscitation, secure airway control is paramount.
- Special clinical situations: Such as congenital diaphragmatic hernia, extremely low birth weight (<1000 g), or elective intubation for surfactant administration (Wyckoff et al., 2020).

Endotracheal intubation is a procedure that requires a minimum of two trained personnel to ensure its successful completion. One individual is responsible for performing the procedure, while another provides assistance and monitors the neonate. It is imperative that the procedure be completed within 30 seconds to minimize the risk of hypoxia. During the attempt, free-flow oxygen should be provided to the patient. All necessary equipment, including appropriately sized tubes, must be prepared in advance to ensure a seamless and efficient process (Wyllie et al., 2015).

Equipment and Sizing

- *Laryngoscope blades:* Laryngoscopes are classified into three sizes, designated as size 0 for preterm neonates, size 1 for term neonates, and size 00 for extremely preterm infants.
- *Endotracheal tubes:* Cuffed tubes are generally avoided in neonates. Uncuffed tubes are sized according to gestational age and weight (Table 2) (Oygür et al., 2018).

Table 2. Appropriate ETT sizes based on birth weight and gestational age

Tube Size (Inner Diameter, mm)	Weight (g)	Gestational Age (weeks)
2.5	Less than 1000 g	Below 28 weeks
3.0	1000–2000 g	28–34 weeks
3.5	2000–3000 g	34–38 weeks
3.5–4.0	Over 3000 g	Above 38 weeks
ETT: Endotracheal Tube		

1. *Positioning:* The neonate should be placed in a supine position with the neck slightly extended to align the oral, pharyngeal, and tracheal axes.
2. *Intubation Technique:* The laryngoscope is to be held in the left hand, with the blade inserted along the right side of the mouth, in order to sweep the tongue to the left. The blade is then to be advanced to the vallecula in order to visualize the vocal cords. The endotracheal tube is then to be inserted through the cords until the vocal cord marker aligns with the cords.
3. *Confirmation of Tube Placement:* It is imperative to assess for rapid improvement in heart rate post-intubation. Bilateral breath sounds should be auscultated, and symmetrical chest rise should be observed. The position must be confirmed using end-tidal CO_2 detection or a chest X-ray.

Table 3. Endotracheal tube insertion depth for orotracheal intubation

Gestational Age (weeks)	Endotracheal Tube Insertion Depth from Lip Line (cm)	Infant Weight (g)
23–24	5.5	500–600
25–26	6.0	700–800
27–29	6.5	900–1000
30–32	7.0	1000–1400
33–34	7.5	1500–1800
35–37	8.0	1900–2400
38–40	8.5	2500–3100
41–43	9.0	3200–4200

Fixation: The tube is secured at the upper lip using appropriate depth estimation methods, such as measuring the length from the nose to the tragus, with an additional 1 centimeter, or by utilizing gestational age-based depth charts (Table 3) (Madar et al., 2021).

In the event that visualization of the vocal cords has not been achieved, the following measures should be taken:

- In the case that the blade has not been advanced sufficiently, it is necessary to gradually advance the blade until the epiglottis becomes visible.
- If the blade has been advanced too far, it is necessary to withdraw it gently until the epiglottis reappears.
- If the blade is misaligned, it is necessary to center the blade and adjust its position based on anatomical landmarks.

Laryngeal Mask

The laryngeal mask airway (LMA) is indicated for use in cases where face mask ventilation or endotracheal intubation has been unsuccessful or deemed unfeasible. Its efficacy in facilitating ventilation in neonates, both term and preterm, with a weight of at least 1500 g (equivalent to 34 weeks of gestation), has been well-documented, contingent upon the appropriate sizing of the LMA for the infant's laryngeal inlet (Monsieurs et al., 2015). The LMA is a device designed to create a seal around the glottis. It consists of a soft silicone cuff that is designed to fit over the glottis. The device is inserted into position by sliding it along the hard palate with the index finger, and no additional instruments are required. Once in place, the cuff is inflated to create a seal against the hypopharynx. The LMA features a standard 15-mm connector that is compatible with positive pressure ventilation (PPV) devices.

Chest Compressions

In cases where the heart rate remains below 60 beats per minute (bpm) despite the administration of effective positive pressure ventilation (PPV), the initiation of chest compressions in conjunction with PPV is recommended. The recommended location for compressions is the lower third of the sternum, just below the line passing through the nipple level. Among the available techniques, the two-thumb technique is preferred over the two-finger technique for delivering chest compressions, as it provides more effective and consistent pressure (Oygür et al., 2018). During chest compressions, the depth of compression should result in a decrease of the anterior-posterior diameter of the chest by approximately one-third. Subsequent to each compression, pressure is released to allow the heart to refill. It is imperative to avoid direct pressure on the xiphoid process, as it may result in hepatic injury.

In the context of neonatal resuscitation, chest compressions are invariably accompanied by positive pressure ventilation (PPV), with a ratio of three compressions to one ventilation maintained (90 compressions and 30 ventilations per minute). Subsequent to the initiation of compressions, the oxygen concentration is to be augmented to 100%. Following the restoration of a satisfactory heart rate and the cessation of compressions, the oxygen concentration should undergo a gradual reduction, contingent upon the targeted SpO_2.

A brief pause in compressions, lasting approximately 60 seconds, is recommended to allow reassessment of heart rate. This interval facilitates evaluation using various methods such as electrocardiogram (ECG) monitoring, auscultation, or pulse oximetry, each with its inherent limitations.

- *Auscultation:* May prolong the pause in compressions during resuscitation.
- *Pulse oximetry:* May fail to detect the pulse accurately if circulation is severely compromised.
- *ECG monitoring:* Provides real-time electrical activity and reduces pause durations, but it may still show electrical activity (pulseless electrical activity) in the absence of effective cardiac output.

The performance of chest compressions is discontinued once the heart rate reaches a minimum of 60 beats per minute. Positive pressure ventilation (PPV) is continued at a rate of 40 to 60 breaths per minute as required. (Foglia et al., 2019).

Medications Used in Neonatal Resuscitation

Although the majority of newborns requiring resuscitation exhibit a positive response to adequate ventilation and chest compressions, a small subset (approximately 1-3 per 1,000 term and late preterm births) may require pharmacological intervention when the heart rate (HR) remains below 60 beats per minute (bpm). In such cases, inadequate coronary perfusion and insufficient oxygen delivery result in weak cardiac contractions, necessitating the administration of pharmacological agents such as epinephrine (Zaichkin et al., 2016).

Epinephrine

Epinephrine continues to be the drug most frequently recommended for neonatal resuscitation. Its mechanism of action involves the stimulation of alpha-adrenergic receptors, leading to improved systemic vascular resistance, and beta-adrenergic receptors, resulting in increased cardiac output and heart rate. Despite its extensive utilization, there is a paucity of evidence from prospective, placebo-controlled studies conducted in neonatal populations (Perlman et al., 2010).

Indications for Epinephrine

- HR remains <60 bpm after at least 30 seconds of effective positive-pressure ventilation (PPV) and
- 60 seconds of chest compressions combined with 100% oxygen.

Dosage and Administration

- *Concentration:* 1:10,000 (0.1 mg/mL)
- *Intravenous (IV) or Intraosseous (IO):* 0.01–0.03 mg/kg (equivalent to 0.1–0.3 mL/kg).
- *Endotracheal (ET):* If vascular access is not established, a higher dose of 0.05–0.1 mg/kg (0.5–1 mL/kg) is recommended.

- Repeat every 3-5 minutes if the HR remains below 60 bpm, ensuring that prior resuscitation steps have been correctly implemented (Wyckoff et al., 2015).

Volume Expanders

In instances where suspicion of hypovolemia arises, the presence of signs such as pale skin, prolonged capillary refill time, and weak pulses is indicative of the condition. In such cases, the utilization of volume expanders is recommended, particularly in instances where there is a documented history of antepartum or intrapartum blood loss (Lee et al., 2019).

1. *Isotonic Crystalloid Solution (0.9% Sodium Chloride):* The recommended dosage is 10 milliliters per kilogram of body weight, administered over a period of 5–10 minutes.
2. *Ringer Lactate:* Alternative crystalloid solution.
3. *O-negative Packed Red Blood Cells (PRBCs):* Indicated in cases of documented or suspected severe blood loss or anemia.

Medications Not Routinely Recommended

1. *Naloxone:* In the domain of neonatal resuscitation, the utilization of naloxone, a narcotic antagonist, has been advised to be avoided in recommended practices. While maternal opioid exposure has been observed to result in neonatal respiratory depression, the prevailing treatment approach entails the provision of adequate ventilation and oxygenation. The safety, efficacy, and dosing of naloxone for newborns remain subjects of ongoing research and clinical investigation.
2. *Sodium Bicarbonate:* Sodium bicarbonate has not been widely adopted as a standard treatment in neonatal resuscitation. Although its potential benefits in addressing metabolic acidosis are acknowledged, concerns regarding its safety persist. Administration of sodium bicarbonate can lead to adverse effects, including impaired cardiac and cerebral function (Kattwinkel et al., 2010).

Rapid Vascular Access During Neonatal Resuscitation

In the context of neonatal resuscitation, the establishment of expeditious and dependable vascular access is paramount for the administration of emergency medications and volume expanders. The umbilical vein is the most efficacious and readily accessible route for intravenous (IV) drug delivery in newborns, particularly during resuscitation.

Umbilical Venous Catheterization

The umbilical vein offers a direct conduit to the central circulation, thereby establishing itself as the optimal approach for vascular access in neonates necessitating prompt pharmacological intervention (Aziz et al., 2020).

1. *Preparation:* The resuscitation team is responsible for the distribution of tasks, ensuring the maintenance of positive pressure ventilation (PPV) and chest compressions. Concurrently, another team member prepares for catheter insertion under aseptic conditions.
2. *Catheter Placement:* The use of a sterile umbilical venous catheter (UVC) is initiated by gentle insertion into the umbilical vein, which is readily identifiable at the base of the umbilical stump. The catheter should be advanced approximately 2-4 centimeters in term infants (less in preterm infants), stopping at the point where blood is first aspirated to confirm correct positioning (Katheria et al., 2016).
3. *Stabilization and Drug Administration*: Once the catheter is correctly positioned, it must be stabilized by holding it firmly in place to prevent dislodgement. A three-way stopcock is attached to the device to ensure precise and controlled administration of pharmaceutical agents. After administration of drugs (e.g., epinephrine or volume expanders), the catheter is flushed with 0.5-1 mL of normal saline (0.9% NaCl) to ensure effective drug entry into the systemic circulation (Wyckoff et al., 2015).

Alternative Routes for Vascular Access

In cases where umbilical venous access is not immediately feasible, alternative vascular access routes must be considered to ensure timely administration of life-saving drugs and fluids.

1. *Intraosseous Access:* The intraosseous route is a highly effective alternative, particularly when peripheral venous access cannot be established. It allows rapid and reliable administration of drugs such as epinephrine and volume expanders. Studies have shown that intraosseous access can be established more quickly than umbilical venous catheterization and is a viable option in emergencies (Wagner et al., 2018). It has been widely used in neonates during resuscitation and is supported as a bridging technique until more definitive vascular access can be obtained (Scrivens et al., 2019).
2. *Peripheral Venous Access:* Access to peripheral veins, such as those in the hands, feet, or scalp, remains an option. However, this method can be time-consuming and requires considerable skill, particularly in neonates with small and fragile veins. The median time to insert a peripheral venous access is approximately 4-5 minutes under optimal conditions (Wagner et al., 2018).

Resuscitation Failure in Neonates

In exceptional circumstances, neonates do not respond to resuscitation efforts. In such cases, the resuscitation team has an obligation to ensure that all phases of neonatal resuscitation have been carried out in a meticulous and comprehensive manner. Identifying the underlying cause of resuscitation failure is of paramount importance as it facilitates the subsequent management and decision-making process (Weiner & Zaichkin, 2022). Potential causes of resuscitation failure:

- *Failure to Respond to Positive Pressure Ventilation (PPV)*
  - *Mechanical Obstruction Causes:* Meconium aspiration, mucus plugging, choanal atresia, pharyngeal malformations (e.g., Pierre-Robin sequence), laryngeal webs (Saugstad et al., 2012).

   - *Inadequate Pulmonary Function Causes:* Pneumothorax, pleural effusion, congenital diaphragmatic hernia, pulmonary hypoplasia, congenital pneumonia, and surfactant deficiency (hyaline membrane disease) (Sweet et al., 2019).
- *Persistent Cyanosis*
   - *Congenital Heart Disease (CHD):* Critical CHDs, such as transposition of the great arteries, may present as profound cyanosis unresponsive to oxygen and ventilation.
- *Persistent Bradycardia*
   - *Cardiac Causes:* Congenital heart block is a notable cause of unresponsive bradycardia, often associated with maternal autoimmune disease (anti-Ro/SSA antibodies) (Brucato et al., 2010).
- *Apnea*
   - *Neurological Causes:* Hypoxic-ischemic encephalopathy (HIE), congenital neuromuscular disorders, or central nervous system injury. Maternal opioid use or sedative medications during labor may also lead to respiratory depression (Wyckoff et al., 2015).

When to Discontinue Resuscitation

Resuscitation efforts may be stopped if the newborn shows no signs of response after 10 minutes of active intervention, including an Apgar score of 0, no detectable heart rate, or no respiratory effort. However, this recommendation is not universally applicable and should be adapted to the specific circumstances and condition of the newborn at the time. Clinical judgment and consideration of the individual case are crucial in making this decision (Madar et al., 2021).

Post-Resuscitation Care

Neonates requiring resuscitation are at increased risk of multiple organ dysfunction and long-term complications due to hypoxia, acidosis, and other resuscitation-related factors. Managing these risks requires a holistic approach that integrates vigilant monitoring, immediate therapeutic intervention, and ongoing specialized care. This comprehensive strategy not only reduces the potential for further complications but also increases the likelihood of improved neonatal outcomes. To implement this approach effectively, attention must be paid to monitoring and assessment, immediate management, and ongoing care (Ghosh et al., 2017).

Monitoring and assessment are essential to assess the condition of the newborn after resuscitation. Apgar scores should be recorded every five minutes up to 20 minutes if the score remains below 7 at the five-minute mark. In addition, blood gas analysis, including pH and base deficit, can provide valuable information on the degree of hypoxia and acidosis.

Immediate management focuses on the prompt treatment of complications to stabilize the newborn. Pulmonary complications such as persistent pulmonary hypertension or pneumonia must be treated immediately. Intravenous glucose infusion should be started to prevent hypoglycemia. Close monitoring is also necessary to detect and treat seizures, hypotension, fluid-electrolyte imbalances, and temperature instability.

Prolonged care requires neonates who undergo extensive resuscitation to be admitted to a neonatal intensive care unit (NICU) for continuous monitoring of vital signs, including heart rate, blood pressure, and oxygen saturation. In cases of hypoxic-ischemic encephalopathy, therapeutic hypothermia may be indicated to minimize brain injury and improve neurological outcomes (Ghosh et al., 2017).

Conclusion

Neonatal resuscitation is a critical life-saving intervention aimed at reducing neonatal morbidity and mortality. A comprehensive understanding of the basic physiological transitions from fetal to neonatal life is essential to effectively manage respiratory and circulatory challenges during this vulnerable period. The implementation of standardized resuscitation protocols, as outlined in international guidelines, has led to significant improvements in outcomes, particularly in resource-rich settings.

In the context of high-risk deliveries and preterm infants, timely preparation, the integration of a multidisciplinary team approach, and the accessibility of appropriate equipment are of paramount importance. Continued research and innovation in neonatal resuscitation techniques is essential to further improve survival and reduce long-term complications in this vulnerable population, and by addressing knowledge gaps and ensuring equitable access to care, significant progress can be made toward improved neonatal health outcomes worldwide.

References

Aziz, K., Lee, H. C., Escobedo, M. B., Hoover, A. V., Kamath-Rayne, B. D., Kapadia, V. S., Magid, D. J., Niermeyer, S., Schmölzer, G. M., Szyld, E., Weiner, G. M., Wyckoff, M. H., Yamada, N. K., & Zaichkin, J. (2020). Part 5: Neonatal Resuscitation: 2020 American Heart Association Guidelines for Cardiopulmonary Resuscitation and Emergency Cardiovascular Care. *Circulation*, *142*(16_suppl_2), S524-S550. https://doi.org/doi:10.1161/CIR.0000000000000902.

Bajaj, M., Natarajan, G., Shankaran, S., Wyckoff, M., Laptook, A. R., Bell, E. F., Stoll, B. J., Carlo, W. A., Vohr, B. R., & Saha, S. (2018). Delivery room resuscitation and short-term outcomes in moderately preterm infants. *The Journal of Pediatrics*, *195*, 33-38. e32.

Berisha, G., Boldingh, A., Blakstad, E., Rønnestad, A., & Solevåg, A. (2021). Management of the Unexpected Difficult Airway in Neonatal Resuscitation. *Frontiers in Pediatrics*, *9*. https://doi.org/10.3389/fped.2021.699159.

Brucato, A., Ramoni, V., Penco, S., Sala, E., Buyon, J., & Clancy, R. (2010). Passively acquired anti-SSA/Ro antibodies are required for congenital heart block following ovodonation but maternal genes are not. *Arthritis and rheumatism*, *62 10*, 3119-3121. https://doi.org/10.1002/art.27575.

De Almeida, M., Guinsburg, R., Sancho, G., Rosa, I., Lamy, Z., Martinez, F., Da Silva, R., Ferrari, L., De Souza Rugolo, L. M. S., Abdallah, V., & Silveira, R. (2014). Hypothermia and early neonatal mortality in preterm infants. *The Journal of Pediatrics*, *164 2*, 271-275. https://doi.org/10.1016/j.jpeds.2013.09.049.

El-Naggar, W., & McNamara, P. (2012). Delivery room resuscitation of preterm infants in Canada: current practice and views of neonatologists at level III centers. *Journal of Perinatology*, *32*, 491-497. https://doi.org/10.1038/jp.2011.128.

Ersdal, H., Mduma, E., Svensen, E., & Perlman, J. (2012). Early initiation of basic resuscitation interventions including face mask ventilation may reduce birth asphyxia related mortality in low-income countries: a prospective descriptive observational study. *Resuscitation*, *83 7*, 869-873. https://doi.org/10.1016/j.resuscitation.2011.12.011.

Fischer, N., Soraisham, A., Shah, P., Synnes, A., Rabi, Y., Singhal, N., Ting, J., Creighton, D., Dewey, D., Ballantyne, M., & Lodha, A. (2019). Extensive cardiopulmonary resuscitation of preterm neonates at birth and mortality and developmental outcomes. *Resuscitation*, *135*, 57-65. https://doi.org/10.1016/j.resuscitation.2019.01.003.

Foglia, E. E., Ades, A., Sawyer, T., Glass, K. M., Singh, N., Jung, P., Quek, B. H., Johnston, L. C., Barry, J., & Zenge, J. (2019). Neonatal intubation practice and outcomes: an international registry study. *Pediatrics*, *143*(1).

Frugoni, B., & Downey, L. (2018). Neonatal Physiology. *DeckerMed Anesthesiology*. https://doi.org/10.2310/anes.18007.

Ghosh, S., Tran, L., Shuster, J., & Zupanc, M. (2017). Therapeutic hypothermia for neonatal hypoxic ischemic encephalopathy is associated with short-term reduction of seizures after discharge from the neonatal intensive care unit. *Child's Nervous System*, *33*, 329-335. https://doi.org/10.1007/s00381-016-3321-x.

Hooper, S., Kitchen, M., Polglase, G., Roehr, C., & Pas, A. T. (2018). The physiology of neonatal resuscitation. *Current Opinion in Pediatrics*, *30*, 187. https://doi.org/10.1097/MOP.0000000000000590.

Janet, S., Carrara, V., Simpson, J., Thin, N., Say, W., Paw, N. T. M., Chotivanich, K., Turner, C., Crawley, J., & McGready, R. (2018). Early neonatal mortality and neurological outcomes of neonatal resuscitation in a resource-limited setting on the Thailand-Myanmar border: A descriptive study. *PLoS ONE, 13*. https://doi.org/10.1371/journal.pone.0190419.

Kapadia, V., Urlesberger, B., Soraisham, A., Liley, H., Schmölzer, G., Rabi, Y., Wyllie, J., & Wyckoff, M. (2020). Sustained Lung Inflations During Neonatal Resuscitation at Birth: A Meta-analysis. *Pediatrics*, *147*. https://doi.org/10.1542/peds.2020-021204.

Katheria, A., Rich, W., & Finer, N. (2016). Optimizing Care of the Preterm Infant Starting in the Delivery Room. *American Journal of Perinatology*, *33*, 297-304. https://doi.org/10.1055/s-0035-1570385.

Kattwinkel, J., Perlman, J. M., Aziz, K., Colby, C., Fairchild, K., Gallagher, J., Hazinski, M. F., Halamek, L. P., Kumar, P., Little, G., McGowan, J. E., Nightengale, B., Ramirez, M. M., Ringer, S., Simon, W. M., Weiner, G. M., Wyckoff, M., & Zaichkin, J. (2010). Neonatal resuscitation: 2010 American Heart Association Guidelines for Cardiopulmonary Resuscitation and Emergency Cardiovascular Care. *Pediatrics*, *126*(5), e1400-1413. https://doi.org/10.1542/peds.2010-2972E.

Kc, A., Peven, K., Ameen, S., Msemo, G., Basnet, O., Ruysen, H., Zaman, S. B., Mkony, M., Sunny, A., Rahman, Q., Shabani, J., Bastola, R., Assenga, E., Kc, N., Arifeen, E., Kija, E., Malla, H., Kong, S., Singhal, N., … Lawn, J. (2021). Neonatal resuscitation: EN-BIRTH multi-country validation study. *BMC Pregnancy and Childbirth*, *21*. https://doi.org/10.1186/s12884-020-03422-9.

Lakshminrusimha, S., Pediatrician In, C., & Davis, U. (2020). Neonatal Resuscitation. *Definitions*. https://doi.org/10.32388/4v6du9.

Lakshminrusimha, S., & Saugstad, O. (2016). The fetal circulation, pathophysiology of hypoxemic respiratory failure and pulmonary hypertension in neonates, and the role of oxygen therapy. *Journal of Perinatology*, *36*. https://doi.org/10.1038/jp.2016.43.

Lee, J. H., Kim, E. H., Jang, Y. E., Kim, H. S., & Kim, J. T. (2019). Fluid responsiveness in the pediatric population. *Korean J Anesthesiol*, *72*(5), 429-440. https://doi.org/10.4097/kja.19305.

Logan, J., Shepherd, E., & Tobias, J. (2014). Neonatal resuscitation: An update. *18*, 386-396. https://consensus.app/papers/neonatal-resuscitation-an-update-logan-shepherd/d59d5c9129ca561eac33e4ba397ca58e/.

Madar, J., Roehr, C. C., Ainsworth, S., Ersdal, H., Morley, C., Rüdiger, M., Skåre, C., Szczapa, T., Te Pas, A., Trevisanuto, D., Urlesberger, B., Wilkinson, D., & Wyllie, J. P. (2021). European Resuscitation Council Guidelines 2021: Newborn resuscitation and support of transition of infants at birth. *Resuscitation*, *161*, 291-326. https://doi.org/10.1016/j.resuscitation.2021.02.014.

Monsieurs, K. G., Nolan, J. P., Bossaert, L. L., Greif, R., Maconochie, I. K., Nikolaou, N. I., Perkins, G. D., Soar, J., Truhlář, A., & Wyllie, J. (2015). European resuscitation council guidelines for resuscitation 2015: section 1. Executive summary. *Resuscitation, 95*, 1-80.

Nesterenko, T., Pocevic, S., Elgendy, M., Mohamed, M., & Aly, H. (2023). Is it feasible to avoid suction before spontaneous breathing is established? *Journal of neonatal-perinatal medicine*. https://doi.org/10.3233/npm-230080.

Neumann, R. P., & von Ungern-Sternberg, B. S. (2014). The neonatal lung–physiology and ventilation. *Pediatric Anesthesia, 24*(1), 10-21.

Oygür, N., Önal, E. E., & Zenciroğlu, A. (2018). Türk Neonatoloji Derneği ulusal doğum salonu yönetimi rehberi. *Türk Pediatri Arşivi, 53*(1), 3-17.

Perlman, J. M., Wyllie, J., Kattwinkel, J., Atkins, D. L., Chameides, L., Goldsmith, J. P., Guinsburg, R., Hazinski, M. F., Morley, C., & Richmond, S. (2010). Part 11: neonatal resuscitation: 2010 international consensus on cardiopulmonary resuscitation and emergency cardiovascular care science with treatment recommendations. *Circulation, 122*(16_suppl_2), S516-S538.

Ramaswamy, V. V., Abiramalatha, T., Weiner, G., & Trevisanuto, D. (2021). A Comparative Evaluation And Appraisal Of 2020 American Heart Association And 2021 European Resuscitation Council Neonatal Resuscitation Guidelines. *Resuscitation*. https://doi.org/10.1016/j.resuscitation.2021.08.039.

Saugstad, O. D., Sejersted, Y., Solberg, R., Wollen, E. J., & Bjørås, M. (2012). Oxygenation of the newborn: a molecular approach. *Neonatology, 101*(4), 315-325.

Schilleman, K., Siew, M., Lopriore, E., Morley, C., Walther, F., & Pas, A. T. (2012). Auditing resuscitation of preterm infants at birth by recording video and physiological parameters. *Resuscitation, 83 9*, 1135-1139. https://doi.org/10.1016/j.resuscitation.2012.01.036.

Scrivens, A., Reynolds, P., Emery, F., Roberts, C., Polglase, G., Hooper, S., & Roehr, C. (2019). Use of Intraosseous Needles in Neonates: A Systematic Review. *Neonatology, 116*, 305-314. https://doi.org/10.1159/000502212.

Shikuku, D., Milimo, B., Ayebare, E., Gisore, P., & Nalwadda, G. (2018). Practice and outcomes of neonatal resuscitation for newborns with birth asphyxia at Kakamega County General Hospital, Kenya: a direct observation study. *BMC Pediatrics, 18*. https://doi.org/10.1186/s12887-018-1127-6.

Singh, Y., & Tissot, C. (2018). Echocardiographic Evaluation of Transitional Circulation for the Neonatologists. *Frontiers in Pediatrics, 6*. https://doi.org/10.3389/fped.2018.00140.

Soraisham, A., & Srivastava, A. (2021). Recent Update on Neonatal Resuscitation. *Indian Journal of Pediatrics*. https://doi.org/10.1007/s12098-021-03796-4.

Sweet, D. G., Carnielli, V., Greisen, G., Hallman, M., Ozek, E., Te Pas, A., Plavka, R., Roehr, C. C., Saugstad, O. D., & Simeoni, U. (2019). European consensus guidelines on the management of respiratory distress syndrome–2019 update. *Neonatology, 115*(4), 432-450.

Tana, M., Tirone, C., Aurilia, C., Lio, A., Paladini, A., Fattore, S., Esposito, A., De Tomaso, D., & Vento, G. (2023). Respiratory Management of the Preterm Infant: Supporting

Evidence-Based Practice at the Bedside. *Children, 10.* https://doi.org/10.3390/children10030535.

Thakre, R. (2021). Highlights of Newborn Resuscitation Science, 2020. *Journal of Neonatology, 35*, 24-28. https://doi.org/10.1177/09732179211005998.

Vrancken, S., Van Heijst, A., & De Boode, W. (2018). Neonatal Hemodynamics: From Developmental Physiology to Comprehensive Monitoring. *Frontiers in Pediatrics, 6.* https://doi.org/10.3389/fped.2018.00087.

Wagner, M., Olischar, M., O'Reilly, M., Goeral, K., Berger, A., Cheung, P., & Schmölzer, G. (2018). Review of Routes to Administer Medication During Prolonged Neonatal Resuscitation. *Pediatric Critical Care Medicine, 19*, 332. https://doi.org/10.1097/PCC.0000000000001493.

Weiner, G., & Zaichkin, J. (2022). Updates for the Neonatal Resuscitation Program and Resuscitation Guidelines. *Neoreviews, 23 4.* https://doi.org/10.1542/neo.23-4-e238.

Wyckoff, M. (2010). Neonatal Cardiopulmonary Resuscitation: Critical Hemodynamics. *Neoreviews, 11.* https://doi.org/10.1542/NEO.11-3-E123.

Wyckoff, M., Wyllie, J., Aziz, K., De Almeida, M., Fabres, J., Fawke, J., Guinsburg, R., Hosono, S., Isayama, T., Kapadia, V., Kim, H., Liley, H., McKinlay, C., Mildenhall, L., Perlman, J., Rabi, Y., Roehr, C., Schmölzer, G., Szyld, E.,…Weiner, G. (2020). Neonatal Life Support: 2020 International Consensus on Cardiopulmonary Resuscitation and Emergency Cardiovascular Care Science With Treatment Recommendations. *Circulation.* https://doi.org/10.1161/CIR.0000000000000895.

Wyckoff, M. H., Aziz, K., Escobedo, M. B., Kapadia, V. S., Kattwinkel, J., Perlman, J. M., Simon, W. M., Weiner, G. M., & Zaichkin, J. G. (2015). Part 13: neonatal resuscitation: 2015 American Heart Association guidelines update for cardiopulmonary resuscitation and emergency cardiovascular care. *Circulation, 132*(18_suppl_2), S543-S560.

Wyllie, J., Bruinenberg, J., Roehr, C. C., Rüdiger, M., Trevisanuto, D., & Urlesberger, B. (2015). European Resuscitation Council Guidelines for Resuscitation 2015: Section 7. Resuscitation and support of transition of babies at birth. *Resuscitation, 95*, 249-263.

Zaichkin, J., McCarney, L., & Weiner, G. (2016). NRP 7th edition: are you prepared? *Advances in Neonatal Care, 16*(4), 255-263.

Chapter 15

Newborn Trauma

Arif İsmet Çatak*, MD
Department of Pediatrics, Tokat Gaziosmanpaşa University, Turkey

Abstract

Newborn trauma has a wide range of clinical conditions, from self-healing bruises and lacerations to serious hemorrhages or nerve injuries. The incidence varies between 2 and 52 per 1000 live births. There are maternal (maternal obesity and diabetes) and fetal (macrosomia, macrocephaly, malpresentation, and prematurity) risk factors. These factors lead to traumas that cause morbidity and mortality. Recently, newborn traumas have decreased with increased use of cesarean delivery. Newborn traumas can affect every system of the body. Soft tissue injuries are the most common type and include bruising, petechiae, and lacerations. Caput succedaneum and cephalhematoma are superficial lesions of the head. Subgaleal, epidural, subdural, subarachnoid, and intraventricular hemorrhages can be seen. Ocular injuries are also a common type of face injury. Skull and clavicle fractures, facial nerve injury, and brachial plexus injury are traumas with high morbidity.

Keywords: newborn, trauma, risk factors, birth injuries

---

* Corresponding Author's Email: arifcatak@yahoo.com

In: Current Approaches to Newborn Emergencies
Editors: Zuhal Keskin Sarılar and Serap Samut Bülbül
ISBN: 979-8-89530-999-5

Introduction

Newborn trauma is defined as the structural destruction or functional impairment of the body due to perinatal or iatrogenic traumatic causes. There is a wide range of clinical conditions, from self-healing bruises and lacerations to serious hemorrhages or nerve injuries, which can cause morbidity and mortality.

The incidence of newborn traumas varies between 2 and 52 per 1000 live births in Turkey (Bülbül et al., 2013). It is noticed that incidence is decreasing over the last decades due to refinements in obstetrical techniques and the increased use of cesarean delivery (Merriam et al., 2017).

Risk Factors

Maternal Factors

Maternal obesity and maternal diabetes are associated with a higher risk of newborn traumas. It may be because of macrosomia, type of delivery, and the use of instrumentation during delivery.

Primiparity, maternal pelvic anomalies, and small maternal stature are also associated with increased risk of newborn traumas to the head and neck (Boulet et al., 2003).

Type of Delivery

It is unclear whether cesarean or vaginal delivery is more protective against newborn trauma, but the use of forceps or a vacuum device in the vaginal delivery is associated with an increased risk of newborn trauma (Merriam et al., 2017).

Fetal Factors

Macrosomia is a risk factor for newborn trauma when the fetal weight is greater than 4000 g.

Macrocephaly and fetal congenital anomalies are also associated with increased risk.

Oligohydramnios, malpresentation, very low birth weight, and extreme prematurity are also other risk factors for newborn trauma (Wei et al., 2012).

Type of Injuries

Soft Tissue Injuries

The most common type of newborn injuries are associated with soft tissues, which include bruising, petechiae, subcutaneous fat necrosis, and lacerations.

While bruising located at the genitalia can be associated with breech position, petechiae of the neck and head are associated with vertex position. They are mostly self-limiting injuries and managed with well-baby nursery. If petechiae are widespread and continue to develop, thrombocytopenia and thrombocyte dysfunction should be excluded (Alexander et al., 2006).

Ischemic injury to the adipose tissue can cause subcutaneous fat necrosis and is characterized by palpation of nodules in the subcutaneous area. It may take a few weeks to resolve, and hypercalcemia can develop during this period; therefore, serum calcium should be monitored (Alexander et al., 2006).

Fetal laceration is the most common trauma seen in cesarean delivery, and steri-strips are usually enough to repair it.

Head Injuries

Superficial lesions of the head, bone fractures, and extracranial and intracranial hemorrhages can be seen.

Caput succedaneum is subcutaneous edema of the scalp. The edema is between the skin and the periosteum, and swelling crosses suture lines. It can be due to birth canal pressure or vacuum device use. It is usually a benign condition and needs no treatment. Alopecia and scarring can rarely be seen on the swelling area (Pollina et al., 2001).

Fractures of the skull are usually a result of instrumented vaginal delivery. They may be linear or depressed, and intracranial injuries may accompany them. While linear fractures can be asymptomatic, depressed ones are more complicated. If there is a suspicion, imaging methods should be performed (Demissie et al., 2004).

Linear fractures heal within several weeks without any treatment, but if there is a depression greater than 1 cm, surgical intervention should be required.

Cephalhematoma is also usually a result of instrumented vaginal delivery, and bleeding is localized to the subperiosteal area. It is usually unilateral and does not cross the suture lines, unlike caput succedaneum. It also resolves without treatment, but hyperbilirubinemia, calcification, and infection like osteomyelitis can be seen as complications (Krishnan et al., 2024).

Subgaleal hemorrhage is usually a complication of instrumented vaginal delivery, but it can also be seen in spontaneous vaginal deliveries. The bleeding is in the loose areolar tissue space between the galea aponeurotica and periosteum. The injury occurs when traction pulls the scalp away from the stationary bony calvarium, resulting in the shearing of the bridging vessels. Imaging methods should be performed when suspected, and hemoglobin and hematocrit levels should be monitored. Vital signs monitoring and head circumference (occipitofrontal circumference) measurements should also be done because of bleeding hypovolemia (Amar et al., 2003).

Subgaleal hemorrhage has a mortality risk between 10 and 15%. These patients can rarely require surgical intervention for decompression and supportive care; restoration of blood volume with red blood cells or fresh frozen plasma should also be included in treatment (Kilani & Wetmore, 2006).

Epidural hemorrhage is very rare in newborns and is usually due to middle meningeal artery injury with a fracture. Increased intracranial pressure symptoms can be seen, like bradycardia, hypertension, and bulging of the fontanelle. Seizure or hypotonia can also be seen. Imaging methods (CT or MRI) should be performed when suspected (Heyman et al., 2005). Supportive therapy and neurosurgical intervention should be necessary for these babies.

Subdural hemorrhage is mostly seen in instrumented vaginal delivery and is the most common intracranial hemorrhage in newborns (Krishnan et al., 2024). Bleeding is between the arachnoid membrane and the dura mater. Patients may be asymptomatic or present with increased intracranial pressure signs and symptoms. Seizures, apnea, or consciousness problems can also be seen in these babies. Treatment of subdural hemorrhage depends on the bleeding site of the brain and the extent of bleeding. Surgical evacuation is mostly needed in posterior fossa subdural hemorrhages (Rooks et al., 2008).

Subarachnoid hemorrhage is the second most common intracranial hemorrhage type. The problem is rupture of bridging veins. Instrumented vaginal delivery is a risk factor like other hemorrhages (Looney et al., 2007). Conservative treatment is usually sufficient.

Intraventricular hemorrhage is associated with prematurity. Instrumented vaginal delivery is also a risk factor (Dani et al., 2010). Maternal factors like maternal inflammation and hypertensive disorder of pregnancy are associated with increased risk of intraventricular hemorrhage (Shankaran et al., 2014). Small blood vessels in the germinal matrix are usually the problematic structures. Patients can be asymptomatic at the beginning, so routine screening with cranial ultrasound for newborns who are smaller than 32 weeks gestational age (Krüse-Ruijter et al., 2022). The hemorrhage is graded according to bleeding location. Maternal indomethacin use is associated with severity (Hammers et al., 2015). Cerebrospinal fluid drainage is needed in these newborns. Serial lumbar punctures, temporary ventricular access devices, or permanent shunting can be needed for the drainage (de Vries et al., 2019; Berger et al., 2000).

Face and Neck Injuries

Ocular injuries are commonly seen, especially subconjunctival hemorrhages, which are benign conditions that resolve without intervention. They are superficial hematomas of the conjunctiva. Instrumented vaginal delivery is a risk factor for corneal abrasions and vitreous hemorrhages (Holden et al., 1992). These conditions should be followed by an ophthalmologist to prevent visual defects.

Facial nerve injuries are also seen mostly with forceps usage or prominent maternal sacral promontory, and the mandibular branch is mostly affected. There is a diminished movement on the affected side of the face. It usually resolves without intervention in a few weeks.

Clavicular fracture is the most common fracture seen in newborns. Operative delivery, macrosomia, shoulder dislocation, and increased maternal age are risk factors. Asymmetrical appearance, lack of movement of the affected side, and abnormal crying can be seen in these newborns. They can also be asymptomatic. Plain radiographs should be performed when suspected (Hsu et al., 2002). It should be kept in mind that brachial plexus palsy can accompany a clavicular fracture.

The brachial plexus is a complicated network of nerve fusions and divisions with an important function, which provides innervation of the upper extremity, shoulder, and upper chest.

Neonatal brachial plexus palsy (NBPP) is a condition that has been recognized since the 18th century. In the 1800s, clinicians identified that weakness in the upper arm - particularly affecting muscles like the deltoid and biceps - was linked to damage at the fifth and sixth cervical nerve roots. This form, which later became known as Erb's palsy, is now understood to be the most frequently encountered type of brachial plexus injury. Conversely, a distinct variant involving the lower part of the brachial plexus was described in the late 19th century, characterized by significant weakness in hand function while proximal muscle strength remains intact. This presentation, often accompanied by signs of Horner's syndrome on the same side, is associated with injury to the C8 and T1 nerve roots. One of the leading causes of NBPP is shoulder dystocia during childbirth, which increases the likelihood of excessive traction on the infant's neck and shoulder region (McGillicuddy, 2011).

Treatment generally begins with physiotherapy aimed at improving motor function, though surgical options may be considered in more severe or persistent cases.

Conclusion

Although many cases of newborn trauma resolve spontaneously, certain injuries - such as intracranial hemorrhages or brachial plexus palsy - require prompt medical or surgical intervention. A multidisciplinary approach involving neonatology, neurosurgery, orthopedics, and rehabilitation services is critical for optimal recovery. Timely diagnosis and individualized treatment plans significantly improve functional outcomes and quality of life for affected infants.

References

Amar, A. P., Aryan, H. E., Meltzer, H. S., & Levy, M. L. (2003). Neonatal subgaleal hematoma causing brain compression: report of two cases and review of the literature. *Neurosurgery, 52*(6),1470–1474. https://doi.org/10.1227/01.neu.0000065180.07961.54.

Alexander, J. M., Leveno, K. J., Hauth, J., Landon, M. B., Thom, E., Spong, C. Y., Varner, M. W., Moawad, A. H., Caritis, S. N., Harper, M., Wapner, R. J., Sorokin, Y., Miodovnik, M., O'Sullivan, M. J., Sibai, B. M., Langer, O., & Gabbe, S. G. (2006).

Fetal injury associated with cesarean delivery. *Obstetrics and Gynecology, 108*(4), 885–890. https://doi.org/10.1097/01.aog.0000237116.72011.f3.

Berger, A., Weninger, M., Reinprecht, A., Haschke, N., Kohlhauser, C., & Pollak, A. (2000). Long-term experience with subcutaneously tunneled external ventricular drainage in preterm infants. *Child's nervous system : ChNS : official journal of the International Society for Pediatric Neurosurgery, 16*(2), 103–110. https://doi.org/10.1007/s003810050022.

Boulet, S. L., Alexander, G. R., Salihu, H. M., & Pass, M. (2003). Macrosomic births in the united states: determinants, outcomes, and proposed grades of risk. *American journal of obstetrics and gynecology, 188*(5), 1372–1378. https://doi.org/10.1067/mob.2003.302.

Bülbül, A., Sözeri, Ş., Selalmaz, M., Kunt, A., vd. (2013). Yenidoğan Bebeklerde Doğum Travması Sıklığı ve İlişkili Risk Faktörleri. Journal of Turgut Ozal Medical Center, 20(4), 326-330.

Dani, C., Poggi, C., Bertini, G., Pratesi, S., Di Tommaso, M., Scarselli, G., & Rubaltelli, F. F. (2010). Method of delivery and intraventricular haemorrhage in extremely preterm infants. *The journal of maternal-fetal & neonatal medicine : the official journal of the European Association of Perinatal Medicine, the Federation of Asia and Oceania Perinatal Societies, the International Society of Perinatal Obstetricians, 23*(12), 1419–1423. https://doi.org/10.3109/14767051003678218.

Demissie, K., Rhoads, G. G., Smulian, J. C., Balasubramanian, B. A., Gandhi, K., Joseph, K. S., & Kramer, M. (2004). Operative vaginal delivery and neonatal and infant adverse outcomes: population based retrospective analysis. *BMJ (Clinical research ed.), 329*(7456), 24–29. https://doi.org/10.1136/bmj.329.7456.24.

de Vries, L. S., Groenendaal, F., Liem, K. D., Heep, A., Brouwer, A. J., van 't Verlaat, E., Benavente-Fernández, I., van Straaten, H. L., van Wezel-Meijler, G., Smit, B. J., Govaert, P., Woerdeman, P. A., Whitelaw, A., & ELVIS study group (2019). Treatment thresholds for intervention in posthaemorrhagic ventricular dilation: a randomised controlled trial. *Archives of disease in childhood. Fetal and neonatal edition, 104*(1), F70–F75. https://doi.org/10.1136/archdischild-2017-314206.

Heyman, R., Heckly, A., Magagi, J., Pladys, P., & Hamlat, A. (2005). Intracranial epidural hematoma in newborn infants: clinical study of 15 cases. *Neurosurgery, 57*(5), 924–929. https://doi.org/10.1227/01.neu.0000180026.73246.bf.

Holden, R., Morsman, D. G., Davidek, G. M., O'Connor, G. M., Coles, E. C., & Dawson, A. J. (1992). External ocular trauma in instrumental and normal deliveries. *British journal of obstetrics and gynaecology, 99*(2), 132–134. https://doi.org/10.1111/j.1471-0528.1992.tb14471.x.

Hsu, T. Y., Hung, F. C., Lu, Y. J., Ou, C. Y., Roan, C. J., Kung, F. T., Changchien, C. C., & Chang, S. Y. (2002). Neonatal clavicular fracture: clinical analysis of incidence, predisposing factors, diagnosis, and outcome. *American journal of perinatology, 19*(1), 17–21. https://doi.org/10.1055/s-2002-20169.

Kilani, R. A., & Wetmore, J. (2006). Neonatal subgaleal hematoma: presentation and outcome--radiological findings and factors associated with mortality. *American journal of perinatology, 23*(1), 41–48. https://doi.org/10.1055/s-2005-923438.

Krishnan, V., Jaganathan, S., Choudhary, A. K., Ou, X., Choudhary, R., Choudhary, A., Na, X., Mankad, K., Ramakrishnaiah, R., & Jayappa, S. (2024). Birth-related subdural hemorrhage in asymptomatic neonates: evolution over time and differentiation from traumatic subdural hemorrhage. *Pediatric radiology*, *54*(10), 1631–1642. https://doi.org/10.1007/s00247-024-06003-6.

Krüse-Ruijter, M. F., Boswinkel, V., Consoli, A., Nijholt, I. M., Boomsma, M. F., de Vries, L. S., van Wezel-Meijler, G., & Leijser, L. M. (2022). Neurological Surveillance in Moderate-Late Preterm Infants-Results from a Dutch-Canadian Survey. *Children (Basel, Switzerland)*, *9*(6), 846. https://doi.org/10.3390/children9060846.

Looney, C. B., Smith, J. K., Merck, L. H., Wolfe, H. M., Chescheir, N. C., Hamer, R. M., & Gilmore, J. H. (2007). Intracranial hemorrhage in asymptomatic neonates: prevalence on MR images and relationship to obstetric and neonatal risk factors. *Radiology*, *242*(2), 535–541. https://doi.org/10.1148/radiol.2422060133.

McGillicuddy J. E. (2011). Neonatal brachial plexus palsy - historical perspective. *Journal of pediatric rehabilitation medicine*, *4*(2), 99–101. https://doi.org/10.3233/PRM-2011-0161.

Merriam, A. A., Ananth, C. V., Wright, J. D., Siddiq, Z., D'Alton, M. E., & Friedman, A. M. (2017). Trends in operative vaginal delivery, 2005-2013: a population-based study. *BJOG : an international journal of obstetrics and gynaecology*, *124*(9), 1365–1372. https://doi.org/10.1111/1471-0528.14553.

O'Sullivan, M. J., Sibai, B. M., Langer, O., Gabbe, S. G., & National Institute of Child Health and Human Development Maternal-Fetal Medicine Units Network (2006). Fetal injury associated with cesarean delivery. *Obstetrics and gynecology*, *108*(4), 885–890. https://doi.org/10.1097/01.AOG.0000237116.72011.f3.

Pollina, J., Dias, M. S., Li, V., Kachurek, D., & Arbesman, M. (2001). Cranial birth injuries in term newborn infants. *Pediatric neurosurgery*, *35*(3), 113–119. https://doi.org/10.1159/000050403.

Rooks, V. J., Eaton, J. P., Ruess, L., Petermann, G. W., Keck-Wherley, J., & Pedersen, R. C. (2008). Prevalence and evolution of intracranial hemorrhage in asymptomatic term infants. *AJNR. American journal of neuroradiology*, *29*(6), 1082–1089. https://doi.org/10.3174/ajnr.A1004.

Shankaran, S., Lin, A., Maller-Kesselman, J., Zhang, H., O'Shea, T. M., Bada, H. S., Kaiser, J. R., Lifton, R. P., Bauer, C. R., Ment, L. R., & Gene Targets for Intraventricular Hemorrhage Study (2014). Maternal race, demography, and health care disparities impact risk for intraventricular hemorrhage in preterm neonates. *The Journal of pediatrics*, *164*(5), 1005–1011.e3. https://doi.org/10.1016/j.jpeds.2014.01.036.

Wei, C., Stevens, J., Harrison, S., Mott, A., & Warner, J. (2012). Fractures in a tertiary Neonatal Intensive Care Unit in Wales. *Acta paediatrica (Oslo, Norway: 1992)*, *101*(6), 587–590. https://doi.org/10.1111/j.1651-2227.2012.02640.x.

Chapter 16

Neonatal Respiratory Stress

Fatma Kocael*, MD

Department of Pediatrics, Dörtçelik Children's Hospital, Bursa, Turkey

Abstract

Neonatal respiratory distress syndrome (RDS) is a critical respiratory failure syndrome that typically occurs within the first hours of life, most often immediately after delivery, and is predominantly observed in premature newborns. RDS is a result of surfactant deficiency, leading to alveolar collapse, impaired oxygenation, increased work of breathing, and systemic hypoxemia.

The incidence of RDS is inversely proportional to gestational age; as prematurity increases, the risk and severity of RDS also escalate. Although rare in term infants, the incidence can increase in the presence of contributing factors such as maternal diabetes, cesarean delivery, or perinatal asphyxia.

Modern perinatal care strategies, such as antenatal corticosteroid administration, exogenous surfactant therapy, and advanced respiratory support techniques (e.g., continuous positive airway pressure, high-frequency oscillatory ventilation, and invasive mechanical ventilation), have significantly reduced the morbidity and mortality associated with RDS. However, this condition remains a leading cause of neonatal death, particularly among highly preterm infants.

Contemporary treatment of RDS aims to provide adequate respiratory support while minimizing the need for invasive interventions. In this context, noninvasive ventilation methods, such as continuous positive airway pressure (CPAP) and high-flow nasal cannula (HFNC), as well as minimally invasive surfactant administration techniques, including less-

* Corresponding Author's Email: fatma.irioglu@gmail.com

In: Current Approaches to Newborn Emergencies
Editors: Zuhal Keskin Sarılar and Serap Samut Bülbül
ISBN: 979-8-89530-999-5

invasive surfactant administration (LISA) and minimally invasive surfactant therapy (MIST), are increasingly being prioritized.

Keywords: respiratory stress syndrome, premature, newborn

Introduction

Neonatal respiratory distress syndrome (RDS) is the most common cause of respiratory failure in preterm infants, primarily due to pulmonary immaturity and surfactant deficiency. Surfactant, a substance that reduces surface tension and prevents alveolar collapse, is a crucial pathophysiological component of RDS. In recent years, the prognosis for RDS has improved significantly with the application of antenatal corticosteroids, noninvasive respiratory support strategies, and surfactant therapy. This progress in RDS management should encourage optimism about the future of neonatal care. However, it is crucial to remember that early diagnosis and effective clinical management remain essential in neonatal medicine. Noninvasive post-extubation ventilation strategies and evidence-based protocols for antenatal corticosteroid administration are particularly crucial, as both have a significant impact on patient outcomes.

This chapter provides a comprehensive review of the mechanisms, risk factors, diagnostic methods, current treatment strategies, and complications associated with RDS.

Epidemiology and Risk Factors

RDS is among the most common causes of respiratory failure in preterm infants, and its incidence increases inversely with gestational age. Although the incidence reaches approximately 98% in newborns born at 24 weeks of gestation, it decreases to 5% at 34 weeks and drops below 1% at 37 weeks of gestation.

Key risk factors influencing the development of RDS include prematurity (especially before 34 weeks of gestation), male sex, maternal diabetes, elective cesarean section without labor onset, perinatal asphyxia, and genetic mutations involving surfactant proteins (e.g., SP-B, SP-C). Maternal diabetes has been shown to delay fetal lung maturation by inhibiting surfactant synthesis (Piper, Xenakis, & Langer, 1998).

Pathophysiology

The fundamental pathophysiological mechanism underlying respiratory distress syndrome (RDS) is a combination of surfactant deficiency and lung immaturity.

Role of Surfactant in Lung Function

Surfactant is a lipoprotein complex synthesized by type II alveolar epithelial cells that serves to reduce alveolar surface tension and prevent collapse. A surfactant deficiency initiates a cascade of pathological events, as detailed below.

The pathophysiological basis of respiratory distress syndrome (RDS) is a deficiency in pulmonary surfactant, a vital lipoprotein substance necessary to reduce surface tension within the alveoli. In the absence of sufficient surfactant supply, the tension at the alveolar surface increases, leading to alveolar instability and increased susceptibility to collapse, particularly during expiration. This collapse disrupts efficient gas exchange, culminating in a ventilation-perfusion (V/Q) mismatch, where oxygenation is compromised despite adequate pulmonary perfusion. As a result, affected newborns exhibit hypoxemia and hypercapnia, which ultimately leads to respiratory acidosis. The persistent imbalance in gas exchange may also facilitate the development of pulmonary edema, thus exacerbating respiratory failure and increasing the risk of morbidity and mortality.

Laplace's law elucidates this phenomenon: $P = \frac{2T}{R}$, where P denotes the pressure required to maintain an alveolus in an open state, T represents the surface tension, and R signifies the radius of the alveolus. In the absence of surfactant, an escalation in surface tension results in smaller alveoli collapsing into larger ones, thereby contributing to the onset of atelectasis. This progression consequently affects gas exchange, resulting in hypoxemia, hypercapnia, and respiratory acidosis (Fernsler & Zasadzinski, 2009).

In advanced stages, pulmonary edema and the formation of hyaline membranes are frequently observed, further compromising oxygenation due to a ventilation-perfusion imbalance. Ultimately, the condition may evolve to include hypoxemia, hypercapnia, pulmonary edema, and secondary respiratory acidosis. Without adequate management, this can result in pulmonary hypertension and respiratory failure.

The primary risk factor for RDS is premature birth. Additional contributing factors that increase the risk include male sex, Caucasian ethnicity, multiple gestation, particularly in the case of second-born twins, macrosomia (high birth weight), cesarean section performed before the onset of labor, maternal diabetes, and the presence of intrahepatic cholestasis during pregnancy. Secondary surfactant deficiency can arise in association with conditions such as intrapartum asphyxia, pulmonary infections, pulmonary hemorrhage, meconium aspiration syndrome, congenital diaphragmatic hernia, and pulmonary hypoplasia. Furthermore, external factors such as hypothermia, hypoxia, and acidosis can adversely affect surfactant synthesis and secretion, thus exacerbating the severity of RDS. Genetic mutations that result in partial or complete deficiency of surfactant protein B (SP-B) can also contribute to the development of RDS, even in full-term neonates (Jackson, 2012). On the contrary, certain conditions have been associated with a reduced risk of RDS, including intrauterine growth restriction, prolonged membrane rupture, and maternal substance abuse (Cekinmez et al., 2013).

Clinical Findings

The main clinical findings of RDS are summarized in Table 1.

Table 1. Clinical findings in RDS

Symptom	Description
Tachypnea	The respiratory rate exceeds 60 breaths per minute.
Nasal flaring	A compensatory response designed to minimize the effort required for ventilation.
Expiratory grunt	Preserves alveolar pressure to prevent collapse.
Cyanosis	Cyanosis is characterized by bluish discoloration of the skin, resulting from oxygen deficiency.
Subcostal/intercostal retractions	Indicates an excessive level of activity in the respiratory muscles.

Diagnostic Methods for Neonatal Respiratory Distress Syndrome (RDS)

The diagnosis of Neonatal Respiratory Distress Syndrome (RDS) is achieved through the meticulous evaluation of postnatal respiratory distress symptoms, along with imaging and laboratory data. The prompt identification of this condition is not merely critical; it is imperative to facilitate timely interventions (Reuter et al., 2014).

Clinical Evaluation

RDS typically presents within the first few hours following birth. Proficiency in clinical evaluation is essential for establishing a diagnosis. Observed signs provide vital clinical insight and indicate the need for additional testing in suspected cases. The ability to conduct clinical assessments is crucial in diagnosing RDS.

Chest radiography is widely recognized as the primary imaging modality for diagnosing respiratory distress syndrome (RDS). Radiographic findings may vary depending on the stage and severity of the condition. A characteristic feature is the reticulogranular or ground-glass pattern, which denotes diffuse granularity and indicates a deficiency of surfactant. Additionally, the presence of air bronchograms, where air-filled bronchi are prominently displayed against a backdrop of collapsed alveoli, is another critical finding. Low lung volume, frequently attributed to atelectasis and decreased lung compliance, is a common radiographic indicator, particularly in premature infants. In advanced or severe cases of RDS, imaging may reveal increased lung opacity, along with poorly defined diaphragmatic borders, indicating deteriorated aeration and disease progression. Chest X-rays also play a crucial role in differentiating RDS from other neonatal respiratory disorders (Reuter et al., 2014).

Arterial blood gas (ABG) analysis serves as a crucial instrument to assess respiratory status and the severity of respiratory distress syndrome (RDS). Common abnormalities observed in ABG results include hypoxemia, characterized by a reduction in the partial pressure of oxygen (PaO_2); hypercapnia, indicated by an elevation in the partial pressure of carbon dioxide ($PaCO_2$); and respiratory acidosis, demonstrated by a decrease in blood pH level. These parameters underscore the impairment of gas exchange and compromised respiratory function in affected neonates. In cases of severe hypoxemia, oxygen saturation levels may drop below 85%, necessitating prompt initiation of mechanical ventilation to maintain adequate oxygenation and prevent further deterioration.

Lung ultrasound (LUS) has been recognized as an exceptionally valuable, noninvasive, and radiation-free imaging modality for the early diagnosis and monitoring of neonatal respiratory conditions, including respiratory distress syndrome (RDS). It is particularly preferred in neonatal intensive care settings due to its safety and ease of bedside accessibility. In the context of RDS, LUS reveals several characteristic findings. The "white lung" pattern, characterized by a homogeneously hyperechoic appearance, signifies widespread atelectasis resulting from surfactant deficiency. Another significant feature is thickening of the pleural line, which serves as an indicator of lung immaturity, especially in preterm neonates. Additionally, decreased lung sliding is frequently observed, which reflects impaired alveolar expansion and surfactant insufficiency. In addition to its diagnostic utility in RDS, LUS is instrumental in differentiating RDS from transient tachypnea of the newborn (TTN), which presents with distinct ultrasonographic features and typically resolves more quickly (Raimondi et al., 2021; Popa et al., 2024).

Pulse oximetry and transcutaneous carbon dioxide ($TcCO_2$) monitoring represent critical noninvasive methods for the real-time evaluation of oxygenation and ventilation in newborns suffering from respiratory distress syndrome (RDS). These modalities have significant value in the prompt identification of hypoxemia, thereby facilitating timely clinical interventions that can prevent further respiratory complications. In addition, they provide vital information to evaluate oxygen needs and evaluate the efficacy of therapeutic interventions, including additional oxygen or mechanical ventilation. TCO_2 monitoring provides an indirect yet continuous assessment of carbon dioxide levels, which complements arterial blood gas analysis without requiring frequent blood sampling. Such tools are particularly beneficial for preterm infants receiving respiratory support, as vigilant monitoring is imperative to avert complications such as oxygen toxicity or permissive hypercapnia (Reuter et al., 2014).

Given that several neonatal conditions may clinically resemble RDS, supplementary laboratory evaluations are often required for accurate diagnosis and appropriate treatment planning. For example, when bacterial pneumonia is suspected as a possible differential diagnosis, specific assessments such as blood cultures and C-reactive protein (CRP) levels prove essential to identify infectious agents and assess the presence of systemic inflammation.

Furthermore, a complete blood count (CBC) with particular emphasis on neutrophil counts offers critical information on infant immunological status and helps identify infectious or inflammatory processes. These investigations are instrumental in distinguishing RDS from other etiologies of neonatal respiratory distress, ensuring timely and targeted interventions (Barnett & Klein, 2016).

In the differential diagnosis of neonatal respiratory distress, it is imperative to exclude cardiac and metabolic etiologies that may present with or contribute to clinical manifestations similar to respiratory distress syndrome (RDS). Echocardiography functions as an essential instrument to assess congenital heart disease and pulmonary hypertension, both of which can present with respiratory compromise in neonates. Concurrently, a thorough metabolic panel and assessment of serum electrolytes are pivotal in detecting systemic disorders such as metabolic acidosis, hypoglycemia, or other biochemical imbalances that may underlie or exacerbate respiratory symptoms. These diagnostic approaches are critical to ensure that RDS is not misdiagnosed, thus facilitating timely and appropriate interventions. The increasing inclination towards non-invasive imaging techniques, such as lung ultrasound and echocardiography, also illustrates a clinical commitment to minimizing radiation exposure in this vulnerable population (Hermansen & Mahajan, 2015).

Prenatal Care and Antenatal Corticosteroids

The most critical factor in preventing respiratory distress syndrome (RDS) is the avoidance of preterm delivery. For pregnancies identified as at risk for early delivery, it is advisable to refer the patient to a facility equipped with neonatal intensive care and, whenever possible, facilitate in utero transport. In cases where preterm birth is unavoidable, the utilization of antenatal corticosteroids should be considered.

Antenatal corticosteroids are administered to expedite fetal lung maturation and reduce the risk of respiratory distress syndrome (RDS) and other complications linked to prematurity. Frequently employed agents, such as betamethasone and dexamethasone, act to increase surfactant production within the alveoli and facilitate lung development (McGoldrick et al., 2020; Daskalakis et al., 2023).

The administration of antenatal corticosteroids serves as a widely endorsed and evidence-based intervention designed to promote fetal lung maturation in pregnancies deemed at risk of preterm delivery. These corticosteroids, particularly betamethasone and dexamethasone, elicit various physiological responses that significantly mitigate the incidence and severity of respiratory distress syndrome (RDS). They stimulate the production of surfactant, which prevents alveolar collapse; improve intraalveolar fluid resorption, thereby facilitating effective pulmonary clearance at the time of birth; increase lung compliance, which in turn enhances ventilation and gas exchange; and decrease pulmonary vascular resistance, consequently reducing the likelihood of persistent pulmonary hypertension in neonates (McGoldrick et al., 2020). From a clinical perspective, antenatal corticosteroids are recommended for pregnant women between 24 and 34 weeks of gestation who face an imminent risk of preterm birth. The main indications include threatened preterm labor, marked by cervical dilation and regular uterine contractions; preterm premature rupture of membranes (PPROM); planned cesarean delivery before 34 weeks; and high-risk situations, including multiple gestations or early delivery necessitated by preeclampsia or placental insufficiency. Availability of corticosteroids in these circumstances is associated with improved neonatal respiratory outcomes and reduced morbidity (McGoldrick et al., 2020).

Administration Protocols

Common antenatal corticosteroid regimens are summarized in Table 2.

Antenatal corticosteroids show maximum efficacy 24 hours after administration, with benefits lasting approximately 7 days. This intervention significantly reduces the incidence of neonatal respiratory complications, such as respiratory distress syndrome (RDS) (Walters et al., 2022). If the risk of premature delivery persists beyond 14 days, a rescue dose may be administered if delivery is expected within 7 days. The practice of repeat dosing is approached with clinical caution due to the limitations in long-term data regarding neonatal outcomes; therefore, potential benefits must be meticulously evaluated (Williams et al., 2022). Antenatal corticosteroids decrease the incidence of RDS by up to 50% by enhancing fetal lung maturation. Additionally, they mitigate the risks associated with bronchopulmonary dysplasia (BPD), reduce the need for mechanical ventilation, and decrease the incidence of intraventricular hemorrhage (IVH) and necrotizing enterocolitis (NEC), thereby improving the survival rates of preterm neonates. Despite their recognized safety, the use of corticosteroids requires the exercise of clinical judgment, particularly in cases of maternal sepsis or chorioamnionitis, due to the potential for immunosuppression. Significant contraindications include hypersensitivity and poorly controlled diabetes, with associated risks such as maternal hyperglycemia and fetal growth restriction. While transient hypoglycemia may occur in neonates, the advantages remain substantial when corticosteroids are administered several hours before delivery, ideally 24 hours in advance (McGoldrick et al., 2020). Current guidelines advocate for the administration of antenatal corticosteroids to women between 24 and 34 weeks of gestation who are at risk for preterm birth. Betamethasone and dexamethasone may be utilized interchangeably. The decision to administer a rescue dose should be guided by the ongoing risk of preterm delivery and concerns regarding fetal growth. It is imperative to monitor maternal glucose levels diligently, particularly among diabetic patients, and to maintain vigilance for intrauterine infections, as corticosteroid administration in the context of chorioamnionitis may be contraindicated. Although early intervention before 24 weeks has not been extensively studied, it can still confer benefits in high-risk pregnancies (McGoldrick et al., 2020).

Postnatal Stabilization of Preterm Infants

Stabilization of preterm infants immediately after birth is crucial to mitigate complications and reduce mortality rates. Primary objectives include ensuring optimal respiratory function and thermoregulation. Delayed cord clamping for at least 60 seconds is recommended to facilitate the neonatal circulatory transition, enhance hematocrit levels, and increase iron stores.

For infants who spontaneously breathe and are born before 32 weeks of gestation, early use of continuous positive airway pressure (CPAP) at 6–8 cmH_2O is essential to prevent atelectasis due to surfactant deficiency and to reduce dependence on mechanical ventilation.

Table 2. Common antenatal corticosteroid regimens

Drug	Dose	Route and Frequency	Total Dose
Betamethasone	12 mg IM	2 doses, 24 hours apart	24 mg
Dexamethasone	6 mg IM	4 doses, 12 hours apart	24 mg

Invasive mechanical ventilation should be reserved exclusively for infants experiencing severe respiratory failure. When possible, non-invasive strategies such as CPAP or Nasal Intermittent Positive Pressure Ventilation (NIPPV) should be employed. Providing thermal care with plastic wraps and heated, humidified gases is vital to prevent hypothermia, a significant risk factor associated with increased morbidity and mortality.

These stabilization strategies are evidence-based interventions that have been shown to improve outcomes for preterm neonates (Mahmoud et al., 2022).

Surfactant Therapy and Its Importance

Surfactant deficiency leads to alveolar collapse, reduced lung compliance, and hypoxemia. Replacement of deficient surfactant is a fundamental aspect of managing respiratory distress syndrome (RDS), as it significantly reduces morbidity and the need for mechanical ventilation (Sweet et al., 2023).

Indications

In the clinical management of RDS, timely identification of neonates that require increased respiratory support is essential to improve outcomes. Endotracheal intubation may be necessary immediately in the delivery room to achieve initial stabilization, particularly in infants who demonstrate inadequate respiratory effort, apnea, or severe desaturation. During the early management of continuous positive airway pressure (CPAP), the requirement for a fraction of inspired oxygen (FiO_2) exceeding 30% at pressures equal to or greater than 6 cmH_2O is a widely accepted threshold indicating inadequate lung recruitment and the potential need for exogenous surfactant therapy or mechanical ventilation. Furthermore, characteristic imaging findings, including reticulogranular patterns or a white lung appearance on chest radiography or lung ultrasound, substantiate the diagnosis of RDS and underscore the need for therapeutic escalation. A prompt response to these clinical and diagnostic indicators ensures optimal support for lung function and reduces the risk of secondary complications such as barotrauma or bronchopulmonary dysplasia (Table 3).

Table 3. Types of surfactant and dose strategies

Type	Source	Initial dose (mg/kg)	Repeat Dose	Strategy
Poractant alfa (Curosurf®)	Porcine	200	100	A higher initial dose improves the results.
Beractant (Survanta®)	Bovine	100	100	Enhanced response with repeated doses
Calfactant (Infasurf®)	Bovine	100	100	Equitable distribution through the pulmonary circulation.
Lucinactant (Surfaxin®)	Synthetic	175	175	Reduce the likelihood of inflammation while following a protein-free diet.

(Jeon, 2019; Qiu et al., 2020).

Surfactant Administration Techniques

The method of surfactant delivery plays a crucial role in improving outcomes and minimizing complications in newborns diagnosed with RDS. Various administration strategies have been developed to maintain a balance between efficacy and minimal invasiveness. The Less Invasive Surfactant Administration (LISA) or Minimally Invasive Surfactant Therapy (MIST) technique involves the delivery of surfactant through a slender catheter while the infant remains on continuous positive airway pressure (CPAP). Research indicates that this approach significantly reduces the incidence of bronchopulmonary dysplasia (BPD) and considerably decreases the need for mechanical ventilation, making it the preferred and most effective method in contemporary neonatal practice (Silveira et al., 2024; Ng & Shah, 2021). Another technique, INSURE, an acronym for Intubation-Surfactant-Extubation, involves a brief intubation for surfactant administration, followed by prompt extubation back to noninvasive support. This method also proves effective in mitigating ventilator-induced lung injury, although it is somewhat more invasive than LISA. The nebulized surfactant represents a promising noninvasive alternative currently undergoing clinical investigation; however, further studies are required to substantiate its efficacy and establish standardized protocols. The choice of delivery method should be determined by institutional resources, clinical experience, and the clinical condition of the newborn.

Repeat Doses and Clinical Outcomes

In circumstances where an infant requires a fraction of inspired oxygen (FiO2) greater than 30% after the initial administration of surfactant, it is recommended to administer an additional dose. Poractant alfa exhibits improved early oxygenation outcomes when a high initial dosage protocol is utilized. Surfactant therapy is correlated with a decrease in the risks of bronchopulmonary dysplasia (BPD), intraventricular hemorrhage (IVH), and pulmonary hemorrhage.

Mechanical Ventilation and Oxygen Support

The primary objective is to minimize the need for mechanical ventilation by adopting non-invasive ventilation (NIV) as the initial approach. Continuous Positive Airway Pressure (CPAP) is considered the preferred method, while Non-Invasive Positive Pressure Ventilation (NIPPV) may be utilized as an alternative in instances where CPAP proves ineffective. High-flow nasal cannula (HFNC), although less effective than CPAP, may be employed in circumstances where CPAP is poorly tolerated. In cases that require ventilation, the tidal volume should be maintained within the range of 4 to 6 ml/kg. The application of inhaled nitrous oxide (iNO) may confer benefits in cases of hypoxic pulmonary hypertension (National Guideline Alliance, 2019).

Oxygen Targets: Oxygen saturation (SpO2) should be maintained within the range of 90% to 94%. Levels below 85% present a risk of hypoxic injury, while levels greater than 95% increase the probability of retinopathy of prematurity (ROP) (Saugstad & Aune, 2014).

Complications of Respiratory Distress Syndrome (RDS)

Respiratory distress syndrome (RDS) in newborns, while often manageable with timely intervention, is associated with a variety of early and late complications that can significantly impact both short-term outcomes and long-term morbidity. Early complications typically include pulmonary hemorrhage, a life-threatening condition characterized by alveolar bleeding resulting from capillary stress and inflammation. Furthermore, the persistence of a patent ductus arteriosus (PDA) is frequently observed, particularly in preterm infants, and may exacerbate respiratory compromise by increasing pulmonary blood flow and affecting gas exchange. The development of pulmonary hypertension can also occur, complicating oxygenation and increasing the risk of right heart failure. Regarding late complications, bronchopulmonary dysplasia (BPD) represents a major chronic sequela, particularly in infants who require prolonged oxygen therapy or mechanical ventilation; this condition reflects arrested lung development and ongoing inflammation (Bhandari & McGrath-Morrow, 2013). Intraventricular hemorrhage (IVH), which involves bleeding into the brain's ventricular system, constitutes another significant complication of prematurity often associated with hemodynamic instability observed in severe RDS. Furthermore, prematurity retinopathy (ROP), a condition characterized by abnormal retinal vascular development, can be precipitated by prolonged exposure to additional oxygen, a common necessity in the treatment of RDS (Ovalı, 2007). It is essential to maintain awareness of these complications to facilitate early detection, intervention, and implementation of preventive strategies in high-risk newborns.

Conclusion

Respiratory distress syndrome (RDS) is a significant factor in neonatal morbidity and mortality, particularly among preterm infants. The prompt identification of this condition, in conjunction with evidence-based interventions, is imperative to enhance both short- and long-term outcomes. The implementation of antenatal corticosteroids, the early initiation of continuous positive airway pressure (CPAP), and minimally invasive surfactant administration (LISA) have considerably revolutionized the management of RDS by mitigating the severity of respiratory distress and reducing the dependency on invasive mechanical ventilation. Despite these advances, RDS persists as a clinical challenge, especially in infants born at extremely premature gestation. Ongoing research on innovative therapeutic approaches, such as nebulized surfactant and gene-based interventions, offers promise for further improvements in neonatal respiratory care and reduction in complication rates. Continuous progress in personalized medicine, non-invasive monitoring, and preventive strategies will be vital for optimizing outcomes for this vulnerable population.

References

Bhandari, A., & McGrath-Morrow, S. (2013). Long-term pulmonary outcomes in patients with bronchopulmonary dysplasia. *Seminars in Perinatology, 37*(2), 132–137. https://doi.org/10.1053/j.semperi.2013.01.010.

Daskalakis, G., Pergialiotis, V., Domellöf, M., Ehrhardt, H., Di Renzo, G. C., Koç, E., ... Jacobsson, B. (2023). European guidelines on perinatal care: Corticosteroids for women at risk of preterm birth. *The Journal of Maternal-Fetal & Neonatal Medicine, 36*(1), 2160628. https://doi.org/10.1080/14767058.2022.2160628.

Jeon, G. W. (2019). Surfactant preparations for preterm infants with respiratory distress syndrome: Past, present, and future. *Korean Journal of Pediatrics, 62*(5), 155–161. https://doi.org/10.3345/kjp.2019.62.5.155.

Mahmoud, R. A., Schmalisch, G., Oswal, A., & Roehr, C. (2022). Non-invasive ventilatory support in neonates: An evidence-based update. *Paediatric Respiratory Reviews, 44*, 11–18. https://doi.org/10.1016/j.prrv.2022.09.001.

McGoldrick, E., Stewart, F., Parker, R., & Dalziel, S. R. (2020). Antenatal corticosteroids for accelerating fetal lung maturation for women at risk of preterm birth. *Cochrane Database of Systematic Reviews, 12*, CD004454. https://doi.org/10.1002/14651858.CD004454.pub4.

National Guideline Alliance (UK). (2019). *Evidence reviews for respiratory support: Specialist neonatal respiratory care for preterm babies*. National Institute for Health and Care Excellence (NICE).

Ng, E. H., & Shah, V. (2021). Guidelines for surfactant replacement therapy in neonates. *Paediatrics & Child Health, 26*(1), 35–49. https://doi.org/10.1093/pch/pxaa116.

Ovalı, F. (2007). Prematüre retinopatisi: Epidemiyoloji ve risk faktörleri. *Türk Pediatri Arşivi, 42*(4), 157–163.

Piper, J. M., Xenakis, E. M., & Langer, O. (1998). Delayed appearance of pulmonary maturation markers is associated with poor glucose control in diabetic pregnancies. *The Journal of Maternal-Fetal Medicine, 7*(3), 148–153. https://doi.org/10.1002/(SICI)1520-6661(199805/06)7:3<148::AID-MFM9>3.0.CO;2-K.

Popa, A. E., Popescu, S. D., Tecuci, A., Bot, M., & Vladareanu, S. (2024). Current trends in the imaging diagnosis of neonatal respiratory distress syndrome (NRDS): Chest X-ray versus lung ultrasound. *Cureus, 16*(9), e69787. https://doi.org/10.7759/cureus.69787

Qiu, C., Ma, C., Fan, N., Zhang, X., & Zheng, G. (2020). Comparative efficacy of pulmonary surfactant in respiratory distress syndrome in preterm infants: A Bayesian network meta-analysis. *Archives of Medical Science, 19*(5), 1446–1453. https://doi.org/10.5114/aoms.2020.97065.

Raimondi, F., Migliaro, F., Corsini, I., Meneghin, F., Dolce, P., Pierri, L., Perri, A., Aversa, S., Nobile, S., Lama, S., Varano, S., Savoia, M., Gatto, S., Leonardi, V., Capasso, L., Carnielli, V. P., Mosca, F., Dani, C., Vento, G., & Lista, G. (2021). Lung Ultrasound Score Progress in Neonatal Respiratory Distress Syndrome. *Pediatrics, 147*(4), e2020030528. https://doi.org/10.1542/peds.2020-030528.

Reuter, S., Moser, C., & Baack, M. (2014). Respiratory distress in the newborn. *Pediatrics in Review, 35*(10), 417–429. https://doi.org/10.1542/pir.35-10-417.

Saugstad, O. D., & Aune, D. (2014). Optimal oxygenation of extremely low-birth-weight infants: A meta-analysis and systematic review of oxygen saturation target studies. *Neonatology, 105*(1), 55–63. https://doi.org/10.1159/000357431.

Silveira, R. C., Panceri, C., Munõz, N. P., Carvalho, M. B., Fraga, A. C., & Procianoy, R. S. (2024). Less invasive surfactant administration versus intubation-surfactant-extubation in the treatment of neonatal respiratory distress syndrome: A systematic review and meta-analyses. *Jornal de Pediatria, 100*(1), 8–24. https://doi.org/10.1016/j.jped.2023.05.008.

Sweet, D. G., Carnielli, V. P., Greisen, G., Hallman, M., Klebermass-Schrehof, K., Ozek, E., Te Pas, A., Plavka, R., Roehr, C. C., Saugstad, O. D., Simeoni, U., Speer, C. P., Vento, M., Visser, G. H. A., & Halliday, H. L. (2023). European Consensus Guidelines on the Management of Respiratory Distress Syndrome: 2022 Update. *Neonatology, 120*(1), 3–23. https://doi.org/10.1159/000528914.

Walters, A., McKinlay, C., Middleton, P., Harding, J. E., & Crowther, C. A. (2022). Repeat doses of prenatal corticosteroids for women at risk of preterm birth for improving neonatal health outcomes. *Cochrane Database of Systematic Reviews, 4*, CD003935. https://doi.org/10.1002/14651858.CD003935.pub5.

Williams, M. J., Ramson, J. A., & Brownfoot, F. C. (2022). Different corticosteroids and regimens for accelerating fetal lung maturation for babies at risk of preterm birth. *Cochrane Database of Systematic Reviews, 8*, CD006764. https://doi.org/10.1002/14651858.CD006764.pub4.

Chapter 17

Neonatal Jaundice

Nihal Aydın[*], MD
Department of Pediatrics, Samsun University, Samsun Training and Research Hospital, Samsun, Turkey

Abstract

Jaundice is a common finding in newborn infants. It is regarded as a typical physiological state, generally considered to be benign and transient. Nevertheless, in a minority of newborns, the levels may reach a point that could potentially result in irreversible severe brain damage. The incidence of acute bilirubin encephalopathy and kernicterus can be reduced if cases are diagnosed and treated promptly.

Keywords: newborn, jaundice, hyperbilirubinemia, phototherapy, exchange transfusion

Introduction

Unless the serum total bilirubin (STB) level exceeds 5 mg/dl, jaundice is not seen clinically (Kaplan et al., 2015). Jaundice is a common finding in newborns and can be observed in 60-80% of healthy term and late preterm infants. In most cases, jaundice resolves spontaneously; however, in some infants, hyperbilirubinemia may reach severe levels (Kaplan et al., 2015; Cayabyab & Ramanathan, 2019). Infants with severe hyperbilirubinemia

[*] Corresponding Author's Email: nihalcayonu@gmail.com

In: Current Approaches to Newborn Emergencies
Editors: Zuhal Keskin Sarılar and Serap Samut Bülbül
ISBN: 979-8-89530-999-5

(STB > 20 mg/dL) may experience severe neurological sequelae, including acute bilirubin encephalopathy or chronic bilirubin encephalopathy (kernicterus), which is defined as bilirubin-induced neurological dysfunction (BIND). In severe cases, the infant may even die if not treated promptly and appropriately (Kaplan et al., 2015; Cayabyab & Ramanathan, 2019). To minimize the risk of neurological damage, it is imperative to rapidly and appropriately lower high bilirubin levels (Johnson & Bhutani, 2011; American Academy of Pediatrics, 2004).

In a healthy term newborn, the TSB level should be evaluated in the nomogram displaying the percentile distribution of bilirubin according to age in hours. The risk zone should be determined, and it should be established whether treatment is necessary.

Categories of Clinically Significant Hyperbilirubinaemia

Significant Hyperbilirubinemia

Unconjugated bilirubin concentration requiring treatment with phototherapy that varies with postnatal age and cause of the condition (typically total serum bilirubin [TSB] ≥12 mg/dL).

Severe Hyperbilirubinemia

Bilirubin concentrations at or near exchange transfusion threshold based on postnatal age and cause of the condition (typically TSB ≥20 mg/dL) or any elevated TSB associated with the early signs of mild acute bilirubin encephalopathy.

Extreme Hyperbilirubinemia

Bilirubin concentrations at exchange transfusion threshold (typically TSB ≥25 mg/dL) or any elevated TSB associated with signs of mild to moderate acute bilirubin encephalopathy

Hazardous or Critical Hyperbilirubinemia

Bilirubin concentrations at exchange transfusion threshold (typically TSB ≥30 mg/dL) or any elevated TSB associated with signs of moderate to severe acute bilirubin encephalopathy.

Approach to a Jaundiced Infant and Prevention of Jaundice

Primary Protection

Adequate and Successful Breastfeeding

A robust correlation has been established between the likelihood of hyperbilirubinemia and exclusive breastfeeding (Preer & Philipp, 2011). The advantages of breast milk are well documented, and mothers should be encouraged to breastfeed their infants. It is recommended that breastfeeding be initiated as soon as possible, preferably within the first hour after birth. An increase in the frequency of breastfeeding has been demonstrated to reduce the likelihood of developing significant hyperbilirubinemia. It is therefore recommended that mothers should breastfeed their infants at least 8-12 times per day during the first few days of life (American Academy of Pediatrics, 2004). An infant who is adequately fed will typically wet 5 or more diapers per day during the first 72 hours (Flaherman & Maisels, 2017).

Avoiding Water and Sugar Water Supplementation

The administration of water or dextrose solution to infants with jaundice does not prevent hyperbilirubinemia or reduce bilirubin levels (Smith and Becker, 2016). Accordingly, the administration of water or sugar water to newborns with jaundice is not indicated (Flaherman & Maisels, 2017; Smith & Becker, 2016).

Secondary Protection

Determination of Blood Groups

It is advisable to exercise caution when determining the risk of severe hyperbilirubinemia in newborns (American Academy of Pediatrics, 2004).

- It is recommended that blood group determination be performed in all pregnant women and that an indirect Coombs test be conducted in Rh(-) pregnant women.
- In the event that the maternal blood group is unknown or if the maternal blood group is O or Rh(-), it is advised that the cord blood be tested for direct Coombs test, ABO, and Rh(D) blood group.

Clinical Assessment

It is advised that all newborns be monitored for the development of jaundice. The examination should include a visual assessment of the infant's skin color, as well as a determination of whether there are any associated changes in the infant's skin. The presence of jaundice in the skin and conjunctiva should be evaluated at 8- to 12-hour intervals in conjunction with vital signs. A visual assessment of jaundice should be conducted in a well-lit environment, preferably in natural light, with the infant unclothed. The color of the skin should be evaluated after gently pressing the skin with a finger to create a fading effect. The initial presentation of jaundice is typically observed on the face and subsequently spreads to the trunk and extremities. Nevertheless, estimation of bilirubin levels based on the spread of jaundice is not a reliable method (American Academy of Pediatrics, 2004). It is therefore recommended that bilirubin be assessed in all infants within the first 12 hours of admission or prior to discharge. A total bilirubin test is of paramount importance for infants exhibiting jaundice. The sclera and conjunctiva lack melanin pigmentation, rendering them highly susceptible to bilirubin-induced discoloration. As bilirubin accumulates in the bloodstream, the whites of the eye, namely the conjunctiva and sclera, undergo a change in coloration, becoming yellow and manifesting the condition known as conjunctival jaundice. The absence of conjunctival jaundice may be useful in excluding significant hyperbilirubinemia (Azzuqa & Watchko, 2017).

Jaundice developing in the first 24 hours should be considered pathological until proven otherwise. It is imperative to assess the serum bilirubin levels of these infants and investigate the possibility of hemolytic disease and other pathological causes.

Evaluation as a Laboratory Procedure

It is recommended that bilirubin levels be monitored in all jaundiced infants. In cases where a neonate develops hyperbilirubinemia at a level requiring treatment, exhibits a decline in bilirubin levels in repeated measurements, and no underlying cause for the jaundice is identified through history or physical examination, the neonate is evaluated according to the criteria outlined in Table 1 (American Academy of Pediatrics, 2004). It is imperative that each bilirubin value be interpreted in accordance with the bilirubin nomogram, which has been prepared according to the age of the infant in hours (Figure 1) (Bhutani et al., 1999). The utilization of the nomogram in accordance with postnatal age enables the monitoring of the trajectory of repeated bilirubin values and the prediction of the infant who will subsequently develop hyperbilirubinemia. This nomogram, known as the "Bhutani nomogram," has been in use since 1999 and remains a topic of ongoing debate.

The probability of hyperbilirubinemia can be estimated by assessing TSB or TcB levels in conjunction with identified risk factors while the infant is under maternal observation. A blood sample can be obtained concurrently with metabolic screening. The evaluation of TSB or TcB in the bilirubin nomogram enables the risk of developing severe hyperbilirubinemia to be determined. A follow-up plan is devised based on the evaluation of the risk of jaundice development, incorporating risk zones and clinical risk factors (see Figures 1 and 3). In infants in whom bilirubin levels are obtained at more than one different time point, these values are marked on the nomogram, and the rate of bilirubin increase is evaluated. Should the bilirubin level approach the upper percentile curves, hemolysis is deemed a potential cause and subject to further investigation and monitoring (Bhutani et al., 1999; Maisels et al., 2009).

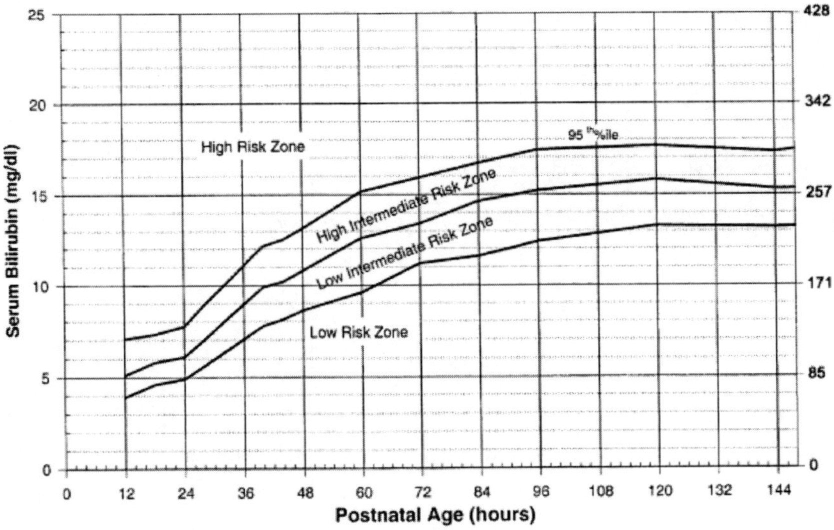

Figure 1. Nomogram created to determine the risk status of infants according to postnatal age and total bilirubin values (American Academy of Pediatrics, 2004).

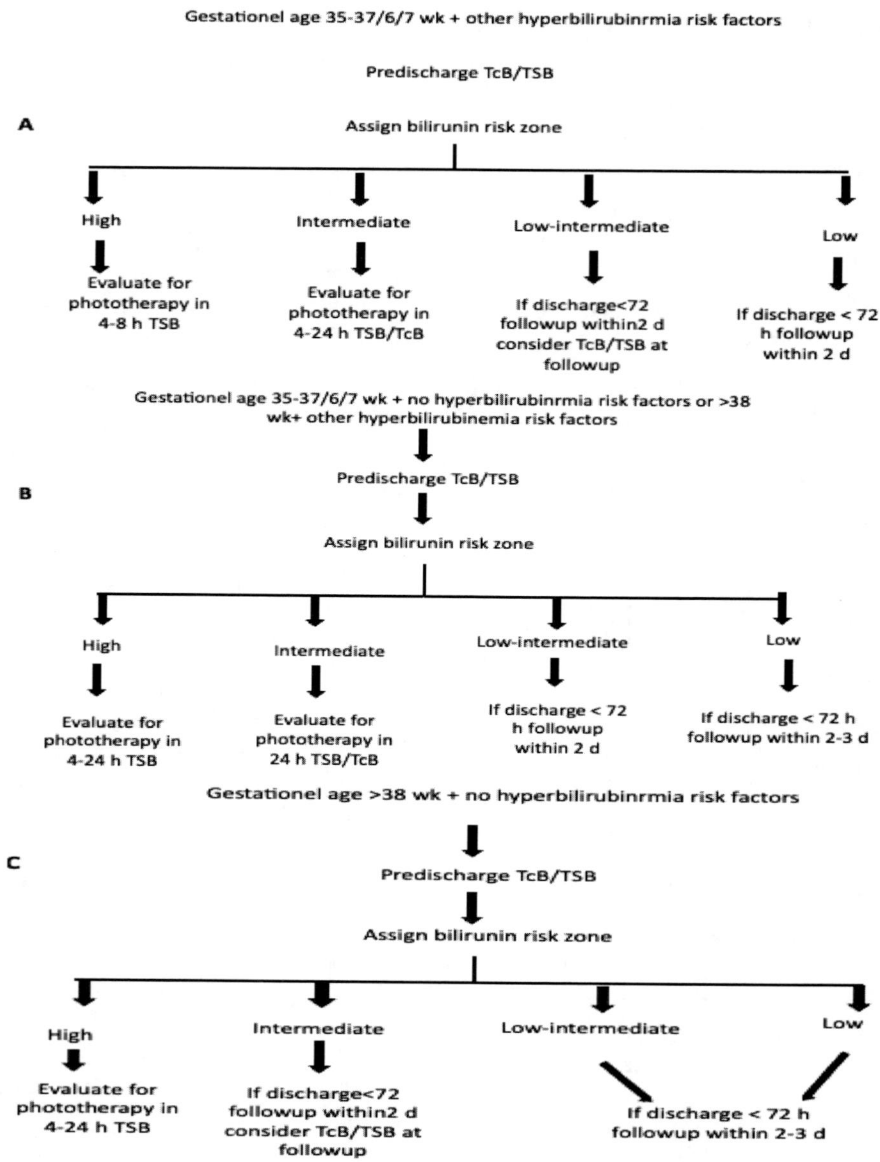

Figure 2. Algorithm providing recommendations for management and follow-up according to predischarge bilirubin measurements, gestation, and risk factors for subsequent hyperbilirubinemia (Maisels et al., 2009)

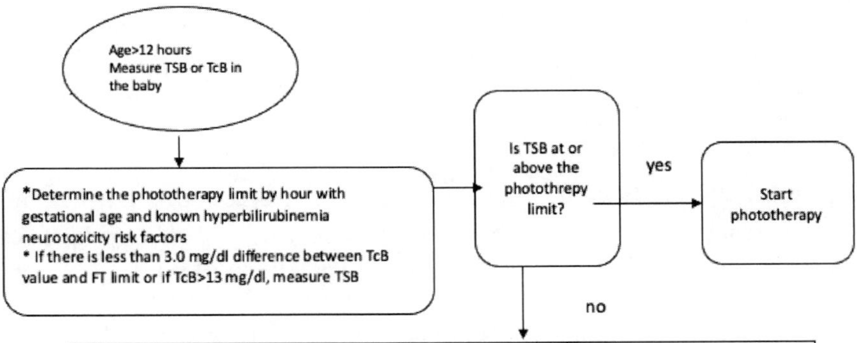

Phototherapy limit - TcB or TSB value		Discharge Recommendations
0,1-1.9 mg /dL	Age < 24 hour	Measure TSB in 4-8 hours, think phototherapy, delayed discharge
	Age≥ 24 hour	Measure TSB in 4-24 hour a Options: *Delay discharge and consider phototherapy *Discharge without applying phototherapy with close follow-up
2.0-3.4 mg /dL	Regardless of age or time of discharge	Measure TSB in 4-24 hour a
3.5-5.4 mg /dL	Regardless of age or time of discharge	Measure TSB or TcB in 1-2 days
5.5-6.9 mg /dL	Discharge < 72 hour	Followup within 2 days; TSB or TcB according to clinical evaluationb
	Discharge ≥ 72 hour	Clinical evaluationb
≥ 7.0 mg /dL	Discharge < 72 hour	Followup within 3 days; TSB or TcB
	Discharge≥ 72 hour	according to clinical evaluationb

A) The time interval between 4-24 hours is decided by clinical assessment. **B)** Clinical assessment decisions include physical examination, risk factors for developing hyperbilirubinemia (Table 4), risk factors for neurotoxicity (gestational age < 3 g/dL, isoimmune hemolytic disease (positive direct Coombs test), G6PD deficiency, or other hemolytic conditions, sepsis, severe clinical disorder in the last 24 hours), nutritional deficiency, weight monitoring, and family support.

Figure 3. Flow chart for post-discharge follow-up in infants who did not receive phototherapy during hospitalization (Kemper et al., 2022).

In the 2022 update of the AAP guideline, a novel scheme for post-discharge follow-up was proposed (Kemper et al., 2022). The difference between the bilirubin level measured in the period closest to discharge and the phototherapy threshold at the time of this measurement is calculated, and a follow-up plan is formulated in accordance with the recommendations set forth in Figure 3. This figure can be utilized from 12 hours after birth, at the earliest, in infants who have not undergone phototherapy previously. Furthermore, both the AAP (Figure 4) and Bhutani (Figure 2) discharge schemes can be employed safely.

The Infant Was Admitted to the Hospital for Treatment of Jaundice

The following tests are recommended for parents who present with jaundice and require treatment (American Academy of Pediatrics, 2004).

1. Maternal and infant blood groups
2. Direct Coombs test
3. Complete blood count and peripheral smear
4. Reticulocyte count
5. Total, direct, and indirect bilirubin levels
6. G6PD enzyme level
7. Reducing substance in urine
8. Serum albumin level if TSB is approaching the exchange limit
9. Serum electrolytes if there is pathologic weight loss
10. Complete urine examination, urine culture, and sepsis indicators if there is an increase in direct bilirubin or late-onset jaundice
11. In cases of prolonged jaundice, in addition to the above tests, thyroid function tests should be performed. If direct bilirubin is elevated, further evaluation for cholestasis is warranted.

Bilirubin Assessment Methods

Blood Bilirubin Measurement

Chemical Laboratory Analysis

TB levels are measured directly in serum or plasma by chemical reaction (diazo) or spectrophotometrically. These measurements are considered the gold standard. However, venous blood collection is required (Vreman et al., 1996).

Table 1. Evaluation in newborns with hyperbilirubinemia

Indications	Evaluation
Jaundice appearing within the first 24 hours	Measure TSB
Baby appears more jaundiced than normal	Measure TcB and/or TSB
Jaundice unexplained by history and physical examination, with rapidly rising TSB or undergoing phototherapy	Blood type and direct Coombs test Complete blood count and peripheral smear Direct bilirubin measurement Reticulocyte count, G6PD enzyme, urine for reducing substances* Repeat based on the baby's age and TSB within 4–24 hours
TSB at exchange transfusion levels or unresponsive to phototherapy	Albumin
Direct hyperbilirubinemia	Urinalysis and urine culture, sepsis evaluation (if suggested by history and physical examination), abdominal ultrasound, urine for reducing substances, tandem mass spectrometry (TANDEM-MS)

TSB: Total Serum Bilirubin TcB: Transcutaneous Bilirubin *In infants with hyperbilirubinemia requiring treatment and with an unexplained cause.

Non-chemical Photometric Method

Bilirubin levels are measured spectrophotometrically at the bedside with special measuring devices, and a small amount of blood (heel capillary blood sample) is required. There is a close correlation between bilirubin levels measured by photometric devices and standard chemical bilirubin measurements. However, when bilirubin levels exceed 15 mg/dL, this correlation is disrupted, and TB values are measured lower. In this case, bilirubin should be evaluated by standard laboratory method (Grohmann et al., 2006).

Transcutaneous Bilirubin (TcB) Measurement

The TcB meter is used to measure the total serum or plasma bilirubin at the skin surface. The use of TcB measurement has reduced the number of blood draws required to determine bilirubin values in infants with jaundice. However, it should not be used in infants undergoing phototherapy. TcB measurement is not reliable in infants with dark skin color (Gothwal et al., 2021). Since TcB measurements may yield lower results than TSB measurements at high bilirubin levels, it should be confirmed with standard laboratory methods (Taylor et al., 2015).

TSB is recommended in the following cases (Maisels et al., 2009; Maisels, 2004)

1. Infants with TcB > 13 mg/dL
2. Infants with jaundice in the first 24 hours
3. Newborns for whom a treatment decision has been made
4. Newborns receiving phototherapy treatment
5. Those with bilirubin values above the 75th percentile according to the Bhutani curve
6. Infants with a TcB level of 70% of the recommended FT value.

Risk Factors

Important risk factors for severe hyperbilirubinemia (Maisels et al., 2009):

1. ,Low gestational week (<40 weeks; the lower the week, the higher the risk)
2. Observation of jaundice in the first 24 hours
3. TSB/TcB level close to the phototherapy limit before discharge
4. Hemolysis of any cause or rapid increase in TSB/TcB (rate of increase >0.3 mg/dL in the first 24 hours, then >0.2 mg/dL)
5. Receiving phototherapy before discharge
6. History of phototherapy or exchange transfusion in parents or siblings
7. Family history of inherited erythrocyte disorders such as G6PD deficiency
8. Inadequate exclusive breastfeeding
9. Cephalohematoma or diffuse ecchymosis
10. Down syndrome
11. Macrosomic baby of a diabetic mother.

Risk Assessment Before Discharge

It is imperative that the risk of developing severe hyperbilirubinemia be assessed in every newborn prior to discharge. Furthermore, risk assessment protocols must be established to ensure the safety of these vulnerable patients. It is of particular importance to conduct a risk assessment for newborns who are discharged from the hospital before reaching the 72-hour mark. It is recommended that TSB or TcB be measured in all infants prior to hospital discharge in order to ascertain the risk. This approach facilitates the identification of infants at risk of developing severe hyperbilirubinemia (American Academy of Pediatrics, 2004). In addition to bilirubin measurements, it is recommended that risk factors be determined and used in conjunction with one another (Maisels et al., 2009). It is contraindicated to discharge newborns with bilirubin levels in the high-risk zone (>95th percentile) prior to the recommended timeframe for observation. A follow-up scheme based on bilirubin levels is presented in Figure 2.

Post-Discharge Follow-up

It is recommended that infants discharged from the hospital before 72 hours be seen within two days of discharge. During this appointment, the medical team should assess the infant's jaundice and the necessity of bilirubin measurement. In the case of infants with identified risk factors, a follow-up appointment should be scheduled within 24 hours. For those without identified risk factors, a longer interval between appointments may be appropriate (Figure 2).

In general, infants who are discharged from the hospital prematurely should be seen by a healthcare professional at an earlier point in time (American Academy of Pediatrics, 2004).

- Discharged before 24 hours, 72 hours of life,
- Those discharged between 24-48 hours, 96 hours of life,
- Those discharged between 48-72 hours should be seen at 120 hours of life.

Treatment

The most feared complication of neonatal jaundice is kernicterus. The development of kernicterus is contingent upon the concentration of free bilirubin, which is not bound to bilirubin, and the permeability of the blood-brain barrier. The gestational week has been demonstrated to influence the permeability of the blood-brain barrier. In this regard, birth weight is a more practical indicator, with a correlation between birth weight and maturation observed in the majority of infants. The mean birth weight of term infants is approximately 2500 grams. However, late preterm infants, who are at an elevated risk for jaundice relative to term infants, may also attain this weight. In light of these considerations, gestational week emerges as a more pivotal factor in these borderline cases. Treatment thresholds are determined using both gestational week and birth weight, as indicated in the relevant curves or tables (Bratlid et al., 2011; Newman, 2007; Arlettaz et al., 2007). In infants with a gestational age of 35 weeks or greater, the AAP curves that incorporate both gestational age and risk factors are commonly utilized (American Academy of Pediatrics, 2004).

The reduction of bilirubin levels is a treatment strategy employed in infants with identified risk factors. The following risk factors have been identified as potential contributors to bilirubin neurotoxicity (Kemper et al., 2022; Palma & Arain, 2016):

1. Gestational age <38 weeks; this risk increases with the degree of prematurity
2. Albumin < 3 g/dL
3. Isoimmune hemolytic disease positive direct Coombs test, G6PD deficiency, or other hemolytic conditions
4. Sepsis
5. Severe clinical deterioration in the last 24 hours.

Criteria for Hemolysis in the Newborn

In the event of jaundice and a rapid increase in bilirubin levels within the first 24 hours, it is imperative to conduct an evaluation to ascertain the presence of hemolysis. In evaluating bilirubin levels, it is crucial to ascertain the hourly rate of increase. An hourly rate of increase in bilirubin levels above 0.3 mg/dL in the first 24 hours and above 0.2 mg/dL thereafter is considered an indicator of hemolysis (Kaplan et al., 2008). In patients where hemolysis is a potential diagnosis, a comprehensive evaluation of the patient's blood should be conducted. This evaluation should include, but is not limited to, the following tests: blood group, direct Coombs test, complete blood count, peripheral smear, reticulocyte count, and G6PD enzyme level. In the peripheral smear, the morphology of erythrocytes is evaluated in terms of microspherocytosis (hereditary spherocytosis, ABO incompatibility), elliptocytosis, blister formation, and the presence of deficient erythrocytes (G6PD enzyme deficiency), echinocytes (pyruvate kinase deficiency), and schistocytes (DIC, perinatal asphyxia), as well as Heinz body formation (hemolytic anemia).

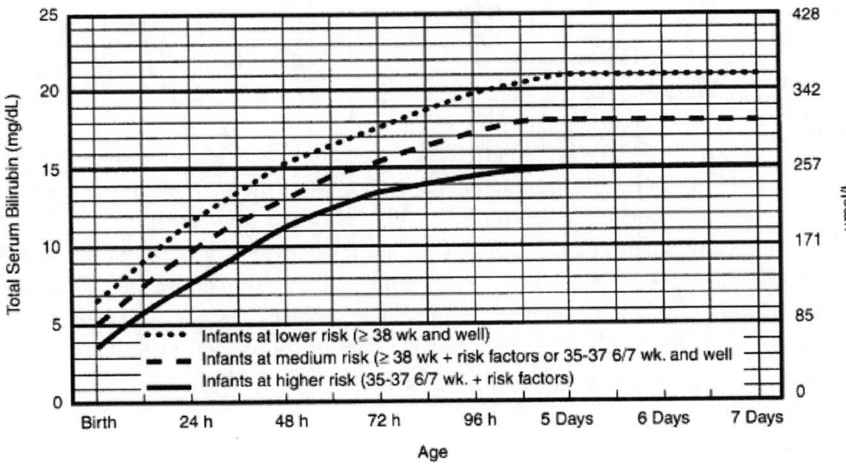

Use total bilirubin. Do not subtract direct reacting or conjugated bilirubin.

Risk factors = isoimmune hemolytic disease, G6PD deficiency, asphyxia, significant lethargy, temperature instability, sepsis, acidosis, or albumin < 3.0 g/dL (if measured)

For well infants 35–37 6/7 wk can adjust TSB levels for intervention around the medium risk line. It is an option to intervene at lower TSB levels for infants closer to 35 wks and at higher TSB levels for those closer to 37 6/7 wk.

It is an option to provide conventional phototherapy in hospital or at home at TSB levels 2–3 mg/dL (35–50 mmol/L) below those shown but home phototherapy should not be used in any infant with risk factors.

Figure 4. Guidelines for phototherapy in hospitalized infants of 35 or more weeks gestation (American Academy of Pediatrics, 2004).

Table 2. Limits of phototherapy and exchange transfusion in infants with gestational age <35 weeks

Gestational age	24 hour	48 hour	72 hour
23 week	4 (8)*	6 (10)	8 (13)
24 week	4 (8)	6 (11)	8 (14)
25 week	4 (8)	6 (11)	9 (15)
26 week	5 (8)	7 (12)	9 (15)
27 week	5 (8)	7 (12)	10 (16)
28 week	5 (9)	7 (12)	10 (16)
29 week	5 (9)	8 (13)	11 (17)
30 week	6 (9)	9 (13)	11 (17)
31 week	6 (9)	9 (13)	12 (18)
32 week	6 (9)	9 (14)	13 (19)
33 week	6 (9)	9 (15)	13 (19)
34 week	6 (10)	10 (15)	14 (20)

*The first number indicates the phototherapy limit, and the number in parentheses indicates the blood exchange limit (mg/dL). Adapted from the NICE guideline (phototherapy and exchange transfusion limits in the NICE guideline are based on reported care practices in neonatal units and consensus opinions) (53). The threshold for initiation of phototherapy in babies with a postnatal age of more than 72 hours is calculated with the following formula according to the gestational week (23): Total bilirubin (mg/dL) = (Gestational week x 0.6) – 6.

Table 3. Phototherapy and exchange criteria according to bilirubin-albumin ratio

Birth weight (g)	Phototherapy				Exchange			
	Standard risk		High risk		Standard risk		High risk	
	TSB	B/A**	TSB	B/A**	TSB	B/A**	TSB	B/A**
<1000	5.8	2.3	5.8	2.3	9.9	3.9	9.9	3.9
1000–1250	8.7	3.5	5.8	2.3	12.8	5.1	9.9	3.9
1250–1500	11.1	3.7	8.7	2.9	15.2	6.1	11.8	5.1
1500–2000	12.8	4.2	11.1	3.7	16.9	6.8	15.2	6.1
2000–2500	14.0	4.6	12.8	4.2	18.1	7.2	16.9	6.8

Indicators of Hemolysis

1. Jaundice in the first 24 hours
2. Direct Coombs test positivity and accompanying laboratory findings
    a. Hemolysis findings in peripheral smear
    b. Elevated reticulocyte count
    c. Decrease in hemoglobin and hematocrit levels.

3. G6PD enzyme deficiency with increased TSB level
4. Bilirubin level increased > 0.3 mg/dL in the first 24 hours and > 0.2 mg/dL thereafter
5. TSB increased or not decreased despite FT.

Phototherapy

The objective of phototherapy is to reduce the indirect bilirubin level, minimize the necessity for exchange transfusion, and avert the emergence of bilirubin encephalopathy. Figure 4 is applicable to infants with a gestational age of 35 weeks or above (American Academy of Pediatrics, 2004), while Table 2 (NICE, 2010) is applicable to infants with a gestational age below 35 weeks. Table 3, based on birth weight, can be used in preterm infants with unknown gestational age (Watchko & Maisels, 2018).

The clinical efficacy of phototherapy is evaluated by measuring the bilirubin level 4–6 hours after the initiation of treatment. A reduction in bilirubin levels by 2-3 mg/dL is anticipated (American Academy of Pediatrics, 2004). The efficacy of phototherapy is contingent upon not only the dosage of light employed but also the severity and underlying cause of hyperbilirubinemia.

In instances of severe hyperbilirubinemia, the aggressive utilization of phototherapy not only diminishes the necessity for exchange transfusion but also mitigates the severity of bilirubin neurotoxicity (Hansen et al., 2009). To gauge the efficacy of phototherapy, repeated measurements of bilirubin levels are employed. It is important to be mindful of the potential for a sudden increase in bilirubin levels (rebound) that may occur following the discontinuation of phototherapy.

To deliver intensive phototherapy, the surface area of the infant's body exposed to phototherapy can be increased, or devices with high-intensity lamps can be utilized. Intensive phototherapy is administered using two distinct phototherapy devices, one positioned beneath the bosom and the other above, or alternatively, through the use of tunnel phototherapy devices. Intensive phototherapy is employed in instances where bilirubin levels are within 3 mg/dL of the exchange limit, whereas unidirectional phototherapy is utilized in cases where bilirubin levels are lower. Although previously advised, recent studies (Chen et al., 2002; Shinwell et al., 2002) have challenged the efficacy of changing the direction of the infant's body every 2-3 hours. Nevertheless, the American Academy of Pediatrics (AAP) continues to recommend that the infant's posture be altered every two to three hours to enhance the area exposed to light (Ahlfors et al., 2009). Phototherapy is deemed efficacious when a reduction in bilirubin levels exceeding 0.5 mg/dL per hour is attained. The most significant reduction in bilirubin levels is observed during the initial 4-6 hours of treatment (American Academy of Pediatrics, 2004).

In cases where bilirubin levels are approaching the exchange limit, phototherapy is administered continuously. There is no scientific rationale for intermittent administration. Once a reduction in bilirubin levels is observed, phototherapy is discontinued for a period of 30 minutes to facilitate maternal-child bonding and enable feeding (American Academy of Pediatrics, 2004).

The infant is then returned to the mother for breastfeeding. The treatment is terminated when the total serum bilirubin level declines by 2-3 mg/dL below the threshold for initiating phototherapy in infants without risk factors (American Academy of Pediatrics, 2004). In circumstances that are considered high-risk, such as hemolysis, or in cases where the infant is readmitted to the hospital after a period of phototherapy, the treatment may be continued for a longer duration (American Academy of Pediatrics, 2004).

Rebound bilirubin refers to an increase in the total serum bilirubin level that occurs after the discontinuation of phototherapy. It is typically not necessary to restart phototherapy. Only 5% of infants require restarting phototherapy within 72 hours after its discontinuation (Arlettaz et al., 2007). The following factors are associated with an increased risk of developing this condition: gestational age below 38 weeks, breastfeeding, a positive direct Coombs test, and the need for phototherapy in the first 72 hours of life (Arlettaz et al., 2007). In these infants, rebound is monitored following the cessation of phototherapy. Nevertheless, there is no requirement for the infant to remain in the hospital for follow-up of rebound bilirubin levels. The infant is discharged and subsequently monitored as an outpatient.

Blood Exchange

The objective is to forestall the development of kernicterus. In the event that the infant displays indications of bilirubin encephalopathy or when the serum bilirubin level reaches the treatment thresholds (Figure 5, Table 2) that have been determined in accordance with the postnatal age of the infant and potential risk factors for bilirubin neurotoxicity despite the administration of intensive phototherapy and IVIG when necessary, an exchange transfusion is performed (American Academy of Pediatrics, 2004). The emergency and intensive treatment approach ("escalation of care") in bilirubin levels approaching the exchange transfusion threshold (below 2 mg/dL) is illustrated in Figure 6 (Kemper et al., 2022).

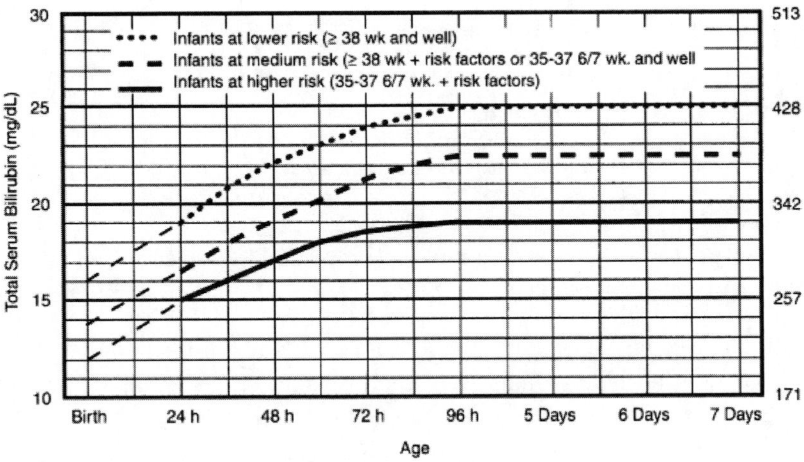

The dashed lines for the first 24 hours indicate uncertainty due to a wide range of clinical circumstances and a range of responses to phototherapy.

Immediate exchange transfusion is recommended if infant shows signs of acute bilirubin encephalopathy (hypertonia, arching, retrocollis, opisthotonos, fever, high pitched cry) or if TSB is ≥ 25 mg/dL (85 µmol/L) above these lines.

Risk factors – isoimmune hemolytic disease, G6PD deficiency, asphyxia, significant lethargy, temperature instability, sepsis, acidosis.

Measure serum albumin and calculate B/A ratio (See legend).

Use total bilirubin. Do not subtract direct reacting or conjugated bilirubin.

If infant is well and 35–37 6/7 wk (median risk) can individualize TSB levels for exchange based on actual gestational age.

Figure 5. Guidelines for exchange transfusion in infants 35 or more weeks gestation (American Academy of Pediatrics, 2004).

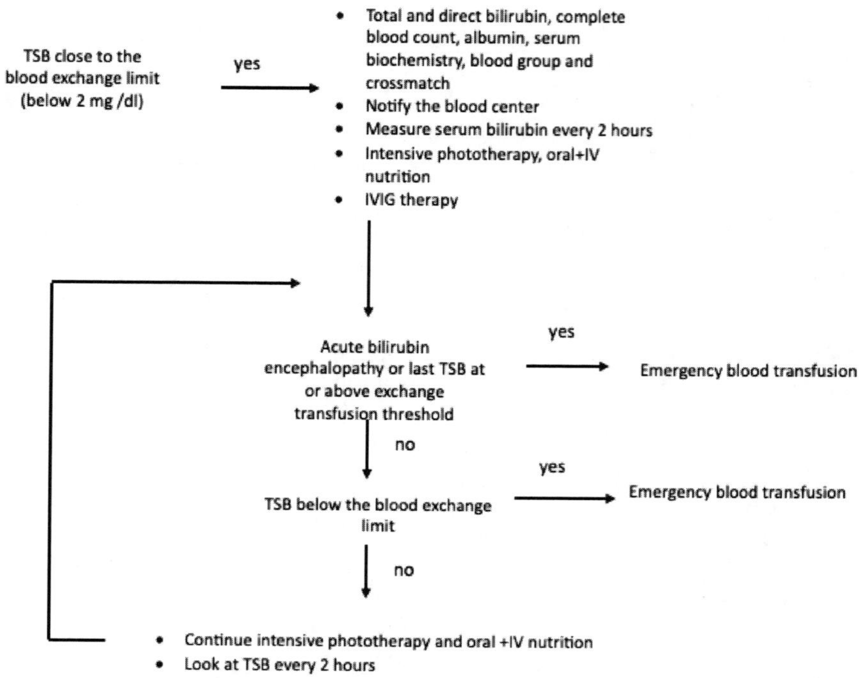

Figure 6. Emergency and intensive treatment approach for TSB levels close to exchange transfusion (Escalation of care).

In infants who have been discharged from the home setting, if the bilirubin value exceeds the levels indicated for exchange transfusion, intensive phototherapy is initiated while preparing for exchange transfusion. The bilirubin level is then monitored every 2-3 hours, and if it remains above these levels for 6 hours despite intensive phototherapy, exchange transfusion is performed. Exchange transfusion is indicated for infants who are hospitalized after birth and whose bilirubin levels exceed the threshold for exchange transfusion despite intensive phototherapy. Given that free bilirubin levels are elevated in the presence of low albumin levels, there is an increased risk of kernicterus at lower bilirubin levels. It is not advised to perform routine albumin infusion (NICE, 2010).

Blood Products to Be Selected and Their Properties

Blood Groups

Typically, the blood bank combines erythrocytes and plasma with the objective of reducing the hematocrit level to approximately 50%. In Rh incompatibility, an O-negative erythrocyte suspension with low A and B antigens and AB plasma is utilized; in ABO incompatibility, an O erythrocyte suspension compatible with the Rh group of the mother and the infant and often AB plasma are employed. Group A or B plasma may also be utilized, contingent upon the blood group of the infant (Falciglia & Greenwood, 2013; Girelli et al., 2015; Chang, 2008).

In the absence of incompatibility, a blood exchange should be conducted with blood from the same group as that of the child's blood group. In instances of subgroup incompatibility, the use of a blood type that is negative for the antigen responsible for the incompatibility is recommended. In the event that whole blood is utilized for an exchange transfusion, it is imperative that the blood be fresh, with a maximum age of 24 hours. In cases where blood exchange with the infant is required with minimal delay in the delivery room and intrauterine transfusion has already been performed, matching with the maternal blood is conducted. In all other instances, matching with the infant's blood is performed (American Academy of Pediatrics, 2004). The erythrocyte suspension is prepared with the utmost care, using the freshest possible material, with a maximum storage period of five days (Girelli et al., 2015; Chang, 2008). The appropriate blood for exchange, according to the blood groups of the infant and mother, is detailed in Table 4. The blood to be utilized for blood exchange is irradiated, filtered, and heated in a blood warmer or at room temperature (American Academy of Pediatrics, 2004; Falciglia & Greenwood, 2013). Double volume blood exchange is employed in the treatment of hyperbilirubinemia (American Academy of Pediatrics, 2004; Falciglia & Greenwood, 2013).

The estimated blood volume is 85 mL/kg in term infants and 100 mL/kg in preterm infants. Accordingly, the calculation is as follows:

- In a term infant, 2x 85 mL x weight (kg)
- In a preterm infant, 2x 100 mL x weight (kg).

Table 4. ABO erythrocyte suspension and plasma groups to be used during blood exchange

Newborn blood group	Mother blood group	First choice Erythrocyte suspension/full blood	Second choice Erythrocyte suspension	Plasma
A	O	O		A, AB
A	A	A	O	A, AB
A	B	O		A, AB
A	AB	A/fullblood	O	A, AB
B	O	O		B, AB
B	A	O		B, AB
B	B	B	O	B, AB
B	AB	B/fullblood	O	B, AB
O	O	O/fullblood		O, A, B, AB
O	A	O/fullblood		O, A, B, AB
O	B	O/fullblood		O, A, B, AB
AB	A	A	O	AB
AB	B	B	O	AB
AB	AB	AB/fullblood	A, B, O	AB
A, B, O, AB	?	O		AB

With double volume, 86% of the baby's blood is replaced. The duration of the blood exchange process is estimated to be between one and two hours. The maximum volume of blood that can be transfused at one time is 5 mL/kg.

Vital signs are monitored for 4–6 hours following the transfusion. The infant is not fed for a period of three hours, and when feeding is initiated, the infant is monitored closely for any signs of abdominal distension, vomiting, and necrotizing enterocolitis (Falciglia & Greenwood, 2013). Monitoring and treatment of thrombocytopenia, hypocalcemia, and hypoglycemia are conducted as necessary.

Pharmacological Treatment

Fenofibrate or Clofibrate

The efficacy of this treatment has been demonstrated in both term and preterm infants (Sharafi et al., 2010; Awad et al., 2021). It is not recommended that this be used as a routine treatment (Gholitabar et al., 2012).

Phenobarbital

It has been demonstrated that this substance increases the conjugation of bilirubin, as well as its excretion and bile flow. It can be employed in the diagnosis and treatment of Crigler-Najjar syndrome (Dennery, 2002). The routine use of this medication in the treatment of hyperbilirubinemia is not advised.

Reduction of Enterohepatic Circulation

The optimal approach is to initiate breastfeeding as soon as possible and to breastfeed frequently.

Metalloporphyrins

Tin (Sn) and zinc (Zn) protoporphyrin and mesoporphyrin have been demonstrated to reduce bilirubin production by competitively inhibiting both the oxygenase enzyme and heme metabolism. Nevertheless, they remain outside the scope of routine clinical practice (Dennery, 2002).

Intravenous Immunoglobulin (IVIG)

It is postulated that this mechanism prevents hemolysis by blocking Fc receptors in the reticuloendothelial system. Despite the ongoing controversy surrounding IVIG administration, numerous guidelines continue to recommend its use (Bratlid et al., 2011; Newman, 2007; NICE, 2010; Morioka & Nakamura, 2021; Morioka, 2018). In infants with Coombs (+) Rh or ABO incompatibility, standard IVIG (0.5-1 g/kg in 2 hours) may be administered in the presence of elevated serum bilirubin levels despite intensive phototherapy or bilirubin levels approaching the exchange limit (2-3 mg/dL). This treatment may be repeated after 12 hours if necessary (American Academy of Pediatrics, 2004; Bratlid et al., 2011; Newman, 2007; NICE, 2010; Morioka & Nakamura, 2018).

Table 5. Bilirubin values (mg/dL) for exchange transfusion limits in the first 24 hours in infants below 38 weeks of gestational age (NICE, 2010)

Gestational age	6 hour	12 hour	18 hour
23–28	5	6	7
29–33	6	7	8
34–37	6	7	9

Treatment Principles for Jaundice in the First 24 Hours

Jaundice occurring within the first 24 hours is invariably indicative of a pathological process. A TSB level is obtained, and a blood exchange is initiated. The indications for blood exchange in infants are as follows:

- In infants with a gestational age of 38 weeks or greater: In the event that cord bilirubin is examined and the bilirubin level is found to exceed 5 mg/dL, the infant will undergo intensive phototherapy in preparation for an exchange transfusion. The rate of bilirubin increase will then be monitored. The specified limit is 9 mg/dL at the sixth hour, 12 mg/dL at the 12th hour, and above 15 mg/dL at the 18th hour (NICE, 2010).
- In infants with a gestational age of less than 38 weeks: The values presented in Table 5 serve as the basis for further analysis.
- In the event of an elevation in bilirubin levels exceeding 0.5 mg/dL per hour, despite the implementation of intensive phototherapy, an exchange transfusion is conducted.
- In the event that the rate of bilirubin elevation is below 0.5 mg/dL, the course of intensive phototherapy is continued.
- IVIG is given if necessary.

Monitoring

It is recommended that these infants be monitored for hearing, vision, and neurodevelopmental outcomes. Neonatal hearing screening (ABR: auditory brainstem evoked responses) should be repeated before discharge, even in cases where the screening was performed on babies undergoing exchange transfusion. In infants with hyperbilirubinemia, clinical ABR evaluation should be conducted before the sixth month of age (American Academy of Pediatrics, 2007).

Conclusion

In conclusion, the objective of neonatal jaundice treatment is to mitigate the risk of bilirubin neurotoxicity. To this end, newborns should undergo jaundice evaluation prior to discharge, and mothers should receive comprehensive nutrition education. Furthermore, a follow-up plan should be established.

References

Ahlfors, C. E., Amin, S. B., & Parker, A. E. (2009). Unbound bilirubin predicts abnormal automated auditory brainstem response in a diverse newborn population. *Journal of Perinatology, 29*(4), 305–309. https://doi.org/10.1038/jp.2008.199.

American Academy of Pediatrics Subcommittee on Hyperbilirubinemia. (2004). Management of hyperbilirubinemia in the newborn infant 35 or more weeks of gestation. *Pediatrics, 114*(1), 297–316. https://doi.org/10.1542/peds.114.1.297.

American Academy of Pediatrics, Joint Committee on Infant Hearing. (2007). Year 2007 position statement: Principles and guidelines for early hearing detection and intervention programs. *Pediatrics, 120*(4), 898–921. https://doi.org/10.1542/peds.2007-2333.

Arlettaz, R., Blumberg, A., Buetti, L., Fahnenstich, H., Mieth, D., & Roth-Kleiner, M. (2007, July). Assessment and treatment of jaundice in newborn infants 35 0/7 or more weeks of gestation. *Swiss Society of Neonatology, 1*, 1–4.

Awad, M. H., Amer, S., Hafez, M., Nour, I., & Shabaan, A. (2021). Fenofibrate as an adjuvant to phototherapy in pathological unconjugated hyperbilirubinemia in neonates: A randomized control trial. *Journal of Perinatology, 41*(4), 865–872. https://doi.org/10.1038/s41372-020-00861-2.

Azzuqa, A., & Watchko, J. F. (2017). Conjunctival icterus: An important but neglected sign of clinically relevant hyperbilirubinemia in jaundiced neonates. *Current Pediatric Reviews, 13*(3), 169–175. https://doi.org/10.2174/1573396313666170718145535.

Bhutani, V. K., Johnson, L., & Sivieri, E. M. (1999). Predictive ability of a predischarge hour-specific serum bilirubin for subsequent significant hyperbilirubinemia in healthy term and near-term newborns. *Pediatrics, 103*(1), 6–14. https://doi.org/10.1542/peds.103.1.6.

Bratlid, D., Nakstad, B., & Hansen, T. W. (2011). National guidelines for treatment of jaundice in the newborn. *Acta Paediatrica, 100*(4), 499–505. https://doi.org/10.1111/j.1651-2227.2010.02104.x.

Cayabyab, R., & Ramanathan, R. (2019). High unbound bilirubin for age: A neurotoxin with major effects on the developing brain. *Pediatric Research, 85*(2), 183–190. https://doi.org/10.1038/s41390-018-0224-4.

Chang, T. T. (2008). Transfusion therapy in critically ill children. *Pediatrics and Neonatology, 49*(2), 5–12. https://doi.org/10.1016/S1875-9572(08)60004-2.

Chen, C. M., Liu, S. H., Lai, C. C., Hwang, C. C., & Hsu, H. H. (2002). Changing position does not improve the efficacy of conventional phototherapy. *Acta Paediatrica Taiwanica, 43*(5), 255–258.

Dennery, P. A. (2002). Pharmacological interventions for the treatment of neonatal jaundice. *Seminars in Neonatology, 7*(2), 111–119. https://doi.org/10.1053/siny.2002.0098.

Falciglia, H. S., & Greenwood, C. S. (2013, October). Double volume exchange transfusion: Review of the "ins and outs." *NeoReviews, 14*(10), e513–e520. https://doi.org/10.1542/neo.14-10-e513.

Flaherman, V. J., Maisels, M. J., & Academy of Breastfeeding Medicine. (2017). ABM Clinical Protocol #22: Guidelines for management of jaundice in the breastfeeding infant 35 weeks or more of gestation - Revised 2017. *Breastfeeding Medicine, 12*(5), 250–257. https://doi.org/10.1089/bfm.2017.29042.vjf.

Gholitabar, M., McGuire, H., Rennie, J., Manning, D., & Lai, R. (2012). Clofibrate in combination with phototherapy for unconjugated neonatal hyperbilirubinaemia. *Cochrane Database of Systematic Reviews, 12*(12), CD009017. https://doi.org/10.1002/14651858.CD009017.pub2.

Girelli, G., Antoncecchi, S., Casadei, A. M., Del Vecchio, A., Isernia, P., Motta, M., Regoli, D., Romagnoli, C., Tripodi, G., & Velati, C. (2015). Recommendations for transfusion therapy in neonatology. *Blood Transfusion, 13*(3), 484–497. https://doi.org/10.2450/2015.0113-15.

Gothwal, S., Singh, N., Sitaraman, S., Choudhary, R., Meena, K. K., Bairwa, G. S., Bairwa, M., & Jeevan, A. (2021). Efficacy of transcutaneous bilirubinometry as compared to serum bilirubin in preterm newborn during phototherapy. *European Journal of Pediatrics, 180*(8), 2629–2636. https://doi.org/10.1007/s00431-021-04148-2.

Grohmann, K., Roser, M., Rolinski, B., Kadow, I., Müller, C., Goerlach-Graw, A., Nauck, M., & Küster, H. (2006). Bilirubin measurement for neonates: Comparison of 9 frequently used methods. *Pediatrics, 117*(4), 1174–1183. https://doi.org/10.1542/peds.2005-0590.

Hansen, T. W., Nietsch, L., Norman, E., Bjerre, J. V., Hascoet, J. M., Mreihil, K., & Ebbesen, F. (2009). Reversibility of acute intermediate phase bilirubin encephalopathy. *Acta Paediatrica, 98*(10), 1689–1694. https://doi.org/10.1111/j.1651-2227.2009.01409.x.

Johnson, L., & Bhutani, V. K. (2011). The clinical syndrome of bilirubin-induced neurologic dysfunction. *Seminars in Perinatology, 35*(3), 101–113. https://doi.org/10.1053/j.semperi.2011.02.003.

Kaplan, M., Merlob, P., & Regev, R. (2008). Israel guidelines for the management of neonatal hyperbilirubinemia and prevention of kernicterus. *Journal of Perinatology, 28*(6), 389–397. https://doi.org/10.1038/jp.2008.20.

Kaplan, M., Wong, R. J., Sibley, E., & Stevenson, D. K. (2015). Neonatal jaundice and liver diseases. In R. J. Martin, A. A. Fanaroff, & M. C. Walsh (Eds.), *Fanaroff & Martin's neonatal-perinatal medicine: Diseases of the fetus and infant* (10th ed., pp. 1618–1673). Elsevier Saunders.

Kemper, A. R., Newman, T. B., Slaughter, J. L., Maisels, M. J., Watchko, J. F., Downs, S. M., Grout, R. W., Bundy, D. G., Stark, A. R., Bogen, D. L., Holmes, A. V., Feldman-Winter, L. B., Bhutani, V. K., Brown, S. R., Maradiaga Panayotti, G. M., Okechukwu, K., Rappo, P. D., & Russell, T. L. (2022). Clinical practice guideline revision: Management of hyperbilirubinemia in the newborn infant 35 or more weeks of gestation. *Pediatrics, 150*(3), e2022058859. https://doi.org/10.1542/peds.2022-058859.

Maisels, M. J. (2004, July). Use TcB as a screening tool for jaundiced newborns. *AAP News, 25*(1), 9–23.

Maisels, M. J., Bhutani, V. K., Bogen, D., Newman, T. B., Stark, A. R., & Watchko, J. F. (2009). Hyperbilirubinemia in the newborn infant ≥35 weeks' gestation: An update with clarifications. *Pediatrics, 124*(4), 1193–1198. https://doi.org/10.1542/peds.2009-0329.

Morioka, I. (2018). Hyperbilirubinemia in preterm infants in Japan: New treatment criteria. *Pediatrics International, 60*(8), 684–690. https://doi.org/10.1111/ped.13635.

Morioka, I., & Nakamura, H. (2021). Treatment criteria for infants with hyperbilirubinemia in Japan. *Seminars in Perinatology, 45*(1), 151352. https://doi.org/10.1016/j.semperi.2020.151352.

National Institute of Child Health and Clinical Excellence. (2010, May). Jaundice in newborn babies under 28 days. *NICE Clinical Guideline*. https://www.nice.org.uk/guidance/cg98.

Newman, J. (2007). Re: Guidelines for detection, management and prevention of hyperbilirubinemia in term and late preterm newborn infants (35 or more weeks' gestation) - Summary. *Paediatrics & Child Health, 12*(7), 613. https://doi.org/10.1093/pch/12.7.613.

Olusanya, B. O., Kaplan, M., & Hansen, T. W. R. (2018). Neonatal hyperbilirubinaemia: A global perspective. *The Lancet Child & Adolescent Health, 2*(8), 610–620. https://doi.org/10.1016/S2352-4642(18)30139-1.

Palma, J. P., & Arain, Y. H. (2016). Development of a web-based decision support tool to operationalize and optimize management of hyperbilirubinemia in preterm infants. *Clinics in Perinatology, 43*(2), 375–383. https://doi.org/10.1016/j.clp.2016.01.009.

Preer, G. L., & Philipp, B. L. (2011). Understanding and managing breast milk jaundice. *Archives of Disease in Childhood. Fetal and Neonatal Edition, 96*(6), F461–F466. https://doi.org/10.1136/adc.2010.184416.

Sharafi, R., Mortazavi, Z., Sharafi, S., & Parashkouh, R. M. (2010). The effect of clofibrate on decreasing serum bilirubin in healthy term neonates under home phototherapy. *Iranian Journal of Pediatrics, 20*(1), 48–52.

Shinwell, E. S., Sciaky, Y., & Karplus, M. (2002). Effect of position changing on bilirubin levels during phototherapy. *Journal of Perinatology, 22*(3), 226–229. https://doi.org/10.1038/sj.jp.7210678.

Smith, H. A., & Becker, G. E. (2016). Early additional food and fluids for healthy breastfed full-term infants. *Cochrane Database of Systematic Reviews, 2016*(8), CD006462. https://doi.org/10.1002/14651858.CD006462.pub4.

Taylor, J. A., Burgos, A. E., Flaherman, V., Chung, E. K., Simpson, E. A., Goyal, N. K., Von Kohorn, I., Dhepyasuwan, N., & Better Outcomes Through Research for Newborns Network. (2015). Discrepancies between transcutaneous and serum bilirubin measurements. *Pediatrics, 135*(2), 224–231. https://doi.org/10.1542/peds.2014-1919.

Vreman, H. J., Verter, J., Oh, W., Fanaroff, A. A., Wright, L. L., Lemons, J. A., Shankaran, S., Tyson, J. E., Korones, S. B., Bauer, C. R., Stoll, B. J., Papile, L. A., Donovan, E. F., Ehrenkranz, R. A., & Stevenson, D. K. (1996). Interlaboratory variability of bilirubin measurements. *Clinical Chemistry, 42*(6 Pt 1), 869–873.

Watchko, J. F., & Maisels, M. J. (2018). Treatment of hyperbilirubinemia in newborns. In G. Buonocore, R. Bracci, & M. Weindling (Eds.), *Neonatology* (2nd ed., pp. 1185–1206). Springer International Publishing.

Chapter 18

Neonatal Fever

Ömer Yusuf Erdurmuş*, MD
Department of Emergency Service, Ordu State Hospital, Ordu, Turkey

Abstract

The neonatal period in infants covers the first month after birth. Although the cause of fever seen during this period is generally thought to be due to infection, it can also develop due to reasons such as increased ambient temperature, fluid loss, central nervous system damage, and hyperthyroidism. In addition, high fever due to the incomplete development of the immune system in the neonatal period is very important, and the baby should be evaluated urgently, and necessary treatments should be applied within the indication. Many studies conducted on newborns and infants admitted to the hospital with fever indicate that no bacterial agent is found in the etiology of fever and that viral etiologies cause this condition in 60-72% of the cases. Although the etiology is mostly viral in newborns admitted to the hospital with fever, serious bacterial infections can also be seen. The most common bacterial infection detected in newborns is urinary tract infection, and the most common pathogenic agent is *Escherichia coli* bacteria. There is no common protocol accepted worldwide regarding the management of newborns admitted to the hospital with fever. However, the general approach is to evaluate babies with physical examination and tests and, if necessary, to administer antibiotics and antipyretic treatment in the hospital or at home.

Keywords: bacterial infection, fever, neonatal

---

* Corresponding Author's Email: yerdurmus@icloud.com

In: Current Approaches to Newborn Emergencies
Editors: Zuhal Keskin Sarılar and Serap Samut Bülbül
ISBN: 979-8-89530-999-5

Introduction

The neonatal period in babies includes the first month after birth. Although infection is generally considered the cause of fever seen during this period, it can develop due to reasons such as increased ambient temperature, dehydration, central nervous system damage, and hyperthyroidism. Sudden changes in body temperature affect enzyme activity and cause the metabolism to not function properly. Thus, damage to cells, tissues, and organs, and in severe cases, death can occur. For all these reasons and especially due to the fact that the immune system of neonatal babies is not fully developed, high fever is a very important symptom and should be evaluated and treated urgently (Bülbül et al., 2017).

There is no common protocol worldwide regarding the management of neonates admitted to hospitals with fever. However, the general approach is to evaluate babies with physical examination and tests and, if indicated, to administer antibiotics and antipyretic treatment in the hospital or at home (Rehm, 2001). Especially in bacterial infections, when early diagnosis and treatment are not applied, mortality and morbidity rates are considerably higher than in other age groups, and the anxiety it creates in parents makes neonates special compared to other age groups. Therefore, after the necessary tests and examinations are frequently performed, neonatal babies should be hospitalized and monitored within the indication. However, it is known that hospitalizing all neonatal babies with fever and applying antibiotic treatment causes emotional stress in the families of the babies, the development of iatrogenic complications related to hospitalization, and a significant increase in unnecessary hospitalizations. Therefore, in light of current literature, various low-risk criteria are routinely used to identify serious bacterial infections. The purpose of these criteria is to monitor neonates in the hospital without antibiotics or to monitor them as outpatients without hospitalization (Jain et al., 2014).

Despite all this information, the fact that the developed protocols and criteria are valid, especially for the first three months of life, and are not criteria applied only to the neonatal period has caused the failure to establish an accepted consensus in the treatment and examination of patients.

Definition and Measurement Methods of High Fever in Neonates

Although the exact mechanism is not fully determined, it is thought that fever is caused by the mismatch between heat production and consumption. Normal body temperature in neonatal babies is between 36.6 and 37.5°C, and in the literature, a body temperature value measured rectally in the neonatal period is considered a high fever when it is ≥38°C. Although body temperature assessments made by touching, from the axillary region or from the tympanic membrane, are less accurate than rectal measurements, it is known that they correlate with rectal measurements at a rate of 80%. However, rectal measurements are still the most accurate and precise measurement, especially in neonates (Katz-Sidlow et al., 2009).

Before rectal measurement, the baby should be laid in the prone position, while the baby's waist area is fixed with one hand, the thermometer with lubricating gel should be slowly pushed approximately 2 cm into the anus opening, the thermometer should be held between the 2nd and 3rd fingers, and the baby's gluteal region should be supported with the palm of the hand, and after waiting for 2 minutes, the thermometer should be removed and the body temperature should be assessed. It should be known that in measurements made from the axillary region, body temperature is approximately 1°C lower than in rectal measurements and that 30-40% of febrile babies may be missed in body temperature measurements made from the tympanic membrane. In measurements made from the axillary region, the thermometer should be placed at the top of the axilla, and at least 3 minutes should be waited (Smith, 2014).

Diagnosis and Evaluation

After detecting high fever in neonates, the second step is to evaluate the baby clinically. If it is observed that the baby is overdressed before the clinical evaluation, and it is thought that the high body temperature may be due to this situation, the baby's excess clothing should be removed, and the body temperature should be measured again after 30 minutes. If a high fever is detected in the first measurement or in cases such as the aforementioned issue and similar situations, the physical examination of the babies should be performed carefully. Physical examination is very important in this evaluation performed in neonates. The neonates's current systemic findings should be carefully examined, and a focused physical examination should be performed in light of this information. If signs of infection are detected in babies as a result of the clinical evaluation, the patients should be included in the risk group (Pantell et al., 2021).

Etiology of Fever in Neonates

Although the mechanisms that cause fever in neonates have not been fully elucidated in the light of current literature, the most logical explanation is that fever results from a disorder between heat production and consumption. According to this hypothesis, the normal thermal set point in the hypothalamus is pulled upwards by the effect of various immunogenic pyrogens, primarily prostaglandin E2, and as a result, the current body temperature is first maintained through peripheral vasoconstriction and then stabilized by increasing heat production, providing the body temperature target value (Rehm, 2001).

In neonates, there may be an increase in body temperature due to reasons other than immunogenic pyrogens in the fever response. These reasons are listed as follows:

1. Since the sweating mechanism is not effective in neonatal babies, heat loss is low, and body temperature can increase rapidly due to reasons such as excessive environmental temperature or excessive dressing.
2. In healthy, exclusively breastfed babies, there may be an increase in body temperature due to dehydration caused by low breast milk production on the 3rd or 4th postnatal day. This diagnosis should be considered, especially in babies receiving fluid therapy, if the fever drops.
3. In babies with hypoxic-ischemic encephalopathy, an increase in body temperature may be observed in the presence of hypothalamic damage.
4. In the case of status epilepticus, an increase in the baby's metabolic activity may also cause an increase in body temperature.
5. Although the exact cause is not known, an increase in body temperature is observed in the first hours postnatally in babies of mothers who received epidural anesthesia at birth, and it is reported

that these babies are evaluated more frequently for sepsis, and antibiotic use is higher.

6. An increase in body temperature can be observed in the postnatal follow-up of babies with malformations/masses in other parts of the central nervous system and intracranial hemorrhage.

Sepsis, which can be seen in neonates, is a rare cause of high fever. In neonates with serious bacterial infections, there may be no increase in body temperature; on the contrary, paradoxically, hypothermia is more common in neonates with sepsis. However, fever may be the only clinical finding in neonates with serious bacterial infections. Other findings that may accompany sepsis, such as decreased activity and sucking, restlessness, and convulsions, should definitely be questioned in the anamnesis. In the physical examination, causes such as cellulitis, septic arthritis, osteomyelitis, omphalitis, and the presence of a central venous catheter should be carefully evaluated in terms of the source of infection (İmamoğlu, 2018). In the case of fever seen in the early postnatal period, it should be questioned in the history whether the mother has received epidural anesthesia. The baby's weight loss and fluid intake should be evaluated, and the diagnosis of dehydration fever should not be neglected. The temperature of the environment where the baby is located and whether the baby is dressed in thicker clothes than normal should be evaluated. In the event of an increase in body temperature secondary to an increase in ambient temperature, there may be redness all over the body and an increase in temperature in the hands and feet (Bülbül et al., 2017).

Physical Examination in Neonates with Fever

Since their immune systems are not fully developed, and physical examination findings may be vague, all neonates with fever should definitely be evaluated for infection, even if their general condition is good. The risk of bacterial infection in neonates increases in the presence of sick appearance, rectal body temperature of 38.6°C and above, prematurity (early birth before 37 weeks of gestation), concomitant congenital anomaly, chromosomal anomaly, chronic disease, history of antibiotic use in the last week, and a history of antepartum fever, premature membrane rupture, genital HSV infection, and culture positivity in the mother, and the source of infection should definitely be investigated. It is thought that the higher the fever, the higher the risk of secondary fever due to bacterial infection (Jain et al., 2014).

During the physical examination of neonates, the baby's clothes should be completely removed. Vital signs should be evaluated completely. The presence of tachypnea or hypoxemia in the baby can usually suggest a lower respiratory tract infection in the preliminary diagnosis, and in this case, lung auscultation and imaging methods should definitely be used. In the event that the baby is constantly crying and restless, meningitis should definitely be included in the preliminary diagnosis, and a detailed neurological examination should definitely be performed. Bulged fontanelle cases with meningitis can also be seen, but meningeal irritation signs such as neck stiffness are generally not detected in this age group (Bülbül et al., 2017).

Laboratory Tests and Imaging Methods

Laboratory tests and imaging methods, if indicated, have an important place in determining the etiology of fever in neonates and in the approach to diagnosis and treatment. In general, the tests requested from infants are complete blood count, C-reactive protein (CRP), procalcitonin, absolute neutrophil count, absolute band count, and blood culture (Bilavsky et al., 2010). However, these tests should not be requested routinely but should be evaluated in light of the information obtained from the patient's anamnesis and physical examination, and should be evaluated within the indication. Depending on the etiology, urine analysis can also be performed on patients, and sampling is usually performed via bladder catheterization or suprapubic aspiration. Urine analysis has low sensitivity and specificity in detecting urinary tract infection in the neonatal and early infancy (Nosrati et al., 2014). In some studies, evaluating bacterial infections in neonates, urinary tract infection is frequently stated as an overlooked diagnosis. Therefore, as stated in the literature, advanced urine analysis is recommended instead of standard urine analysis in determining the infection because the sensitivity and specificity of advanced urine analysis are higher in determining urinary tract infection (Bressan et al., 2010).

Cerebrospinal fluid (CSF) sampling can be performed in patients suspected of having a central nervous system infection. Especially in neonatal babies with high fever and diarrhea, stool analysis should be added to the requested laboratory tests, and in this test, stool cell count and stool culture can be examined (Nosrati et al., 2014). Apart from these tests, there are also tests that can be requested, although rarely, according to etiology. For example, if a local infection focus is detected in a febrile neonate (cellulitis, otitis, arthritis, etc.), local fluid cell count, gram staining, and fluid culture can be taken. Due to the difficulty of application, viral culture is not routinely performed in neonatal babies, but these tests can be requested depending on the etiology. Especially, RSV and influenza nasal swab kits are frequently used in infancy, and there is not enough information in the literature regarding the routine use of these tests in the neonatal period (Bressan et al., 2010).

In defining serious bacterial infection in neonates, studies have reported that absolute neutrophil count and absolute band count values have higher accuracy rates than leukocyte count. In another study on the subject, it has been reported that CRP value has higher accuracy rates than leukocyte count, absolute neutrophil count, and procalcitonin values. However, a CRP study that includes only febrile neonatal infants in defining serious bacterial infection could not be determined as a result of the literature evaluation (Bressan et al., 2010).

Imaging methods are quite limited in neonates where fever etiology is investigated, and the evaluation should be made according to the benefit-harm principle. Direct lung radiography is recommended, especially in infants with respiratory tract pathological findings, and has a very important place in determining the cause of high fever and in managing the treatment and follow-up of infants admitted to intensive care. Ultrasonography (USG) and magnetic resonance imaging (MRI) can be considered advanced examinations within the indication and can be used in treatment management and differential diagnosis (Jain et al., 2014).

Bacterial Infection in Neonates

In many studies conducted on neonates and infants who presented to the hospital with fever, it was determined that no bacterial agent was found in the etiology of fever and that this condition was caused by viral etiologies in 60-72% of the cases. Among viral pathogens, rhinovirus is the most frequently detected, followed by respiratory syncytial virus (RSV), influenza virus, and parainfluenza virus. Viral infections in neonates occur through vertical transmission from the mother during birth or through transmission from family members or health care personnel in the postnatal period. Viruses that can cause serious illness in neonates are herpes simplex virus (HSV), varicella-zoster virus, enterovirus, influenza virus, adenovirus, and respiratory syncytial virus. Due to the inadequacy of the T cell-mediated immune response, viral infections can cause serious illness in neonates compared to other age groups.

Neonates with viral infections may also develop bacterial infections, which further increases the risk (Garcia et al., 2012).

Viral antigen testing is important in the diagnosis of viral infection. While rapid viral antigen tests are quite reliable in infancy, there is not enough information about the reliability of this test in the neonatal period. However, rapid viral antigen testing in infants with viral upper respiratory tract symptoms is quite useful in differential diagnosis, and the level of recommendation has increased in recent studies. Therefore, in recent years, rapid immunoassay method RSV and Influenza A/B virus antigen testing has been recommended in infants with respiratory tract infections, and PCR screening of fluids in infants with a preliminary diagnosis of enterovirus has been recommended, and it has been stated that the test should be used more frequently (Aronson et al., 2015).

Although the etiology is mostly viral in neonatal babies who apply to the hospital with fever, serious bacterial infections can also be seen. The most common cause of these bacterial infections is urinary tract infection. Urinary tract infection (UTI) is diagnosed by producing a single pathogenic agent >1000 colonies/ml in suprapubic aspiration or >10000 colonies/ml in urine obtained by catheterization. When studies are examined, it is reported that the frequency of urinary tract infection is seen in 3-14% of all febrile babies. When the distribution of urinary tract infection among bacterial infection agents is examined, it is known that it is seen with a frequency of 15-90% (Hui et al., 2012).

The frequency of bacterial meningitis and/or aseptic meningitis, another etiological cause in febrile infants aged 3 months and under, has been reported to be between 0.2% and 14.0%. In studies that only included infants in the neonatal period, the frequency of bacterial meningitis has been reported as 0.5% and 4.4% (Jain et al., 2014). The need for lumbar puncture in febrile infants continues to be an important topic of discussion in the literature. Lumbar puncture application criteria, routine application methods, or the rate at which lumbar puncture is performed, especially in febrile infants, have not been specified. However, studies have shown that meningitis diagnosis is missed in febrile neonates who have a low risk of meningitis and who do not undergo lumbar puncture. Therefore, lumbar puncture is very important in the evaluation of etiology, and neonates should be evaluated meticulously in terms of this examination. The presence of 20 or more leukocytes per mm^3 in direct examination of the cerebrospinal fluid (CSF), CSF glucose being less than 2/3 of the simultaneous blood glucose level, and CSF protein value being over 100 mg/dl in term infants and over 150 mg/dl in preterm infants are evaluated in favor of meningitis (Aronson et al., 2015).

When the agents that generally cause serious bacterial infections in febrile neonates are evaluated, it is reported that *Escherichia coli* bacteria are the most frequently isolated bacteria in culture growths, and their frequency is around 60%. *Escherichia coli* bacteria are found to be the causative agent in 68% of urinary tract infections, 24.3% of bacteremia, and 8% of bacterial meningitis. Group B Streptococcus and Streptococcus pneumoniae are the most common agents in both bacteremia and pneumonia cases, while Staphylococcus aureus is known to be the most common agent in local infections (Bülbül et al., 2017).

Criteria and Frequency of Serious Bacterial Infection

As a result of our literature review, serious bacterial infection criteria are generally grouped under two main headings. These are:

1. The production of bacteria that are considered pathogenic in one or more cultures.
2. The presence of infections that are usually detected together with bacterial agents.

Soft tissue infections other than these can be diagnosed with physical examination findings, regardless of bacterial pathogen production. Similarly, pneumonia diagnosis in neonatal babies can be made by detecting new infiltration on chest X-ray in babies with typical clinical findings and evaluating the findings. It is known that the prevalence of serious bacterial infection in febrile babies younger than three months is between 7.1% and19.7% (Bülbül et al., 2017). In the subgroup distribution of febrile infants, the prevalence of serious bacterial infection in the neonatal period is reported as 9-28%, while this frequency is stated to be 7.1% in 2-3 month old infants. In studies conducted on febrile neonatal infants, it was determined that serious bacterial infection was seen in 31.9% of neonatal infants aged 7-14 days, 3.3% in neonatal infants aged 15-21 days, and 18.3% in infants older than 21 days (Katz-Sidlow et al., 2009). As a result of the studies, it has been determined that the frequency of serious bacterial infections in febrile babies in the neonatal period is higher than in febrile babies in early infancy, which reveals how important this issue is.

Criteria for Exclusion of Serious Bacterial Infection

Rochester criteria are widely used to exclude serious bacterial infection in febrile infants and to prevent unnecessary examination and treatment (Dagan et al., 1985). Alternatively, Boston and Philadelphia criteria can be used. The age distributions for which the protocols are applied differ, and this should be taken into consideration when evaluating infants. Philadelphia criteria are used for infants aged 29-60 days, Rochester criteria for infants aged 60 days and under, and Boston criteria for infants aged 28-89 days. Studies have shown that when the protocols are applied to infants younger than 28 days and older than 28 days, the sensitivity of Boston and Philadelphia protocols is lower in infants younger than 28 days (Jaskiewicz et al., 1994). Rochester Criteria should be used as exclusion criteria in febrile neonates because they provide more accurate results in detecting cases with a low risk of serious bacterial infection. As a result of the studies conducted, the sensitivity of the Rochester criteria was determined as 92%, specificity as 55%, positive predictive value (PPV) as 12.2%, and negative predictive value (NPV) as 98.9% (Aronson et al., 2015). Babies who have 1 or more of these criteria are at high risk for serious bacterial infection, while babies who do not meet any of the criteria are at very low risk for serious bacterial infection (Table 1). However, studies have shown that the false-positive rate for identifying serious bacterial infections is significantly higher in neonatal babies than in older babies (Jaskiewicz et al., 1994). There is a need for new studies that include only neonatal babies on the subject, as the current protocols for approaching febrile babies in infancy are not valid in the evaluation of febrile babies in the neonatal period, and these protocols cannot be used for neonatal babies (Yarden-Bilavsky et al., 2014).

Table 1. Rochester Criteria

Age ≤ 60 days
Rectal temperature ≥ 38 degrees Celsius in emergency department or parental history of equivalent rectal temperature
Infant appears generally well
Born at term
No evidence of focal infection (skin, soft tissue etc.)
No antibiotics at the time of presentation or any time in life
No chronic or underlying illness

No previous hospitalizations
Not treated for unexplained hyperbilirubinemia
Not hospitalized longer than the mother after delivery
No perinatal antibiotics
Normal lab values -WBC 5,000-15,000 mm^3 -Band neutrophils $\leq$ 1,500 mm^3 -Urine WBC $\leq$ 10 WBC/hpf -If diarrhea is present, fecal leukocytes $\leq$ 5 WBC/hpf

Treatment

In neonates with high fever, symptoms such as weakness, not sucking, tendency to sleep, syncope, change in respiratory rate, restlessness, excessive crying or not crying at all, pale skin color, and less activity can be observed. The first thing to do in neonate with high fever with these symptoms is to take off the baby's clothes and adjust the room temperature to 21-22°C. The baby should be dressed in thin clothes that will increase his/her comfort. If the body temperature continues to be above 38°C despite these applications, antipyretic drugs should be applied. Acetylsalicylic acid, one of the antipyretic agents, has been used as the first-line treatment method for a long time as a traditional treatment method. However, the positive relationship between acetylsalicylic acid and Reye Syndrome in studies has decreased the prevalence of use in children. Other options stand out as paracetamol and ibuprofen. In cases of fever of 39°C and above that do not respond to antipyretics, bathing with warm water of 29-30°C is recommended (Jain et al., 2014).

In infants with poor general condition and clinically unstable conditions, antimicrobial treatment should be started rapidly without waiting for the results of the examination. In the presence of septic shock, intravenous fluid treatment should be performed according to the patient's values and by calculating the fluid deficit. After blood, urine, and CSF samples are taken, antibiotic treatment can usually be started empirically in the light of preliminary diagnoses until the culture results are available. In the presence of a clinical vesicular rash, convulsions, toxic appearance, lethargy, increased cells in CSF, elevated transaminases, or a history of maternal genital HSV infection, and especially if these symptoms and findings occur within the first 3 postnatal weeks, HSV infection should definitely be considered in the differential diagnosis of a febrile neonate. HSV is detected as the causative agent in 0.3% of febrile infants. Intravenous acyclovir treatment should be added to empirical treatment by sending viral culture/PCR from suspicious lesions and HSV type 1 and type 2 PCR from blood/CSF samples. Enteroviruses are one of the common viral infection agents, especially in cases of fever in neonates encountered in summer and autumn, and in case of clinical suspicion, enterovirus PCR examination from blood and CSF samples is recommended. However, there is no effective antiviral agent against enteroviruses, and symptomatic treatment is applied (Rehm, 2001).

Conclusion

High fever is a common finding in neonates and determining the cause is very important. In particular, the possibility of serious bacterial infection should be carefully evaluated, and diagnostic tests and treatment should be started quickly. Until an acceptable common protocol is developed for diagnosis and treatment, tests should be requested within the indications after the evaluation of the babies in light of anamnesis and physical examination, and a treatment plan should be implemented. Urinary tract infection is the most common bacterial infection detected in neonates, and the most frequently detected pathogenic agent is *Escherichia coli* bacteria. There is no commonly accepted consensus in the evaluation, examination, and treatment planning of febrile neonatal babies. The low-risk criteria in the Rochester, Philadelphia, and Boston protocols are not sufficient to exclude serious bacterial infection in febrile neonates, and there is a need for criteria that include only neonatal babies on the subject.

References

Aronson, P. L., Thurm, C., Williams, D. J., Nigrovic, L. E., Alpern, E. R., Tieder, J. S., Shah, S. S., McCulloh, R. J., Balamuth, F., Schondelmeyer, A. C., Alessandrini, E. A., Browning, W. L., Myers, A. L., Neuman, M. I., & Febrile Young Infant Research Collaborative. (2015). Association of clinical practice guidelines with emergency department management of febrile infants ≤56 days of age. *Journal of Hospital Medicine*, *10*(6), 358–365. https://doi.org/10.1002/jhm.2329.

Bilavsky, E., Yarden-Bilavsky, H., Amir, J., & Ashkenazi, S. (2010). Should complete blood count be part of the evaluation of febrile infants aged ≤2 months? *Acta Paediatrica (Oslo, Norway: 1992)*, *99*(9), 1380–1384. https://doi.org/10.1111/j.1651-2227.2010.01810.x.

Bressan, S., Andreola, B., Cattelan, F., Zangardi, T., Perilongo, G., & Da Dalt, L. (2010). Predicting severe bacterial infections in well-appearing febrile neonates: Laboratory markers accuracy and duration of fever. *The Pediatric Infectious Disease Journal*, *29*(3), 227–232. https://doi.org/10.1097/INF.0b013e3181b9a086.

Bülbül, A., Kıray Baş, E., & Uslu, S. (2017). Management of febrile neonate. *SiSli Etfal Hastanesi Tip Bulteni/The Medical Bulletin of Sisli Hospital*, 26–31. https://doi.org/10.5350/SEMB.20161225114041.

Dagan, R., Powell, K. R., Hall, C. B., & Menegus, M. A. (1985). Identification of infants unlikely to have serious bacterial infection although hospitalized for suspected sepsis. *The Journal of Pediatrics*, *107*(6), 855–860. https://doi.org/10.1016/S0022-3476(85)80175-X.

Garcia, S., Mintegi, S., Gomez, B., Barron, J., Pinedo, M., Barcena, N., Martinez, E., & Benito, J. (2012). Is 15 days an appropriate cut-off age for considering serious bacterial infection in the management of febrile infants? *The Pediatric Infectious Disease Journal*, *31*(5), 455–458. https://doi.org/10.1097/INF.0b013e318247b9f2.

Hui, C., Neto, G., Tsertsvadze, A., Yazdi, F., Tricco, A. C., Tsouros, S., Skidmore, B., & Daniel, R. (2012). Diagnosis and management of febrile infants (0-3 months). *Evidence Report/Technology Assessment*, *205*, 1–297.

İmamoğlu, E. Y. (2018). Yenidoğanda Ateş ve Hipotermiye Yaklaşım (Approach to fever and hypothermia in the newborn). *Klinik Tıp Aile Hekimliği*, *10*(4), Article 4.

Jain, S., Cheng, J., Alpern, E. R., Thurm, C., Schroeder, L., Black, K., Ellison, A. M., Stone, K., & Alessandrini, E. A. (2014). Management of febrile neonates in US pediatric emergency departments. *Pediatrics*, *133*(2), 187–195. https://doi.org/10.1542/peds.2013-1820.

Jaskiewicz, J. A., McCarthy, C. A., Richardson, A. C., White, K. C., Fisher, D. J., Dagan, R., Powell, K. R., Korones, D. N., Bracikowski, A., Deveikis, A., Stutman, H., Lohr, J. A., Carlson, D. W., Kennedy, R. M., Beach, P. S., Krause, P. J., Gudnason, T., Li, M., & Matsell, D. (1994). Febrile infants at low risk for serious bacterial infection - An appraisal of the Rochester criteria and implications for management. *Pediatrics*, *94*(3), 390–399.

Katz-Sidlow, R. J., Rowberry, J. P., & Ho, M. (2009). Fever determination in young infants: Prevalence and accuracy of parental palpation. *Pediatric Emergency Care*, *25*(1), 12–14. https://doi.org/10.1097/PEC.0b013e31819dac6.

Nosrati, A., Ben Tov, A., & Reif, S. (2014). Diagnostic markers of serious bacterial infections in febrile infants younger than 90 days old. *Pediatrics International*, *56*(1), 47–52. https://doi.org/10.1111/ped.12191.

Pantell, R. H., Roberts, K. B., Adams, W. G., Dreyer, B. P., Kuppermann, N., O'Leary, S. T., Okechukwu, K., Woods, C. R., Jr, & Subcommittee On Febrile Infants. (2021). Clinical Practice Guideline: Evaluation and Management of Well-Appearing Febrile Infants 8 to 60 Days Old. *Pediatrics*, *148*(2), e2021052228. https://doi.org/10.1542/peds.2021-052228.

Rehm, K. P. (2001). Fever in infants and children. *Current Opinion in Pediatrics*, *13*(1), 83–88. https://doi.org/10.1097/00008480-200102000-00016.

Smith, J. (2014). Methods and Devices of Temperature Measurement in the Neonate: A Narrative Review and Practice Recommendations. *Neonatal and Infant Nursing Reviews*, *14*(2), 64–71. https://doi.org/10.1053/j.nainr.2014.03.001.

Yarden-Bilavsky, H., Ashkenazi, S., Amir, J., Schlesinger, Y., & Bilavsky, E. (2014). Fever survey highlights significant variations in how infants aged ≤60 days are evaluated and underline the need for guidelines. *Acta Paediatrica (Oslo, Norway: 1992)*, *103*(4), 379–385. https://doi.org/10.1111/apa.12560.

Chapter 19

Neonatal Dehydration and Electrolyte Disorders

Tuba Günebak*, PhD
Department of Nutrition and Dietetics, Istanbul Health and Technology University, Istanbul, Turkey

Abstract

Water constitutes the most prevalent substance within the human body, representing a fundamental component of bodily fluids. This vital element is indispensable for maintaining cellular homeostasis, accounting for approximately 75% of body weight in term infants. Water plays a pivotal role in a multitude of physiological processes. Dynamic alterations in body composition and fluid distribution are observed during the intrauterine period, labor, and the early postnatal period. The equilibrium of body fluid balance and distribution is contingent on the balance between water intake and loss. Dehydration is a prevalent issue in neonates, associated with considerable morbidity and mortality rates, and failure to promptly identify and manage this condition can result in severe complications. Dehydration is classified into three forms according to serum osmolality: hypernatremic, normonatremic (isonatremic), and hyponatremic dehydration. Sodium, potassium, magnesium, calcium, and phosphorus are vital for the maintenance of normal biochemical reactions and homeostatic functioning. Newborns in need of fluid electrolyte support should be evaluated by physical examination and other parameters (low urine volume, high urine density, high serum Na^+), and treatment should be started rapidly.

* Corresponding Author's Email: drtubagunebak@tubagunebak.com

In: Current Approaches to Newborn Emergencies
Editors: Zuhal Keskin Sarılar and Serap Samut Bülbül
ISBN: 979-8-89530-999-5

Keywords: neonatal dehydration, electrolyte disorders

Introduction

Water represents the most common substance in the human body, constituting a primary component of body fluids (Blackmer, 2018). Water is essential for cellular homeostasis and comprises approximately 75% of body weight in term infants (Powers, 2017; Taş, 2024). In the absence of water, humans would die within a few days. The human body has an efficient mechanism of physiologic controls to maintain fluid and ion equilibrium, including the sensation of dehydration, which is signaled by thirst (Powers, 2017). Water plays a key role in numerous physiological processes, including digestion, absorption, and metabolism of nutrients, distribution, excretion, and maintenance of hemodynamic equilibrium (Blackmer, 2018). Total body fluid is considered as a whole of intracellular fluid and extracellular fluid components (Bülbül & Uslu, 2012). Body fluid balance and fluid distribution in the body is a function of the balance between water intake and loss. Extracellular fluid is also composed of intravascular and interstitial fluid compartments (İnce et al., 2018İnce et al., 2018; Bülbül & Uslu, 2012). Dynamic alterations in body composition and fluid distribution are observed in the intrauterine period, during labor, and in the early postnatal period. Factors such as fetal growth rate, the presence of pregnancy-related complications, mode of delivery, the type and amount of fluid therapy administered to the mother during labor, renal function of the newborn, inadequate breastfeeding, and postnatal nutrition fluid intake can influence the distribution of fluid within the body (İnce et al., 2018; Taş, 2024). In term infants, total body fluid constitutes 75% of body weight, and approximately half of it is in the intracellular space. In preterm babies, total body fluid is higher than in term babies, and this excess is largely due to the increase in extracellular fluid (İnce et al., 2018). A neonate may lose fluid via two distinct mechanisms: insensible fluid loss, which comprises the evaporation of fluid from the skin and mucous membranes, and sensible fluid loss, which encompasses the excretion of fluids in the form of urine and feces (Bülbül & Uslu, 2012).

Alterations in the distribution of total body fluid persist during labor. Arterial blood pressure rises a few days before labor. This is due to the increase in catecholamine, vasopressin, and cortisol levels and the passage of blood from the placenta to the fetus. Due to the increase in capillary permeability due to hypoxia during labor, some fluid passes from the intravascular space to the interstitial space, and the intravascular volume decreases by approximately 25% (İnce et al., 2018). Fluid balance in newborns must be considered in the context of the transition to extrauterine life and their rapid growth (Blackmer, 2018). There are some mechanisms providing body fluid balance, which can be summarized as cardiac function, baroreceptors and osmoreceptors in the atria, kidneys (with renal blood flow-diuresis), skin structure (since skin maturation is completed in approximately 28 days after birth, fluid losses from the skin can be seen significantly during this period), and hormones (renin-angiotensin-aldosterone system, vasopressin, bradykinin, prostaglandin, and catecholamines play an active role in maintaining fluid balance in newborn babies) (Bülbül & Uslu, 2012).

After birth, capillary membrane integrity is restored as a result of the increase in oxygenation and alterations in vasoactive hormones, and the fluid that passes into the interstitial space returns to the intravascular space. Thus, intravascular volume is maintained in the first 24-48 hours postnatally when the infant's oral intake is low (İnce et al., 2018). It is essential to consider the challenges of maintaining adequate nutrition and water intake, preventing dehydration, and avoiding the accumulation of excess fluid during the early neonatal period. The postnatal adaptation process is influenced by both intrauterine growth and gestational age (Blackmer, 2018). Atrial natriuretic peptide release is stimulated in response to atrial stretch caused by the maintenance of intravascular volume and the increase in systemic vascular resistance and decrease in pulmonary vascular resistance. Decreased total body water with increased renal excretion of water and sodium (diuresis and natriuresis) is reflected in the clinic as weight loss (İnce et al., 2018). This condition, defined as physiological weight loss, is inversely proportional to the maturity of the infant. While the expected weight loss in term babies in the first week of life is 5-10% of birth weight (which is subsequently regained 10–14 days postpartum), it may be 10-15% in very low birth weight or extremely low birth weight infants. If there is >15% loss of birth weight or physiological weight loss <2% at the end of the first postnatal week, body fluid balance should be carefully evaluated (İnce et al., 2018; Blackmer, 2018; Bülbül & Uslu, 2012; Durrani et al., 2022). The main cause of weight loss is insensible (invisible) fluid loss. Fluid loss occurs through the kidneys, skin, and respiratory tract. Sixty to 65% of the insensible fluid is lost through the skin, and 30-35% is lost through the respiratory tract (Bülbül & Uslu, 2012).

Neonatal Dehydration

Dehydration is a prevalent issue in neonates, associated with considerable morbidity and mortality rates. Failure to promptly identify and manage this condition can result in severe complications (Taş, 2024). Neonatal dehydration can result from a number of factors. Firstly, lactation failure may occur in cases of first-time motherhood. Secondly, maternal illness, inadequate lactation support, early post-delivery discharge, incorrect formula-feeding practices, and neonatal illnesses may also lead to dehydration. The condition can cause a range of complications, including peripheral gangrene, convulsions, central venous and aortic thrombosis, and even death in the acute period. Long-term neurodevelopmental abnormalities have also been reported (Akech et al., 2018).

It is widely accepted that breastfeeding is the superior option to formula feeding, offering numerous health benefits to both infant and mother. The sodium content of human breast milk is typically low, which reduces the likelihood of hypernatremia developing in breastfed neonates. A higher concentration of sodium in breast milk is linked to a reduction in lactation, while a decrease in the frequency of feeding is in conjunction with a notable increase in the sodium content of milk. This association may be related to a reduction in breast milk production, which could be secondary to maternal or neonatal factors. It has been demonstrated that insufficient breast milk production is the primary factor in the induction of neonatal hypernatremic dehydration, which is a potentially lethal condition that can result in cerebral edema, intracranial hemorrhage, seizures, disseminated intravascular coagulation, and ultimately death (Boskabadi et al., 2010).

Dehydration is classified into three forms according to serum osmolality: hypernatremic, normonatremic (isonatremic), and hyponatremic dehydration (Bolat et al., 2013). Normonatremic dehydration is characterized by a sodium level of 130 to 150 mEq/L (130 to 150 mmol/L), which indicates an equal proportion of solute and water loss. Normonatremic dehydration is characterized by a sodium level of 130 to 150 mEq/L (130 to 150 mmol/L), which indicates an equal proportion of solute and water loss. This form of dehydration is most frequently observed in patients presenting with secretory diarrhea, wherein the concentration of the diarrheic solute is equivalent to the plasma solute concentration. Oral rehydration represents a safe and efficacious means of restoring intravascular volume in children with mild-to-moderate normonatremic dehydration. Hyponatremic dehydration, characterized by a sodium concentration below 130 mEq/L (130 mmol/L) (Powers, 2017).

Hyponatremia develops in 3 ways: deficiency of total body water and more deficiency of total body sodium than fluid (it is seen in vomiting, diarrhea, burns, diuretic excess, mineralocorticoid deficiency, and osmotic diuresis), excess total body water (glucocorticoid deficiency, inappropriate vasopressin release, hypothyroidism, pain, and most commonly iatrogenic hypotonic fluid administration), excess total body sodium, and more total body water than sodium (Bülbül & Uslu, 2012). The clinical entity of hypernatremic dehydration, defined as serum sodium levels exceeding 150 mEq/L (150 mmol/L), is distinguished by a greater extent of water loss relative to solute loss. This phenomenon is frequently observed in cases of viral gastroenteritis, such as that caused by rotavirus, and in neonates with inadequate breastfeeding, where diarrheal and insensible water losses are inadequately replaced (Powers, 2017). The hypernatremic type is a potentially lethal form, as it has the capacity to adversely affect the central nervous system, leading to a range of devastating consequences, including intracranial hemorrhage, thrombosis, and even death (Bolat et al., 2013; Das, 2015). Recently, along with a number of other potential causes, early discharge and failure of breastfeeding have been increasingly documented as significant factors in the development of hypernatremic dehydration (Bolat et al., 2013). In Turkey, 5.6% of neonates experience serum sodium concentrations of >145 mmol/L (Das, 2015).

The term hypovolemia is used to describe a state of volume depletion and dehydration. Volume depletion is defined as the loss of salt and water from the intravascular space. The degree of dehydration can be classified as mild, moderate, or severe, corresponding to weight loss of 3–5%, 6–9%, or ≥10%, respectively (Tsegaye, 2023; Powers, 2017). In order to ensure an appropriate assessment and management of dehydration, it is essential to consider the degree of dehydration, the maintenance fluid requirements, and the ongoing fluid losses. The mechanisms of dehydration may be broadly classified into three categories: 1) increased fluid loss, 2) decreased fluid intake, or 3) a combination of the two. Neonatal dehydration is frequently the result of increased output from gastroenteritis, which is characterized by vomiting, diarrhea, or both. Other causes of dehydration may include metabolic diseases, cutaneous losses, or third-space losses. It is of particular concern when the client is vomiting or experiencing a concurrent fever or tachypnea, as these symptoms increase insensible fluid losses (Tsegaye, 2023).

In cases of mild dehydration in infants, the observed effects are frequently insignificant, apart from a reduction in urine output. In addition to a reduction in urine output and lacrimation, children with moderate dehydration frequently present with desiccated mucous membranes, diminished skin turgor, irritation, tachyarrhythmia with delayed capillary refill, and deep respirations. In newborns with at least 5% dehydration, prolonged capillary refill, abnormal skin turgor, and abnormal respiratory patterns may be observed. In cases of severe dehydration, the patient may present with a near-shock to shock state, exhibiting lethargy, tachyarrhythmia, hypotension, hyperpnea, prolonged capillary refill, and cool and mottled extremities. Immediate and aggressive isotonic fluid resuscitation is necessary in such instances. The phenomenon of low blood pressure represents a late indicator of dehydration. This occurs when the compensatory mechanisms that are responsible for maintaining adequate blood perfusion are overwhelmed (Powers, 2017).

Results of laboratory tests are typically normal in neonates with mild dehydration. Laboratory testing is generally indicated only for newborns with greater than 10% dehydration who are requiring intravenous fluid repletion. Assessment of serum bicarbonate, the blood urea nitrogen level, serum sodium, and potassium levels could be essential (Powers, 2017). The evaluation of fluid necessities in neonates presenting with mild or moderate dehydration is contingent upon a fivefold approach: the physical examination, including observations of turgor, edema, the condition of the oral mucosa, ocular examination, and fontanelle measurement. While these parameters offer valuable insight, their reliability is limited in low birth weight infants. Tachycardia, hypotension, capillary refill time >3 seconds, and metabolic acidosis are indicators of intravascular volume depletion. Body weight (to be monitored daily or more frequently), urine output (measured using nappy pads if necessary), urine specific gravity, and laboratory tests - including serum sodium, urea, creatinine, and albumin - should be assessed regularly, with the frequency tailored to the patient's clinical condition (İnce et al., 2018; Bülbül & Uslu, 2012).

The objective of therapy is to ascertain the extent and type of dehydration and to replenish any deficits in water and electrolytes while meeting maintenance requirements and replacing ongoing losses (Powers, 2017; Tsegaye, 2023). In cases of mild and moderate isonatremic dehydration where oral rehydration is the preferred course of treatment, the amount of fluid deficit should be estimated based on either a change in body weight or the presence of clinical signs. The typical replacement rate is 50 to 100 milliliters per kilogram of body weight over a period of two to four hours. The administration of 5 ml should be undertaken using a teaspoon, syringe, or dropper, with the volume increased as tolerated and every few minutes. In cases of severe vomiting or oral ulcers, nasogastric tubes can be employed for continuous volume replacement. It is noteworthy that oral rehydration therapy is unsuccessful in only 4% of cases, necessitating the use of intravenous repletion. The use of oral rehydration is contraindicated in infants and children exhibiting signs of circulatory instability or shock, alterations in mental status, persistent vomiting, bloody diarrhea or ileus, abnormal serum sodium levels, or glucose malabsorption (Powers, 2017).

Neonatal Electrolyte Disorders

Sodium, potassium, magnesium, calcium, and phosphorus are vital for the maintenance of normal biochemical reactions and homeostatic functioning. They act in conjunction to ensure the optimal functioning of cell membranes, nerve conduction, muscle contraction, hormonal activation, bone structure, and fluid and acid-base homeostasis (Blackmer, 2018).

Sodium

Sodium (typical range 135–145 mEq/L) is the most common cation in the body, determining extracellular fluid and plasma volume (İnce et al., 2018; Blackmer, 2018). Sodium is the primary regulator of body water homeostasis, orchestrating the movement of water into and out of cells. This process is governed by intricate interactions between the heart, skin, kidneys, and a network of hormones (Durrani et al., 2022). Sodium fulfills three principal functions: the maintenance of fluid equilibrium, the modulation of osmotic processes, and the sustenance of membrane potential. Rather than sodium intake, sodium excretion primarily regulates sodium homeostasis (Blackmer, 2018). Following birth, term neonates are capable of reabsorbing the filtered sodium through their kidneys. In contrast, preterm infants have immature kidneys with blunted end-organ responsiveness to various hormones, which results in sodium loss being directly related to the degree of prematurity. The maintenance of sodium hemostasis ensures that water balance is constantly maintained between the extracellular fluid and intracellular fluid compartments (Durrani et al., 2022).

Hypernatremia

Hypernatremia is defined as a serum sodium concentration exceeding 145 mEq/L (Blackmer, 2018; İnce et al., 2018). The causes of hypernatremia are numerous and include, but are not limited to, dehydration, gastrointestinal illness, fever, inadequate breastfeeding, and some medications like diuretic therapy and hypertonic saline (Blackmer, 2018). The body's protective mechanisms against hypernatremia are the formation of concentrated urine and a robust thirst sensation mechanism. Inadequate urine concentration capacity and an inability to express thirst are risk factors for hypernatremia in neonates (İnce et al., 2018; Das, 2015). Hypernatremia in healthy neonates usually occurs in the first week of life, typically because of inadequate breastfeeding (Bolat et al., 2013). Adequate milk production occurs in the first four days after birth. It has been reported that hypernatremic dehydration findings occur in the first two weeks of life in breastfed newborns, and this period may be as short as three days and as long as 21 days (Ergin et al., 2013). Physiopathologically, hypernatremia equates to a decrease in intracellular fluid (Bülbül & Uslu, 2012). The clinical manifestations of hypernatremia include increased thirst, fatigue, lethargy, and muscle tenderness. In cases of severe hypernatremia, cerebral cellular dehydration may occur, potentially leading to hemorrhage, neurological complications such as seizures, coma, and even death. The management of hypernatremia hinges on the initial identification of the underlying cause and subsequent correction thereof (Blackmer, 2018). The immediate first question should be: Is hyponatremia due to an excess of water or a deficiency of sodium? Excess water is the most common cause (Bockenhauer & Zieg, 2014). Delayed recognition and treatment of hypernatremia result in severe and prolonged hypernatremia, which is associated with an increased risk of mortality and central nervous system complications, including convulsion, thrombosis, and intracranial hemorrhage (Durrani et al., 2022; Ergin et al., 2013). The brain is the organ most susceptible to damage from hypernatremia (Das, 2015). In hypernatremia, the decrease in brain volume as a result of water transfer from inside to outside the cell to maintain osmotic balance activates adaptation mechanisms. While electrolytes such as sodium, potassium, and chlorine are taken into the cell as an acute response, the later response is the synthesis of osmoprotective amino acids and organic solutes (idiogenic osmoles). If hypernatremia develops very rapidly, intracellular solute increase is insufficient, and the volume of brain cells cannot be maintained and decreases. As a result of this decrease, ruptures in intracerebral veins and bridging blood vessels, subarachnoid, subdural, and parenchymal hemorrhages, convulsions, and coma may occur (İnce et al., 2018). It is of the utmost importance to prevent hypernatremic dehydration. This should be a particular focus in cases of lactation failure. Furthermore, all breastfed neonates should be weighed at least once several days after discharge. In the event of a weight loss exceeding 10%, it is imperative that the infant be weighed on a daily basis until a normal growth velocity can be recorded (Das, 2015).

Hyponatremia

Although hyponatremia is generally defined as a serum sodium level <130 mEq/L, studies in newborns have shown that hyponatremia is an independent risk factor for adverse neuromotor development. Therefore, it would be more accurate to accept a limit of 135 mEq/L (İnce et al., 2018). Hyponatremia is one of the most common electrolyte disturbances (Blackmer, 2018). The initial step is to differentiate between true and pseudohyponatremia (Taş, 2024). Pseudohyponatremia is the underreporting of normal plasma sodium levels due to the measurement technique (not using an ion-selective electrode) (İnce et al., 2018; Bülbül & Uslu, 2012). Sodium is not included in the protein and lipid phases, which are the non-water components of serum. Another cause of pseudohyponatremia is water transfer to the extracellular fluid compartment due to another osmotically active molecule such as glucose, mannitol, or IV contrast agents. In this case, plasma osmolality is high. Each 100 mg/dL increase in glucose decreases the plasma sodium level by approximately 1.6 mEq/L. Sodium concentration normalizes with correction of the underlying cause (İnce et al., 2018). Three categories of hyponatremia, based on plasma osmolality, have been delineated. These are classified as either hypotonic hyponatremia (280–295 mOsm/L) or hypertonic hyponatremia (>295 mOsm/L), the latter of which may be observed on occasion, particularly in premature infants. Hyperglycemia may also be a contributing factor, and hypotonic hyponatremia, defined as a plasma osmolality of less than 280 mOsm/L, can be further categorized into three subtypes based on the patient's extracellular fluid (ECF) volume status: hypovolemic, euvolemic, and hypervolemic (Marcialis et al., 2011). Clinical findings of hyponatremia are primarily neurological and are due to brain edema caused by hypoosmolality. Common findings include decreased sucking, vomiting, lethargy, irritability, convulsions, and coma, and may end with brain stem herniation and respiratory arrest. Clinical findings depend on both the duration and severity of hyponatremia. If hyponatremia develops slowly, the brain tries to adapt to hyponatremia by decreasing intracellular osmolality (İnce et al., 2018). It is imperative that natremia be monitored at two-hourly intervals. In emergency cases, the sodium level must be set at a level that allows the patient to become asymptomatic. Subsequently, a more gradual correction of the electrolyte imbalance is to be applied. It is recommended that plasmatic sodium levels should not increase by more than 8–10 mEq/L in the first 24 hours to avoid both cerebral edema and the risk of myelinolysis. The optimal treatment for chronic hyponatremia is the slow correction of the electrolytic imbalance. In chronic forms, an isotonic saline solution, potentially combined with diuretics, should be the preferred option, as this has been demonstrated to be the most effective treatment for this condition (Marcialis et al., 2011).

Potassium

Potassium is the primary intracellular cation. It regulates the excitability of neuromuscular and cardiovascular tissues. Of the total body potassium, 98% is intracellular and 2% is extracellular. Two mechanisms play a role in the regulation of total body potassium: potassium excretion and potassium transit between intracellular and extracellular compartments. 90-95% of potassium is excreted through the kidneys and approximately 5-10% through the intestines. Serum potassium level may not reflect total body potassium. Each 0.1 unit decrease in extracellular fluid pH increases serum potassium level by 0.6 mEq/L. Serum potassium level should be kept in the range of 3.5-5.0 mEq/L. In neonates, especially small preterm infants, serum potassium levels may be higher in the early postnatal period. The infant may be asymptomatic or may have bradycardia, tachycardia, or shock. Some patients may have fasciculations, weakness, or even paralysis (İnce et al., 2018).

Hyperkalemia

Hyperkalemia is defined as a serum potassium concentration greater than 4.7–5.9 mEq/kg (Blackmer, 2018). Chronic hyperkalemia is better tolerated than acute hyperkalemia (İnce et al., 2018). As potassium is the primary intracellular cation, it is imperative to rule out pseudohyperkalemia before making an assessment (Blackmer, 2018). If there is a true hyperkalemia, electrocardiogram changes should be checked (İnce et al., 2018). Causes of hyperkalemia are decreased renal excretion (low glomerular filtration rate), decreased renal tubular secretion, and potassium extraction from the cell. Besides these, it can be iatrogenic (Bülbül & Uslu, 2012). Hyperkalemia represents one of the most dangerous electrolyte imbalances due to the detrimental effects (changes in cardiac conductivity leading to arrhythmias) it can have on the body (Blackmer, 2018). For the diagnosis of hyperkalemia, firstly, attention should be paid to where the sample was taken (if the sample is taken from the heel or vein with a thin needle, potassium may be falsely elevated due to hemolysis;imilarly, heparin may also cause a high potassium level); secondly, it should be checked how much potassium is given to the baby. Particular attention should be paid to infants receiving diuretic and potassium support due to chronic lung disease (İnce et al., 2018).

Hypokalemia

Serum potassium level lower than 3.5 mEq/L is defined as hypokalemia. Moderate hypokalemia is 2.5-3 mEq/L, and severe hypokalemia is <2.5 mEq/L (İnce et al., 2018). Management includes supplementing potassium either orally or intravenously, depending on severity (Blackmer, 2018). Hypokalemia has effects on nerve conduction, andheart muscle (Bülbül & Uslu, 2012). The clinical signs and symptoms of hypokalemia manifest as a consequence of functional alterations in striated muscle, smooth muscle, and the heart. These include rhabdomyolysis, myoglobinuria, severe muscle weakness, paralysis, respiratory distress, and respiratory arrest. Additionally, fasciculation and tetany are observed in muscles (Sarici & Sarici, 2012). Causes of hypokalemia are intercellular potassium transfer, protein energy malnutrition (inappropriate total parenteral nutrition), extra-renal losses, and excessive losses through the kidney (Bülbül & Uslu, 2012). In the treatment of hypokalemia in preterm infants, 4-7 mEq/kg of potassium may be given. It is aimed not to exceed 40 mEq/L per liter (Bülbül & Uslu, 2012). The primary objective of therapy is to prevent and treat life-threatening cardiac and muscular complications. The secondary objective is to replenish the body's potassium stores (Sarici & Sarici, 2012).

Calcium

Calcium is the most prevalent mineral in the human body, with typical serum levels between 6.2 and 11 mg/dL. Its role is multifaceted, with essential functions encompassing neuromuscular activity, the integrity of cellular membranes, endocrine function, the process of coagulation, and bone metabolism. The parathyroid gland plays a primary role in regulating serum calcium concentrations. In instances where serum concentrations are low, parathyroid hormone is released, which increases bone resorption, renal conservation, and activates vitamin D, thereby improving calcium retention from the gastrointestinal tract (Blackmer, 2018). Early hypocalcemia is usually asymptomatic, and the more immature the infant, the more likely it is to be asymptomatic. When symptomatic, the most common findings are 'jitteriness,' tremors, twitching, exaggerated startle movements or convulsions, which are more common in late hypocalcemia. Lethargy, malnutrition, vomiting, and abdominal distension may also develop. Apnea, cyanosis, tachypnea, tachycardia, vomiting, and heart failure may also occur. Classic findings such as carpopedal spasm and laryngospasm are rare in the newborn (İnce et al., 2018). Neonatal hypocalcemia is a common occurrence in infants with acute critical illness. The etiology of this condition is multifactorial and includes abnormal parathyroid hormone secretion, hypomagnesemia, hypoalbuminemia, sepsis, transfusions, acid–base imbalance, and medications and dietary calcium intake. Infants born to mothers with diabetes, infants born prematurely, and infants who have experienced birth asphyxia are at increased risk of developing early neonatal hypocalcemia, which typically presents within 72 hours of birth (Pajak et al., 2018). In terms of time of onset, 'early hypocalcemia' is typically seen in the first 3 days of life, whereas 'late hypocalcemia' occurs after the first 3 days of life, usually towards the end of the first week, and is rarer (İnce et al., 2018). Depending on the severity of hypocalcemia, treatment involves oral or intravenous calcium supplementation (Blackmer, 2018). Hypocalcemia accompanied by hypomagnesemia cannot be corrected without starting Mg treatment. The baby has high phosphorus levels, low calcium levels, and normal renal function. The aim of treatment is to prevent nephrocalcinosis while keeping plasma calcium levels normal. In hypoparathyroidism, vitamin $1,25(OH)_2D$ (50-100 ng/kg/day, divided into 2-3 doses) and calcium support should be given. Recombinant PTH (teriparatide) can be used in neonates with hypoparathyroidism whose marked hypocalcemia persists despite calcium and vitamin D supplementation (İnce et al., 2018).

A serum calcium level above 11 mg/dL (2.75 mmol/L) or ionized Ca++ level above 5.6 mg/dL (1.4 mmol/L) is defined as hypercalcemia. The most important cause is hypercalcemia secondary to hypophosphatemia, which develops as a result of insufficient phosphorus in parenteral nutrition. Iatrogenic hypercalcemia is caused by giving excess calcium and vitamin D during exchange transfusion or for the treatment of hypocalcemia. If the mother has hypocalcemia and the mother is given too much vitamin D, hypercalcemia may develop in the neonate along with the mother (İnce et al., 2018). In mild to moderate cases of hypercalcemia, fluid therapy is first line and usually effective. For severe cases, intravenous fluid therapy, loop diuretics, and dialysis therapy may be needed to prevent dysrhythmias, kidney failure, and death (Blackmer, 2018).

Hypophosphataemia

The principal intracellular anion, phosphorus (typical range 2.7–9 mg/dL, dependent on age), is of critical importance for the maintenance of cellular function, bone and cell membrane composition, pH, energy, and all physiologic functions requiring energy (İnce et al., 2018). Serum phosphorus levels below 4 mg/dL are defined as hypophosphatemia. It is usually divided into mild (<3.5 mg/dL), moderate (<2.5 mg/dL), and severe (<1.0 mg/dL) (İnce et al., 2018). The underlying factors of hypophosphatemia are inadequate phosphorus intake (decreased intake or absorption or increased intestinal loss), increased excretion due to renal tubular defect, and hyperparathyroidism. Hypophosphatemia in the newborn, especially in preterm infants, is often due to nutritional causes (unfortified breastfeeding, prolonged parenteral nutrition with inadequate phosphorus supplementation). Biochemical signs of phosphorus deficiency are prominent in long-term parenteral nutrition, and rachitic changes may occur (İnce et al., 2018). The clinical implications of hypophosphatemia are the development of multi-system disorders, which primarily affect energy-active organs. These may include heart or respiratory failure, muscle hypotension, neurological symptoms, hematological disorders, insulin-resistant hyperglycemia, or metabolic acidosis (Pajak et al., 2018). Some authors have proposed that the "refeeding syndrome" resulting from aggressive parenteral nutrition may lead to hypophosphatemia, hypercalcemia, and hypokalemia. An analysis of the intake of different macronutrients indicated that the high intake of amino acids during the first week of life was the determining factor in calcium and phosphorus levels (Dik et al., 2018). In the treatment of hypophosphatemia, phosphate should be supplemented. Since calcium is generally low in these babies, calcium should also be supplemented. If calcium support is not given, hypocalcemia may develop (vitamin D should be given for adequate bone mineralization) (İnce et al., 2018).

A serum phosphorus value above 8 mg/dL is defined as hyperphosphatemia. It may be due to incorrect dose/preparation, increased intestinal absorption, decreased renal excretion, and rapid transition from intracellular to extracellular space. One of the most important causes of hyperphosphatemia is medical errors, such as an imbalance of Ca, P, and Mg ions in the parenteral solution or substitution of sodium phosphate for calcium gluconate. Feeding cow's milk (containing 67-81 mg/dL P) to infants with renal failure or hypoparathyroidism may cause hyperphosphatemia. Even in normal term infants, serum Ca decreases and serum phosphorus level increases in cow's milk-fed infants compared to breastfed infants (İnce et al., 2018). The majority of cases of hyperphosphatemia are well-tolerated, with many patients remaining asymptomatic. The management of hyperphosphatemia typically involves the implementation of a low-phosphorus diet, adequate hydration, and the addition of phosphate binders (İnce et al., 2018; Blackmer, 2018).

Magnesium

Magnesium, the fourth most abundant cation in the body, plays a pivotal role in numerous physiological functions (Rigo et al., 2017). Magnesium is involved in the development of bone matrix and is essential for the synthesis of biomacromolecules, including deoxyribonucleic acid, ribonucleic acid, and proteins, which serve as an indispensable cofactor for hundreds of enzymatic reactions, including the metabolism of glucose and fatty acids. Magnesium is required for energy generation and is also employed for electrostatic stabilization in cell systems. Additionally, it participates in regulating the active transport of calcium and potassium ions across cell membranes, which in turn regulates muscle contraction, nerve impulse conduction, vascular tone, and cardiac function. It also constitutes a crucial component of bone (Blackmer, 2018; Rigo et al., 2017). A serum magnesium concentration exceeding 2.4 mg/dL is indicative of hypermagnesemia (Blackmer, 2018). Mild hypermagnesemia is typically well-tolerated; however, when serum magnesium concentrations exceed 3 mg/dL, neurological, neuromuscular, and cardiac symptoms may manifest. In neonates, hypermagnesemia may arise as a consequence of placental transfer of magnesium from mothers who have received a high dose of magnesium sulfate for the purpose of preventing preterm labor. In infants born prematurely, magnesium concentrations should be assessed prior to the administration of magnesium in intravenous fluids or parenteral nutrition. Hypomagnesemia is defined as magnesium concentrations below 1.3 mg/dL and is also associated with other electrolyte derangements, including hypokalemia and hypocalcemia (Blackmer, 2018).

Conclusion

Provision of fluid and electrolyte balance is necessary for normal cell and organ functions in the postnatal development process. Knowledge of physiological changes and provision of appropriate support is one of the important issues of the neonatal period. One of the main causes is inadequate breastfeeding. Morbidity and mortality rates may increase in infants whose fluid-electrolyte disorders are not well managed and not adequately treated. It is important to monitor the weight of the babies and to see biochemical markers in those with high weight loss. Newborns in need of fluid electrolyte support should be evaluated by physical examination and other parameters (low urine volume, high urine density, high serum Na+), and treatment should be started rapidly.

References

Akech, S., Rotich, B., Chepkirui, M., et al., (2018). The prevalence and management of dehydration amongst neonatal admissions to general paediatric wards in Kenya: A clinical audit. *Journal of Tropical Pediatrics, 64*, 516–522. https://doi.org/10.1093/tropej/fmx108.

Blackmer, A. B. (2018). Fluids and electrolytes. In C. J. Rollins, B. A. Hall & T. M. Afolabi (Eds.), *Fluids, electrolytes and nutrition* (pp. 7–26). PedSAP Book 2.

Bockenhauer, D., & Zieg, J. (2014). Electrolyte disorders. *Clinical Perinatology*. https://doi.org/10.1016/j.clp.2014.05.007.

Bolat, F., Oflaz, M. B., Güven, A. S., et al., (2013). What is the safe approach for neonatal hypernatremic dehydration? A retrospective study from a neonatal intensive care unit. *Pediatric Emergency Care, 29*, 808–813.

Boskabadi, H., Maamouri, G., Ebrahimi, M., et al., (2010). Neonatal hypernatremia and dehydration in infants receiving inadequate breastfeeding. *Asia Pacific Journal of Clinical Nutrition, 19*(3), 301–307.

Brener Dik, P. H., Galletti, M. F., Bacigalupo, L. T., et al., (2018). Hypercalcemia and hypophosphatemia among preterm infants receiving aggressive parenteral nutrition. *Archivos Argentinos de Pediatría, 116*(3), 371–377.

Bülbül, A., & Uslu, S. (2012). Yenidoğan döneminde sıvı ve elektrolit dengesi [Fluid and electrolyte balance in the neonatal period]. *Şişli Etfal Hastanesi Tıp Bülteni, 46*(1), 36–42.

Das, J. C. (2015). Hypernatremic dehydration in newborn infants. *The Ulutas Medical Journal, 1*(2), 22–25.

Durrani, N. U. R., Imam, A. A., & Soni, N. (2022). Hypernatremia in newborns: A practical approach to management. *Biomed Hub, 7*, 55–69. https://doi.org/10.1159/000524637.

Ergin, H., Sahin, O., Ozmert, M. D., et al., (2013). Hypernatremic dehydration in breastfed infants. *Güncel Pediatri, 11*, 51–56.

İnce, Z., Yıldızdaş, H. Y., & Demirel, D. (2018). Turkish Neonatal Society guideline on fluid and electrolyte balance in the newborn. *Turkish Archives of Pediatrics, 53*(1), 55–64. https://doi.org/10.5152/TurkPediatriArs.2018.01807.

Marcialis, M. A., Dessi, A., Pintus, M. C., et al., (2011). Neonatal hyponatremia: Differential diagnosis and treatment. *The Journal of Maternal-Fetal & Neonatal Medicine, 24*(1), 75–79.

Pajak, A., Królak-Olejnik, B., & Szafrańska, A. (2018). Early hypophosphatemia in very low birth weight preterm infants. *Advances in Clinical and Experimental Medicine, 27*(6), 841–847.

Powers, K. S. (2017). Dehydration: Isonatremic, hyponatremic, and hypernatremic recognition and management. *Pediatrics in Review, 36*, 274–285. https://doi.org/10.1542/pir.36-7-274.

Rigo, J., Pieltain, C., Christmann, V., & Bonsante, F. (2017). Serum magnesium levels in preterm infants are higher than adult levels: A systematic literature review and meta-analysis. *Nutrients, 9*, 1125. https://doi.org/10.3390/nu9101125.

Sarici, D., & Sarici, S. U. (2012). Neonatal hypokalemia. *Research and Reports in Neonatology, 2*, 15–19.

Taş, M. (2024). Treatment of neonatal dehydration and electrolyte disorders. In I. Fidancı (Ed.), *Neonatal emergencies* (pp. 84–88). 1st ed. Turkey Klinikleri.

Tsegaye, A. D., Pavlinac, P. B., Walson, J. L., & Tickell, K. D. (2023). The diagnosis and management of dehydration in children with wasting or nutritional edema: A systematic review. *PLOS Global Public Health, 3*(11), e0002520. https://doi.org/10.1371/journal.pgph.0002520.

Chapter 20

Exploring the Causes and Management of Neonatal Convulsions

Şefika Aldaş*, MD

Department of Pediatrics, University of Health Sciences,
Mersin City Education and Research Hospital, Mersin, Turkey

Abstract

Neonatal convulsions are among the most common neurologic emergencies encountered in the neonatal period, and the incidence is reported to be 1-5 per 1000 live births. It's known that the convulsion threshold is low due to immaturity of the neonatal brain structure and differences in neurotransmitter systems. The most common cause of convulsions in the neonatal period is hypoxic-ischemic encephalopathy, and the etiology may vary according to the level of development of countries. Based on clinical findings, neonatal seizures are divided into four categories: subtle seizures are the most common form. Other types are clonic, tonic, and myoclonic seizures. However, non-epileptic paroxysmal movements, common in the neonatal period, should not be confused with convulsions. Jitteriness, sleep myoclonus, and hyperekplexia are the most common non-epileptic paroxysmal movements. Infants with convulsions in the neonatal period should be hospitalized and monitored with continuous video EEG, possible underlying metabolic disorders should be rapidly evaluated, and if a specific pathology is detected, treatment should be initiated accordingly. Anticonvulsant treatment is needed to control acute seizures. Despite recent studies, phenobarbital is still the most preferred drug in first-line treatment. In second-line treatment, levetiracetam and phenytoin are

* Corresponding Author's Email: drsefikaaldas@gmail.com

In: Current Approaches to Newborn Emergencies
Editors: Zuhal Keskin Sarılar and Serap Samut Bülbül
ISBN: 979-8-89530-999-5

widely used. Treatment should aim not only to stop acute seizures but also to prevent brain damage, reduce the risk of developing epilepsy in the future, and prevent neurologic sequelae.

Keywords: neonatal, phenobarbital, seizures

Introduction

Newborn care involves the management of their health immediately following birth. Diseases such as convulsions or neurological disorders bring worry to parents of the newborn baby. Late detection of newborns' abnormalities may lead to neonatal convulsions. Therefore, it is important to understand the causes, varieties, preventive measures, and treatments of convulsions. The fast development of nerve cells in the brain is the main reason for the beginning of convulsions in babies. This happens between the first hours after birth and the first month. The neonatal convulsion rate in newborns born after a complete period of nine months is one to five births in a group of 1,000 newborns. Causes such as the degree of the mother's disease, the health treatment of pregnant women, the previous history of the birth of the baby, unhealthy delivery procedures, poor preservation after the birth of the baby, or even the inability of some countries to provide proper medical treatment in time are concerning. It is important to identify newborn convulsions early since the repercussions from the unnoticeable disorder may be fatal. Hence, neonatal convulsions are detected as quickly as possible, and the treatment is crucial.

Understanding Newborn Convulsions

Newborn convulsions can be defined as paroxysmal events with an abnormal motor phenomenon in the neonatal period. These events can induce involuntary movement, autonomic dysfunction, or neurobehavioral change. With increasing age, responses between the involved cortical neurons and the motor function-associated neurons become much more effective, and convulsions occur occasionally (Kim et al., 2022). Newborn convulsion is a clinical phenomenon that shows characteristics similar to convulsions in childhood. However, due to the age-related immaturity of the neonatal brain, there are rapid changes in maturation toward other features differing from those in children and elder patients. Although exact statistics about newborn convulsions are still unavailable now, it is accepted that the recognition and treatment of convulsions in newborns are important because the immature brain makes a critical pattern of convulsion occurrence, and the associated morbidity can be significant. With technological advances, it has been reported that the incidence of illnesses, now being a focus of interest due to technological improvements, has increased, or that it has started to be recognized clearly.

The immature brain in the neonatal period has epidemiologic and pathophysiologic characteristics leading to neonatal seizures different from seizures in older children. Seizures are more prevalent in the neonatal period than at any other period in life, and most neonatal seizures are due to various types of brain injuries, including hypoxia-ischemia, stroke, and metabolic disorders. Many factors, such as the immaturity of the brain, birth asphyxia, intracranial hemorrhage, and meningitis, which are known as risk factors for neonatal seizures, may impair neurodevelopmental outcomes such as morbidity (Almuqbil et al., 2023). Because of these conditions, only the recognition of clinical exacerbation is difficult if all clinical signs are observed. Most newborns with convulsions are more immature when gestational age and birth weight are lower, and more neonates with systemic findings are present. Considering that convulsion-related mortality among neonates under 1500g of body weight or 32 weeks of gestational age is about 50%, this high-risk group requires more caution. Routine newborn EEG monitoring in the initially depressed preterm infant has also been recommended during the first 48 hours of life. Non-randomized studies found that nearly 50% of infants had subclinical seizures. Early recognition of neonatal seizures is important for immediate EEG monitoring and aggressive treatment (Samanta, 2021).

Epidemiology

Newborn seizures in the neonatal period are a frequent cause of referrals to pediatric physicians and are an important indicator of central nervous system dysfunction. Their incidence, ranging from 1 to 5 per 1000 live births, is influenced by risk factors such as prematurity, perinatal asphyxia, intracranial hemorrhage, and infection, with higher rates in low birth weight and premature infants. Epidemiological patterns vary by geography, socioeconomic status, and healthcare accessibility.

Assessing incidence is challenging due to variations in seizure definitions and the subtlety of some presentations. Electroclinical dissociation is frequent, and neonatal brain immaturity affects seizure expression, with widespread neuronal activation rather than focal pathways seen in adults. Advances in neuroimaging and EEG monitoring have improved diagnosis, yet epidemiological data remain heterogeneous, necessitating further prospective studies (Anand et al., 2014; Chakkarapani et al., 2024).

Convulsion Types and Non-Epileptic Paroxysmal Movements in the Neonatal Period

One of the most important things to do when evaluating convulsions is to observe and record clinical signs. Systematic observation has a great impact on identifying the types of convulsions. Convulsions are classified under four main headings according to clinical presentation: subtle, clonic, tonic, and myoclonic seizures.

Subtle Seizure: Sudden facial expressions with eye, tongue, and lip movements, abnormal licking, chewing movements, pedaling, side lying, and vasodilation are observed. This condition is also common in cases where the gestational age is low because the central nervous system is less developed.

Clonic Seizure: It occurs as rhythmic contractions that recur 1 to 3 times per second in any part of the body. It may be focal or multifocal; while focal seizures are localized in a specific body region, multifocal seizures occur in different regions. They usually occur without loss of consciousness. It has been associated with cortical dysplasia and metabolic disorders, and pathologic findings are often detected in EEG examinations.

Tonic Seizure: These are seizures that develop suddenly, usually last less than one minute, and are characterized by an increase in muscle tone. They may occur focally or generalized. In addition to the involvement of an extremity in continuous flexion or extension, asymmetric posture in the trunk and neck may be observed. It is associated with intraventricular hemorrhage and hypoxic-ischemic brain injury. In generalized tonic seizures, there is no significant abnormality on EEG, whereas EEG findings may be observed in focal types.

Myoclonic Seizure: It may be observed as focal or generalized. While the focal form occurs as rapid and isolated contractions in the head or extremities, contractions occur simultaneously in both arms and legs in generalized myoclonic seizures. The main features that distinguish them from clonic seizures are that they are faster, do not include a slow phase, and usually involve flexor muscle groups. Pathologic findings may be detected in some cases in EEG examinations.

Non-Epileptic Paroxysmal Movements

Correct differentiation of non-epileptic paroxysmal movements, which are frequently encountered in the neonatal period and may be confused with epileptic seizures, is of great importance. The most common of these movements are jitteriness, sleep myoclonus, and hyperekplexia.

Jitteriness

It is one of the most common non-epileptic motor movements. It is observed as symmetrical and rapid tremors without autonomic symptoms. The cessation of movements with passive flexion is a distinctive feature. There is no need for any treatment in infants diagnosed with jitteriness.

Sleep Myoclonia

It is a condition that is usually observed during REM sleep and occurs as fragmented myoclonic jerks. The typical feature is that the movements end when the baby is awakened from sleep. It does not cause any problems affecting the general condition of the baby and does not require treatment.

Hyperekplexia

It is characterized by hypertonia and exaggerated startle response triggered by auditory, visual, or tactile stimuli. It is associated with genetic mutations in the α subunit of the glycine receptor and may show autosomal dominant inheritance. While jitteriness and sleep myoclonus are benign conditions that do not require treatment, hyperekplexia may lead to serious complications such as apnea, aspiration, and sudden infant death syndrome. Therefore, clonazepam treatment and home monitoring with an apnea monitor are recommended (Acar et al., 2019; Mohammed, 2025; Zinjani, 2023).

Causes of Newborn Convulsions

Convulsions are symptomatic of internal damage due to various causes that put the brain under duress (Kim et al., 2022; Zinjani, 2023). Any distressing stimuli can have such an effect. Under the influence of a difficult birth, the dome of the skull acquires a convexity; the swollen brain swings from side to side and presses on the bony prominences. The longitudinal laceration in the dura mater is apparent. The aggressive growth of septicemia due to unwashed hands, unsterile materials, and cords also turns it into a case of sepsis. Understanding the causes of convulsions is imperative for proper management.

Neonatal convulsions are common in infants. However, they are rarely reported because of the benign nature of primary seizures and the lack of attention due to treatments. Perhaps two million out of a billion births develop convulsions. Improvements in health care have reduced stillbirths, and a hundred thousand more convulsions a year are being prevented as the scientific basis is understood. Convulsions are most common at the beginning of life, where the stresses of labor and birth cause tissue damage, acute severe intercurrent infection from non-sterile handling, and energy deficiency from relatively low blood glucose, independent of hereditary diseases of the newborn. These cause far more convulsions and deaths than underlying hereditary predispositions. Every time convulsions occur; they damage the cerebral cortex. Some hereditary brain diseases manifest themselves during this period, but more often they occur later. The peculiar susceptibility of the newborn is thought to be due to the active maturation of excitatory neurotransmission (Abdelhaie et al., 2021; Kim et al., 2022; Malik & Quddusi, 2013).

Newborns have numerous causes of convulsions, some of which are hypoxia at birth, various metabolic disorders, and others. Neonatal brain injury occurs frequently, and it is the most common cause of convulsions in a child (Zinjani, 2023). Moreover, given the unique characteristics of the neonate, they are more susceptible to convulsions compared to other patients (Kaminiów et al., 2021). Auspicious is the neonate after the first month, when convulsion is rarely fatal, making epidemiology hard. Thus, recognition of various possible causative factors of neonate convulsions and taking care of patients is important for the pediatrician.

Neonatal Brain Injury

Neonatal brain injury is one of the most serious diseases affecting the babies of the neonatal intensive care unit. The head of a newborn accounts for 1/4 of the total body size. After encountering an external force, injuries of different severity to the head often occur, and they always get severe injuries due to a soft head, immature brain, and negative protection of the skull. Hematocephalus occurs in 2–6 per 1000 live births: 1/3 before delivery, 1/3 at birth, and 1/3 in the neonatal period. Hematocerebra of newborn infants in the absence of active treatment is a significant factor in death and a major cause of subsequent cerebral palsy and developmental disorders. Perinatal events, maternal, prenatal, and neonatal events can be divided into four categories: maternal factors, prenatal factors, delivery factors, and neonatal factors. The convulsions caused by neonatal brain injury result from the abnormal discharge of neurons due to the damage to the neurons or their surrounding tissues. Neonatal brain injuries can lead to the occurrence of cerebral convulsions due to various factors, including severe hypoxia, ischemia, metabolic disorders, or intracranial infections. The abnormal discharge of neurons causes damage to the neurons or their surrounding tissues because the brain does not inhibit the barrier. Epilepsy occurs when newborn seizures multiply and spread (Tataranno et al., 2021).

Hypoxic-ischemic encephalopathy and subarachnoid hemorrhage are currently the main causes of convulsions. Other known etiological causes are ischemic stroke, epilepsy, central nervous system infection, and transient metabolic disorders, while no underlying cause can be identified in 9% of infants.

Brain injuries can not only cause minor or major nerve dysfunction, seizures, cramping, and severe injuries. Mental retardation, abnormal cranial nerves, brain injuries in the nervous diseases, infantile tetanus, and subsequent epilepsy because of the existence of the above factors, then it is necessary to focus on brain injuries.

Multidisciplinary management: Neonatal neurology, neonatology, neurosurgery, pediatrics, imaging, and laboratory technologists need cooperation. The brain is a major part of the central nervous system. Its morphology, nerve cell content, and structure determine the function of the brain. The overall development, nerve function in growth and development, complexity, and strong excitability are in connection with the brain. The basal metabolism of the tissue is relatively high. The head of the baby can be easily injured, and this is the most frequent sudden episode of the disease immediately after delivery. The crystal's bones are not closely interconnected, so the fractures are easily glimpsed. Conception, and a series of physiological and biomechanical changes such as the reduction of blood support and placental infection during the process of production, it is easy to dispel the gray matter in the head of the baby, which is easy to cause injury (Chakkarapani et al., 2024).

Metabolic Disorders

Metabolic disorders are the foremost disorders that cause convulsions in the newborn period (Malik & Quddusi, 2013). Multiple metabolic disorders can cause seizures in the newborn period, either by causing a disturbance in the ionic channels or by causing a disturbance in the metabolic situation of the neurons. The major metabolic disorders include hypoglycemia, electrolyte imbalances, and metabolic encephalopathy (Almannai et al., 2021). The disturbance in metabolic and ionic equilibrium might be caused by various etiologies, resulting in a decrease in electro-neuronal threshold and neuronal hyper-excitability. Therefore, the role of timely and proper evaluation and management of metabolic disorders should be emphasized in the newborn period.

Hypoglycemia is the most common metabolic disorder in newborns that causes seizures. Neonatal hypoglycemia is defined as plasma glucose levels less than 30 mg/dL in the first 24 h, less than 45 mg/dL in the first 48 h, and less than 50 mg/dL after the first 48 h in term neonates. Early and accurate monitoring and management of hypoglycemia can prevent long-term complications; therefore, the plasma glucose levels of at-risk neonates must be checked and managed properly.

In addition, the initial approach of the newborn baby must include serum calcium, phosphorus, sodium, and potassium level tests. Calcium, magnesium, and glucose levels must be monitored closely in newborns with convulsions suspected to be due to hypomagnesemia or hypoglycemia. Magnesium sulfate should be considered for the neurological prophylaxis of preterm babies. A better effect can be achieved by combining phenobarbital with magnesium sulfate. Recurrent seizures can also be observed in late-onset metabolic issues;

therefore, late-onset hypoglycemia, particularly in neonates with symptoms such as fever, vomiting, poor feeding, etc., should be taken into consideration. Untreated metabolic disorders that cause seizures can lead to epilepsy, and chronic epilepsy may lead to cortical and subcortical progressive losses. For these reasons, the diagnosis and management of metabolic disorders that may lead to convulsions in newborns have vital importance in preventing future complications.

Diagnosis of Convulsion in Newborns

It is of great importance to take a detailed history of newborns who are evaluated with suspicion of convulsion. Factors such as infections in the prenatal period, maternal diabetes, or complications during labor may provide critical clues in determining the etiology. Family history is guiding in the differentiation of genetically inherited epileptic syndromes. Dysmorphic features detected on physical examination may indicate metabolic diseases or neurocutaneous syndromes. In addition, abnormal odors in sweat and urine require evaluation of metabolic disorders.

Blood glucose, electrolytes, calcium, and magnesium levels should be assessed urgently to exclude rapidly correctable metabolic disorders. If the infection is suspected, a complete blood count and acute phase reactants should be analyzed, while lumbar puncture may be required to exclude central nervous system infections. Metabolic investigations such as blood gas, lactate level, tandem acylcarnitine profile, and urinary organic acids should be performed in the first stage. Although Magnetic Resonance Imaging (MRI) is considered the diagnostic gold standard, transfontanel ultrasonography (USG) may be preferred in emergencies.

EEG is a critical tool in the evaluation of neonatal convulsions. The fact that clinical seizures cannot always be observed on EEG or are detected only electrographically causes diagnostic difficulties in this age group. Seizures accompanied by both clinical and electrographic findings are defined as 'electroclinical seizures.' The gold standard method for definitive diagnosis is continuous video EEG monitoring.

Studies have shown that clinicians may have difficulty in the diagnosis of convulsions, and only a certain proportion of electrographic seizures can be observed clinically. Although amplitude EEG (aEEG) provides continuous monitoring in NICUs, it plays a limited role in diagnosis due to its low sensitivity compared to conventional EEG and its potential for false positive results. However, it is increasingly preferred in the follow-up of neonatal convulsions due to its practical use (Güngör et al., 2023; Kim et al., 2022; Mohammed, 2025; Muthaffar et al., 2024; Spenard et al., 2024).

Management

Newborn seizures are generally prompted by a mere 5% of natal and perinatal pathologies; nevertheless, they are the most common neurological signs at the beginning of life. Around 85% of these seizures are symptomatic of the fact that they either predominate in natal risk(s), physiopathologically follow them, or foresee a risk of intracranial suffering inducing long-term handicaps. The presence of newborn seizures promptly prognosticates a high risk of neurological or other sequelae rather than the same central nervous system involvement phenomenally represented by other clinical, encephalographic, and neuroimaging signs (Spagnoli et al., 2013).

Recent papers have provided precise anamnestic, clinical, laboratory, electroencephalography, and cerebral imaging profiles. The ideal approach to newborn symptomatic seizures has still not been exhaustively outlined. Meanwhile, the most fitting approach should be a prompt and appropriate antiepileptic treatment starting at the time of clinical suspicion, with an effective and rapidly delivered drug followed by early and serial loading in the event of ineffectiveness. Hence, neonatal seizures must deserve accurate observation by subspecialists in a multi-professional milieu (Spagnoli et al., 2018).

Pharmacological Interventions

Although the diagnosis and treatment of neonatal convulsions is urgent, the aim of treatment is not only to stop acute seizures but also to minimize brain damage and subsequent neurological problems. There is a consensus that both electroclinical seizures and electrographic seizures should be treated.

In an infant with convulsion, firstly, the airway should be kept open, and after this basic intervention, the possible causes of seizures should be systematically evaluated. Especially in cases where simple metabolic disorders are detected, treatment should be given for the cause.

In case of hypoglycemia, 2-4 mL/kg of 10% dextrose is administered intravenously. After this first intervention, 6-8 mg/kg/min dextrose perfusion is started to stabilize blood sugar, and it must be monitored regularly.

When hypocalcemia is detected, 10% calcium gluconate should be administered intravenously at a dose of 2 mL/kg for a minimum of 10-15 minutes, followed by cardiac monitoring.

In the case of hypomagnesemia, 50% magnesium sulfate should be administered intravenously or intramuscularly at a dose of 0.1-0.2 mL/kg, aiming to increase the serum level to the appropriate range.

Hyponatremia and Hypernatremia: If serum sodium level is <125 mEq/L or >150 mEq/L, fluid and electrolyte balances should be corrected. Hyponatremia is treated with slow sodium replacement and hypernatremia with careful fluid therapy.

Anticonvulsant Drugs

Phenobarbital is still the first choice for infants for whom anticonvulsant medication is decided to be initiated. Second-line treatments include phenytoin, levetiracetam, benzodiazepines, and lidocaine.

Phenobarbital: Phenobarbital, which acts by decreasing the sensitivity of GABA α-receptors, is a commonly used drug in the management of neonatal convulsions. The initial loading dose is usually 15-20 mg/kg intravenously (IV), and maintenance is started with 5 mg/kg/day at 12-24 hour intervals. Additional doses (up to 10 mg/kg) can be administered if seizure control cannot be achieved (max. 40 mg/kg/day). However, the neurodevelopmental effects of phenobarbital are still controversial, and caution should be taken. Possible adverse effects such as irritability, sedation, hypotension, respiratory depression, and hepatotoxicity must be followed. The use of different anticonvulsant drugs has come to the agenda as a result of the finding that it causes retardation in cognitive functions at high doses (Acar et al., 2019).

Levetiracetam: Levetiracetam is used as an alternative option when phenobarbital is inadequate or its side effects cannot be tolerated. It acts by binding to synaptic vesicle 2a and decreasing presynaptic neurotransmitter release. The initial dose is 10-20 mg/kg, and the dose can be increased up to 40-60 mg/kg in cases where no response is obtained. In the BSID III evaluation of patients treated with phenobarbital or levetiracetam for neonatal convulsion, Nathalie L. Maitre et al., showed that cognitive, language, and motor development were more affected in the group receiving phenobarbital. In addition, it was determined that phenobarbital increased the risk of cerebral palsy at cumulative doses, but levetiracetam had no such effect. It is increasingly preferred in the neonatal period because it has intensity ranges independent of GABA modulation and has a minimal sedative effect (Maitre et al., 2013).

Fosphenytoin and Phenytoin: Fosphenytoin or phenytoin, which are prodrugs that suppress overstimulation by inhibiting voltage-gated sodium channels, can be used in the setting where no response to phenobarbital and levetiracetam is obtained. The initial dose is usually 15-20 mg/kg, and care should be taken against cardiac side effects. It is known that hypotension, bradycardia, and sedation are the most common side effects related to phenytoin use in the neonatal period (Acar et al., 2019).

Midazolam: It is a benzodiazepine with a GABAergic mechanism of action and is used as a first-line agent in the treatment of acute convulsions in adult and pediatric emergencies, while it is the third-line treatment option in neonatal convulsions. The first dose is usually administered as a 0.05-0.2 mg/kg IV bolus; if seizures cannot be controlled, it can be continued as a 0.06-0.1 mg/kg/hour infusion. However, due to the risk of respiratory depression and hypotension, patients should be carefully monitored, and respiratory support should be provided when necessary (Falsaperla et al., 2024).

Lidocaine: As a class 1b antiarrhythmic, it shows an anticonvulsant effect by blocking voltage-gated sodium channels. The loading dose is 2 mg/kg and is administered by IV infusion over 10 minutes. The maintenance dose is determined according to the patient's weight. In retrospective studies, it has been reported that the response rate varies depending on the gestational week, underlying cause, and time of administration but is effective in an average of 70% of cases. However, current data suggest that lidocaine should be preferred only in resistant seizures (Weeke et al., 2016).

Bumetanide: Bumetanide, a loop diuretic, has been investigated for combined use with phenobarbital by increasing sodium-potassium-chloride cotransporter 1 expression. In studies, it did not stop seizures alone, but in combination with phenobarbital, it has been shown that the efficacy increases. However, in a multicenter study conducted in Europe, the study was terminated early due to side effects including hearing loss, hypotension, and severe hyponatremia (Pressler et al., 2015). Therefore, its use in newborns is not recommended.

Topiramate: Topiramate, which reduces convulsions through AMPA receptor blockade, has been shown to reduce the risk of developing epilepsy in neonates treated for hypoxic-ischemic encephalopathy (HIE). However, since continuous EEG monitoring was not performed in the early period, its effect on acute seizures is not known exactly (Filippi et al., 2018). In addition, the lack of an intravenous form is an important factor limiting its use in neonates.

Management of Resistant Convulsions

If convulsions persist despite dual anticonvulsant treatment, metabolic encephalopathies should be considered. Pyridoxine-dependent and folinic acid-responsive seizures may be treated empirically until the exact cause is determined. In this context, 100 mg/kg pyridoxine is given intramuscularly and can be repeated after 10 minutes if necessary. If seizures persist, 4 mg/kg/day of folinic acid is started after CSF sampling, and a response is expected within 24 hours.

Although many studies have been conducted on neonatal convulsions in recent years, the level of evidence for the recommendations in the World Health Organization (WHO) guidelines is still weak. In addition, the fact that acute symptomatic convulsions may spontaneously regress makes it difficult to determine the efficacy of treatment (Committee, 2011).

Prognosis

Although mortality has decreased with the developments in neonatal intensive care units, neurological sequelae continue to be an important problem. The underlying etiology is the most decisive factor in terms of prognosis. In addition, gestational week, birth weight, APGAR score, onset time, type, and duration of convulsion are among the factors affecting the clinical course. Issues such as which seizures cause brain damage and which frequency and duration of convulsions require treatment remain unclear.

Conclusion

In neonatal convulsions, rapid diagnosis and determination of the etiological cause should be the priority. Video EEG monitoring is an ideal method and should be used in all patients if possible. Phenobarbital is preferred in the first line of treatment, while levetiracetam and phenytoin are commonly used in the second line. However, large-scale controlled studies are required to demonstrate the efficacy and safety of anticonvulsant drugs used in the neonatal period.

References

Abdelhaie, O., Rateb, E., & Hosainy, E. (2021). Neonatal seizures and outcome in NICU. *Benha Journal of Applied Sciences*, *6*(5), 237-241.

Acar, D. B., Bülbül, A., & Uslu, S. (2019). Current overview of neonatal convulsions. *Şişli Etfal Hastanesi Tıp Bülteni*, *53*(1), 1-6.

Almannai, M., Al Mahmoud, R. A., Mekki, M., & El-Hattab, A. W. (2021). Metabolic seizures. *Frontiers in Neurology*, *12*, 640371.

Almuqbil, M., Alrumayyan, Y., Alattas, S., Baarmah, D., AlTuwaijri, W., AlRumayyan, A., … Alsaif, S. (2023). Neonatal seizures: Etiologies, clinical characteristics, and radiological features: A cross-sectional study. *Medicine*, *102*(37), e35185.

Anand, V., Pillai, S. K., & Jayakrishnan, D. (2014). Neonatal seizures: our experience of incidence, etiology and outcome in a tertiary care centre. *Indian Journal of Child Health*, *1*(2), 39-43.

Chakkarapani, A. A., Singh, I., & Balakrishnan, U. (2024). Comprehensive insights into neonatal seizure: etiologies, diagnostic tools, management and future directions. *Paediatrics and Child Health*.

Committee, W. G. A. b. t. G. R. (2011). Guidelines on neonatal seizures. *Geneva: World Health Organization.*

Falsaperla, R., Collotta, A. D., Sortino, V., Marino, S. D., Marino, S., Pisani, F., & Ruggieri, M. (2024). The Use of Midazolam as an Antiseizure Medication in Neonatal Seizures: Single Center Experience and Literature Review. *CNS & Neurological Disorders-Drug Targets-CNS & Neurological Disorders)*, *23*(10), 1285-1294.

Filippi, L., Fiorini, P., Catarzi, S., Berti, E., Padrini, L., Landucci, E., … Boldrini, A. (2018). Safety and efficacy of topiramate in neonates with hypoxic ischemic encephalopathy treated with hypothermia (NeoNATI): a feasibility study. *The Journal of Maternal-Fetal & Neonatal Medicine*, *31*(8), 973-980.

Güngör, O., Turgut, M., Yüzbaşı, B. K., Koyuncu, E., & Özdemir, Ö. M. A. (2023). Retrospective Evaluation of Etiological and Prognostic Factors of Neonatal Convulsions.

Kaminiów, K., Kozak, S., & Paprocka, J. (2021). Neonatal seizures revisited. *Children*, *8*(2), 155.

Kim, E.-H., Shin, J., & Lee, B. K. (2022). Neonatal seizures: diagnostic updates based on new definition and classification. *Clinical and experimental pediatrics*, *65*(8), 387.

Maitre, N. L., Smolinsky, C., Slaughter, J. C., & Stark, A. R. (2013). Adverse neurodevelopmental outcomes after exposure to phenobarbital and levetiracetam for the treatment of neonatal seizures. *Journal of Perinatology*, *33*(11), 841-846.

Malik, A. R., & Quddusi, A. I. (2013). Neonatal seizures, experience at Children Hospital and Institute of Child Health Multan. *Pakistan journal of medical sciences*, *29*(5), 1128.

Mohammed, S. J. (2025). Causes and Treatment Responses for Neonatal Convulsions. *Maaen Journal for Medical Sciences*, *4*(1), 3.

Muthaffar, O. Y., Aldail, A. A., Khojah, I. M., Alyazidi, A. S., Alotibi, T. K., & Makki, L. T. (2024). Etiologies and Seizure Outcome of Neonatal Seizures: A Tertiary University Hospital Experience. *Journal of Clinical Neonatology*, *13*(2), 42-47.

Pressler, R. M., Boylan, G. B., Marlow, N., Blennow, M., Chiron, C., Cross, J. H., ... Jullien, V. (2015). Bumetanide for the treatment of seizures in newborn babies with hypoxic ischaemic encephalopathy (NEMO): an open-label, dose finding, and feasibility phase 1/2 trial. *The Lancet Neurology*, *14*(5), 469-477.

Samanta, D. (2021). Recent advances in the diagnosis and treatment of neonatal seizures. *Neuropediatrics*, *52*(02), 073-083.

Spagnoli, C., Falsaperla, R., Deolmi, M., Corsello, G., & Pisani, F. (2018). Symptomatic seizures in preterm newborns: a review on clinical features and prognosis. *Italian Journal of Pediatrics*, *44*(1), 115.

Spagnoli, C., Pavlidis, E., & Pisani, F. (2013). Neonatal seizures therapy: we are still looking for the efficacious drug. *Italian Journal of Pediatrics*, *39*, 1-3.

Spenard, S., Cerda, C. I. S., & Cizmeci, M. N. (2024). Neonatal seizures in low-and middle-income countries: a review of the literature and recommendations for the management. *Turkish Archives of Pediatrics*, *59*(1), 13.

Tataranno, M. L., Vijlbrief, D. C., Dudink, J., & Benders, M. J. (2021). Precision medicine in neonates: a tailored approach to neonatal brain injury. *Frontiers in Pediatrics*, *9*, 634092.

Weeke, L. C., Toet, M. C., Van Rooij, L. G., Groenendaal, F., Boylan, G. B., Pressler, R. M., ... De Vries, L. S. (2016). Lidocaine response rate in aEEG-confirmed neonatal seizures: retrospective study of 413 full-term and preterm infants. *Epilepsia*, *57*(2), 233-242.

Zinjani, S. (2023). Common Medical Conditions in the Neonates. In *Clinical Anesthesia for the Newborn and the Neonate* (pp. 49-70). Springer.

Chapter 21

Neonatal Hematologic Emergencies

Alper Uygun*, MD

Department of Pediatric Hematology and Oncology, Ondokuz Mayıs University, Faculty of Medicine, Samsun, Turkey

Abstract

Hematologic emergencies in the neonatal period arise from the unique physiological characteristics and developmental immaturity of the neonatal hematopoietic and hemostatic systems. These emergencies encompass a wide range of conditions, including disorders of erythrocytes, platelets, leukocytes, and coagulation, each with distinct diagnostic and therapeutic challenges. Neonates exhibit significant differences in hematologic parameters compared to older children and adults, necessitating age-specific reference values and approaches. Prompt recognition and targeted management are critical to ensuring favorable outcomes in these potentially life-threatening conditions. This chapter provides clinical considerations in managing neonatal hematologic emergencies, emphasizing the importance of a multidisciplinary approach to optimize care and improve survival.

Keywords: pediatric hematology, newborn, emergency

---

* Corresponding Author's Email: auygunitf@gmail.com

In: Current Approaches to Newborn Emergencies
Editors: Zuhal Keskin Sarılar and Serap Samut Bülbül
ISBN: 979-8-89530-999-5

Introduction

The hematopoietic system begins developing during the embryonic period and continues its maturation after birth. The functional levels of many procoagulants, coagulation inhibitors, fibrinolytic components, and platelet-associated factors in neonates differ significantly from those in adults (Cantor, 2015). In addition to these developmental characteristics of hemostasis, numerous inherited bleeding and clotting disorders may manifest during the neonatal period (Davenport & Sola-Visner, 2021).

The neonatal hemostatic system is distinct from that of adults, characterized by hyporeactive platelets and reduced levels of coagulation factors. However, compensatory mechanisms mitigate these differences, resulting in a finely tuned and well-balanced hemostatic system (Reiquam & Smith, 1959).

When evaluating bleeding or thrombosis in neonates (<1 month of age for term babies) or infants (<1 year of age), the first order of business is to recognize that "normative" values are very different from what they are in older children (Roberts & Bain, 2022).

The field of neonatal hematology encompasses a wide range of topics, including epidemiology, pathophysiology, differential diagnosis, and therapeutic approaches to various hematological conditions. However, given the scope of this book, the focus will be limited to the hematological emergencies that arise during the neonatal period, rather than addressing the entirety of neonatal hematology in detail.

Erythrocyte Disorders

Neonatal Anemia

Erythropoiesis, the process of red blood cell formation, plays a fundamental role in early embryonic and fetal development. The regulation of this process in both the fetus and newborn, similar to adults, is predominantly controlled by erythropoietin (EPO), a key cytokine. The synthesis of adult hemoglobin (HbA; $\alpha 2\beta 2$) initiates during the second trimester of gestation but remains minimal until approximately 30–32 weeks post-conception, when its levels begin to increase significantly.

Anemia is typically characterized by a hemoglobin level or hematocrit value that falls at least two standard deviations below the mean or below the 5th percentile based on reference ranges adjusted for age and, when applicable, sex. In neonates, these reference values are influenced by gestational age at birth. For term infants, a hemoglobin level below 14 g/dL is considered abnormal and indicative of anemia, whereas in preterm infants born before 30 weeks of gestation, the lower threshold for normal is 11.5 g/dL (Roberts & Bain, 2022).

The common causes of neonatal anemia are summarized in Table 1. In the evaluation of an anemic neonate, the initial step is to determine the normal hemoglobin range based on the neonate's postnatal age and gestational week, as these values vary significantly during this period. Reference guidelines can be utilized to establish these thresholds (Perk et al., 2021). To investigate the etiology of anemia, a series of initial diagnostic tests should be performed. These include a complete blood count (CBC), direct and indirect Coombs tests, blood group determination, peripheral blood smear, and reticulocyte count. These investigations provide essential insights into the underlying causes and guide further diagnostic and therapeutic interventions.

Table 1. Common causes of neonatal anemia

Neonatal Anemia Causes	
Genetic Disorders	Diamond–Blackfan anemia Congenital dyserythropoietic anemia Mitochondrial cytopathy: Pearson syndrome
Infectious Disorders	Parvovirus B19 infection Neonatal Sepsis
Immune hemolytic disease	Immune–hemolytic disease of the newborn ABO incompatibility Rh incompatibility
Red cell membrane disorders	Hereditary Spherocytosis Hereditary Elliptocytosis
Red cell enzymopathies	Glucose-6-Phosphate Dehydrogenase (G6PD) Deficiency Pyruvate Kinase Deficiency
Hemoglobinopathies	Alpha Thalassemia
Others	Congenital Thrombotic Thrombocytopenic Purpura Congenital Hemolytic Uremic Syndrome

The evaluation of anemia in neonates begins with a thorough history and physical examination, followed by the interpretation of a complete blood count (CBC). If anemia is detected, a reticulocyte count should be performed as the next step. A decreased reticulocyte count suggests conditions such as anemia of prematurity, genetic disorders affecting the erythroid lineage in the bone marrow, or drug-induced suppression of red blood cell production.

In cases with an elevated reticulocyte count, a Coombs test (direct antiglobulin test) should be conducted to investigate the etiology. A positive Coombs test indicates possible causes such as ABO, Rh, or subgroup incompatibilities, necessitating further analysis of direct and indirect Coombs tests. If the Coombs test is negative, hemolysis should be investigated using a peripheral blood smear (Ören et al., 2016).

Neonatal Polycythemia

Polycythemia is defined as a hematocrit (HCT) or hemoglobin (HGB) level above the upper limit of normal (>2 standard deviations) for gestational and postnatal age (Okoye et al., 2017). The most common cause is delayed clamping of the umbilical cord. Other etiologies include the recipient twin in twin-to-twin transfusion syndrome and intrauterine chronic hypoxia. While the majority of neonates remain asymptomatic, complications such as hypoglycemia and hyperbilirubinemia may occur. In symptomatic cases, intravenous hydration can be administered as part of the management.

Management of Emergencies Related to Neonatal Erythrocyte Disorders

The acute management of neonatal erythrocyte disorders primarily involves stabilizing the neonate and addressing the underlying cause. Transfusion therapy is indicated when hemoglobin levels are critically low, such as <7 g/dL in asymptomatic neonates or <10 g/dL in symptomatic cases. Administering packed red blood cells (PRBCs) at a dose of 10–15 mL/kg helps restore adequate oxygen delivery. In neonates with cardiorespiratory instability, supplemental oxygen or ventilatory support may be necessary to ensure sufficient tissue oxygenation. Prompt treatment of the underlying etiology, such as hemolysis, infection, or hemorrhage, is essential for optimal outcomes.

Adjunct therapies may include supplementation with iron, folic acid, or vitamin B12 in cases of nutritional deficiencies or chronic blood loss. These measures support erythropoiesis and prevent recurrence of anemia, ensuring comprehensive management of the condition.

The primary treatment for neonatal polycythemia involves partial exchange transfusion (PET) using isotonic saline or plasma to reduce hematocrit levels below 60%, thereby improving blood flow and minimizing complications. Intravenous hydration is also essential to enhance perfusion and dilute elevated hematocrit levels.

Post-intervention, close monitoring of hematocrit, glucose levels, and overall clinical status is crucial, as hypoglycemia is a common complication that requires prompt correction. For long-term management, identifying and addressing underlying causes such as delayed cord clamping or placental transfusion syndromes is vital to prevent recurrence in subsequent pregnancies.

Platelet Disorders

Neonatal Thrombocytopenia

Neonatal thrombocytopenia, characterized by a platelet count below 150×10^9/L, is a common hematological disorder, especially among preterm and sick infants. This condition can arise from impaired platelet production, increased platelet destruction, or a combination of both. Based on the timing of onset, neonatal thrombocytopenia can be categorized into early-onset (<72 hours) and late-onset (>72 hours) forms. Early-onset thrombocytopenia is often associated with intrauterine growth restriction (IUGR), while late-onset thrombocytopenia is frequently linked to sepsis and necrotizing enterocolitis (NEC) (Roberts & Murray, 2003).

From an etiological standpoint, genetic fetal thrombocytopenia can be attributed to chromosomal abnormalities such as trisomies, congenital infections (including cytomegalovirus, parvovirus, and rubella), congenital malignancies, and genetic disorders like congenital amegakaryocytic thrombocytopenia, in addition to immune-mediated conditions. Early neonatal thrombocytopenia is frequently associated with intrauterine growth restriction, perinatal infections, and alloimmune or autoimmune disorders (such as maternal systemic lupus erythematosus or immune thrombocytopenic purpura). Late-onset neonatal thrombocytopenia most commonly arises from sepsis and necrotizing enterocolitis (Gunnink et al., 2014) (Table 2).

Table 2. Common causes of neonatal thrombocytopenia

Etiological Category	Example Causes	Onset Timing
Genetic Causes	Trisomies (e.g., Trisomy 21), Congenital amegakaryocytic thrombocytopenia	Early-onset (<72 hours)
Congenital Infections	Cytomegalovirus, Parvovirus, Rubella	Early-onset (<72 hours)
Congenital Malignancies	Congenital leukemia	Early-onset (<72 hours)
Immune Causes	Alloimmune thrombocytopenia (FNAIT), Autoimmune thrombocytopenia (e.g., maternal SLE or ITP)	Early-onset (<72 hours)
Intrauterine Growth Restriction (IUGR)	Associated with placental insufficiency	Early-onset (<72 hours)
Perinatal Infections	Sepsis, Necrotizing enterocolitis (NEC)	Late-onset (>72 hours)

When evaluating neonatal thrombocytopenia, it is essential to assess the severity of thrombocytopenia, the timing of its onset, and the presence of associated symptoms. Fetal/neonatal alloimmune thrombocytopenia (FNAIT) is the most common cause of severe thrombocytopenia in otherwise healthy, term infants. This condition arises due to the transplacental transfer of maternal anti-human platelet antigen (HPA) alloantibodies targeting fetal platelet antigens that the mother lacks, resulting in fetal platelet destruction and potentially suppressing fetal megakaryopoiesis.

In cases of severe thrombocytopenia (platelet count $<50{,}000/mm^3$), maternal history should be carefully reviewed for rheumatologic and autoimmune disorders. Investigations for infectious etiologies should also be conducted. Additionally, neonates with severe thrombocytopenia must undergo evaluation for intracranial hemorrhages to ensure prompt diagnosis and management.

Platelet Function Disorders

Platelet function disorders are rarely diagnosed during the neonatal period. They may present with bleeding diathesis and, in some cases, lead to thrombocytopenia at a later stage. A detailed history and thorough physical examination are crucial in differentiating between primary and secondary causes.

Among acquired causes, medications such as indomethacin, prostacyclin, and valproate are prominent contributors. Inherited causes, on the other hand, are often linked to conditions like Glanzmann thrombasthenia and adhesion defects.

Neonatal Thrombocytosis

There is no universally accepted upper limit for the platelet count in neonates. However, a large retrospective study identified an upper limit of 750,000/mm^3. There is no evidence to suggest that higher platelet counts are associated with an increased risk of thrombosis. Infectious causes are the most common etiologies observed (Jeon, 2021).

Thrombocytosis in neonates is typically a reactive process following infection, acute or chronic inflammation, or anemia. It is generally benign, resolves spontaneously, and, unlike in adults, is rarely associated with hemorrhagic or thromboembolic complications (Christensen et al., 2012).

Management of Emergencies Related to Neonatal Platelet Disorders

Platelet transfusion is a cornerstone in managing neonatal thrombocytopenia. Current British Committee for Standards in Haematology (BCSH) guidelines recommend transfusion thresholds based on bleeding risk. (New et al., 2016) For "high-risk" neonates (e.g., <28 weeks' gestation, birthweight <1000 g, clinically unstable, minor bleeding, or coagulopathy), the threshold is 25×10^9/L. For "very high-risk" neonates (e.g., major hemorrhage or high risk of intracranial hemorrhage), the threshold is 50×10^9/L.

Interventions for neonatal thrombocytopenia target the underlying etiology, such as antibiotics for sepsis or intravenous immunoglobulin (IVIG) for immune-mediated thrombocytopenia, including alloimmune, autoimmune, and drug-induced cases. Platelet transfusion remains the primary treatment for neonates with active bleeding or at high risk of significant bleeding, such as those with neonatal alloimmune thrombocytopenia (NAIT) or preterm infants. Prophylactic platelet transfusions are specifically indicated for cases with a high risk of serious complications, including intracranial hemorrhage.

Neonatal Leucocyte Abnormalities

Leukocyte abnormalities in neonates, including leukocytosis and leukopenia, represent critical hematologic issues that require precise diagnosis and timely intervention. These conditions may stem from a variety of physiological, infectious, or pathological causes, and their management is crucial in ensuring favorable neonatal outcomes.

The evaluation of neonatal leukocyte abnormalities involves a detailed clinical and laboratory assessment. A complete blood count (CBC) with differential is the cornerstone of diagnostic workup, providing essential data on leukocyte subtypes, such as neutrophils, lymphocytes, and monocytes. In cases of suspected leukocytosis, peripheral smear analysis and bone marrow aspiration may aid in distinguishing leukemoid reactions from hematologic malignancies. For leukopenia, specific markers like neutrophil counts, along with maternal antibody testing, are critical in identifying immune-mediated mechanisms. C-reactive protein (CRP) and procalcitonin levels are useful adjuncts in the early detection of sepsis-related leukocyte abnormalities. Additionally, blood cultures remain indispensable in confirming infectious etiologies, particularly in neonates presenting with clinical signs of sepsis.

Neonatal Leukocytosis

Neonatal leukocytosis, defined as an elevated white blood cell count, can arise from both physiological and pathological causes. A notable physiological cause is stress-related leukocytosis, which is frequently observed in neonates undergoing treatment with prostaglandin E1 for congenital heart disease. (Arav-Boger et al., 2001) This pharmacological intervention predictably increases leukocyte counts, making it a recognized non-infectious etiology. Similarly, prenatal corticosteroid administration, often used to prevent respiratory distress syndrome, has been associated with transient neonatal leukocytosis. Pathological causes primarily include infections, with conditions such as neonatal sepsis or necrotizing enterocolitis frequently linked to late-onset leukocytosis. Extreme leukocytosis, often termed hyperleukocytosis when counts exceed 100,000/μL, can also indicate hematologic malignancies or severe inflammatory responses. Accurate differentiation between benign leukocytosis and severe pathological causes, such as leukemoid reactions, is essential in guiding appropriate clinical management (Golomb et al., 2022).

Neonatal Leukopenia

Leukopenia in neonates, characterized by abnormally low leukocyte counts, often signifies a compromised immune response and heightened susceptibility to infections. This condition is particularly concerning in preterm neonates or those with very low birth weights, where it correlates strongly with early-onset neonatal sepsis. Maternal factors, such as isoimmunization leading to the transplacental transfer of leukoagglutinins, can also cause neonatal neutropenia, a subtype of leukopenia. In such cases, maternal antibodies target neonatal leukocytes, resulting in transient but significant reductions in white blood cell counts. Beyond infectious and immune-mediated causes, genetic disorders and hematologic diseases may also contribute to leukopenia. These conditions require a thorough diagnostic evaluation to differentiate transient forms from those necessitating long-term management (Shah et al., 2020).

Management of Emergencies Related to Neonatal Leucocyte Abnormalities

The management of neonatal leukocyte abnormalities focuses on addressing the underlying cause while mitigating immediate risks. For leukocytosis linked to infections, prompt initiation of empirical antibiotic therapy is critical, with adjustments based on culture results and clinical response. In severe cases of hyperleukocytosis, leukapheresis or exchange transfusion may be necessary to prevent complications such as leukostasis. Conversely, the management of leukopenia, particularly when associated with neutropenia, involves antimicrobial prophylaxis to prevent life-threatening infections. Granulocyte colony-stimulating factor (G-CSF) may be employed in specific cases to stimulate neutrophil production. In immune-mediated neutropenia, cessation of maternal antibody effects typically results in spontaneous recovery, obviating the need for long-term interventions (Adane et al., 2022).

Neonatal Coagulation Disorders

The neonatal coagulation system exhibits unique characteristics due to developmental immaturity, resulting in significant differences compared to adults (Hochart et al., 2021). At birth, neonates have reduced levels of many coagulation factors, including factors II, VII, IX, and X, as well as natural anticoagulants such as protein C and antithrombin. The vitamin K-dependent factors are particularly affected, as neonatal liver immaturity limits their synthesis. Despite these deficiencies, neonates maintain a delicate hemostatic balance, facilitated by elevated fibrinogen levels, hyperreactive platelets, and increased von Willebrand factor (VWF) activity. However, this balance can be easily disrupted by stressors such as infection, hypoxia, or trauma (Garba et al., 2016; Ostilla et al., 2024).

These developmental differences necessitate specific neonatal reference ranges for coagulation tests. For example, prothrombin time (PT), activated partial thromboplastin time (aPTT), and thrombin time (TT) are prolonged in neonates compared to older children and adults. A proper understanding of these values is essential for interpreting laboratory results and avoiding overdiagnosis or unnecessary interventions (Zou & Xu, 2017).

Hereditary Coagulation Disorders in Neonates

Hereditary coagulopathies in neonates include von Willebrand disease, hemophilia, and other rare genetic causes. Hemophilia A (factor VIII deficiency) and hemophilia B (factor IX deficiency) are X-linked recessive disorders that often manifest during the neonatal period. Although spontaneous bleeding is uncommon at birth, affected neonates may present with intracranial hemorrhage or excessive bleeding after invasive procedures such as circumcision or umbilical cord separation. Diagnosis involves prolonged aPTT with normal PT and confirmation by specific factor assays. Early identification is critical to prevent life-threatening complications. Replacement therapy with factor VIII or IX concentrates is the cornerstone of treatment (Saxonhouse & Manco-Johnson, 2009).

VWD, the most common inherited bleeding disorder, arises from quantitative or qualitative defects in VWF, a protein crucial for platelet adhesion. Neonates with VWD may exhibit mild mucosal bleeding, prolonged oozing from umbilical stump sites, or severe hemorrhage in rare cases.

Laboratory findings include prolonged bleeding time and reduced VWF antigen levels. Management depends on disease severity and ranges from desmopressin to VWF concentrates in severe cases (Katsaras et al., 2022).

Less common hereditary disorders include deficiencies of fibrinogen, factors V, XI, and XIII, and congenital afibrinogenemia. These conditions often present with unusual bleeding patterns, such as umbilical stump hemorrhage or delayed wound healing. Diagnosis requires specific assays, and management involves replacement therapy tailored to the deficient factor.

Acquired Coagulation Disorders in Neonates

Acquired coagulation disorders in neonates represent a critical concern in neonatal medicine, often resulting from a variety of factors, including disseminated intravascular coagulation (DIC) and vitamin K deficiency. These conditions can lead to severe hemorrhagic events and require prompt recognition and treatment to prevent long-term complications.

DIC in neonates is typically secondary to severe underlying conditions such as sepsis, perinatal asphyxia, or severe hypoxia. It is characterized by widespread activation of the coagulation cascade, leading to the consumption of clotting factors and platelets, resulting in a paradoxical state of both thrombosis and hemorrhage. Neonates with DIC often present with petechiae, purpura, oozing from venipuncture sites, and mucosal bleeding. Laboratory findings include prolonged prothrombin time (PT) and activated partial thromboplastin time (aPTT), low fibrinogen levels, and elevated fibrin degradation products (FDPs), including D-dimer levels.

Management of DIC primarily focuses on treating the underlying cause, such as administering antibiotics for sepsis or providing respiratory support for perinatal asphyxia. Replacement therapy with fresh frozen plasma (FFP) and cryoprecipitate is used judiciously to replenish consumed clotting factors, especially in neonates with active bleeding. Early intervention with supportive care improves survival rates and reduces complications (O'Sullivan & Hunt, 2015).

Vitamin K deficiency is a prevalent cause of acquired coagulation disorders in neonates due to the low transplacental transfer of vitamin K and the insufficient vitamin K content in breast milk. Neonates are inherently predisposed to a transient deficiency of vitamin K-dependent clotting factors (II, VII, IX, and X), which can result in Hemorrhagic Disease of the Newborn (HDN). HDN is classified into three forms: early (within 24 hours), classic (2–

7 days), and late (2–12 weeks), with the latter being particularly dangerous due to its association with intracranial hemorrhage.

Clinical manifestations of vitamin K deficiency bleeding (VKDB) include gastrointestinal bleeding, umbilical stump bleeding, and, in severe cases, intracranial hemorrhage. The late form is frequently associated with exclusive breastfeeding without vitamin K supplementation. Laboratory findings in VKDB include prolonged PT and aPTT, with normal platelet counts and fibrinogen levels (Ndour, 2017).

Prophylactic administration of vitamin K is a cornerstone of prevention. A single intramuscular dose of 1 mg vitamin K at birth is highly effective in preventing HDN. However, resistance to prophylaxis or non-compliance in administering vitamin K remains a challenge in some regions. In neonates who develop VKDB, immediate administration of vitamin K, either intravenously or intramuscularly, is essential. In cases of severe bleeding, FFP or prothrombin complex concentrates may be necessary (Puckett & Offringa, 2000).

Neonatal Thrombosis

Neonatal thrombosis, although relatively rare, represents a critical condition with potentially life-threatening and disabling outcomes. The neonatal period is uniquely predisposed to thrombotic events due to the immaturity of the coagulation system, which is characterized by reduced levels of both procoagulant and anticoagulant factors. Thrombotic events in neonates can arise from acquired conditions or hereditary predispositions, often requiring a multidisciplinary approach for management.

Acquired thrombosis in neonates is frequently linked to central venous catheters, which are often essential in neonatal intensive care but significantly increase thrombotic risk. Other major contributors include sepsis, dehydration, perinatal asphyxia, polycythemia, and maternal conditions such as diabetes and preeclampsia. Central venous catheterization remains the most common risk factor, particularly in the context of prolonged usage or improper placement, leading to venous thromboembolism in vessels like the superior vena cava or renal veins (Saxonhouse, 2012).

Acquired infections, particularly sepsis, induce a prothrombotic state by triggering endothelial injury and activation of coagulation cascades. Similarly, perinatal asphyxia results in systemic hypoxia and acidosis, further promoting clot formation. The combination of these factors creates an environment conducive to thrombosis in the already fragile neonatal vasculature (Saracco et al., 2009).

Hereditary thrombophilia, though less common, is increasingly recognized as a significant contributor to neonatal thrombosis. Mutations in genes encoding coagulation inhibitors and clotting factors, such as protein C and protein S deficiency, factor V Leiden mutation, and prothrombin gene mutation (G20210A), are well-documented genetic predispositions. Homozygous Protein C deficiency, for example, is associated with severe neonatal purpura fulminans, characterized by disseminated intravascular thrombosis and skin necrosis (Makatsariya et al., 2020).

Hereditary thrombophilias not only predispose neonates to primary thrombotic events but also complicate recovery from other thrombotic triggers, such as catheter-related thrombosis or neonatal sepsis. Genetic evaluation is critical in neonates with recurrent thrombosis or a strong family history of thrombotic disorders to identify and manage these underlying conditions.

Management of neonatal thrombosis requires a balanced approach, emphasizing anticoagulation to prevent thrombus extension while minimizing the risk of bleeding. Low molecular weight heparin (LMWH) is commonly used due to its predictable pharmacokinetics and ease of administration. In life-threatening situations, thrombolysis may be considered, although this is associated with a high risk of bleeding and is reserved for critical cases such as extensive cerebral venous thrombosis.

For neonates with hereditary thrombophilia, long-term anticoagulation or prophylaxis may be required, particularly in recurrent cases or when high-risk factors persist. Genetic counseling and family screening are essential components of care to address the broader implications of inherited conditions.

Management of Neonatal Coagulation Disorders in Emergencies

The management of disseminated intravascular coagulation (DIC) in neonates is centered on addressing the underlying cause while providing supportive care to stabilize the infant. Blood product replacement is critical in active bleeding cases, with fresh frozen plasma (FFP) and cryoprecipitate used to restore depleted coagulation factors and fibrinogen levels. Platelet transfusions are administered in cases of significant thrombocytopenia or ongoing hemorrhage to reduce bleeding risk. In select cases where thrombosis is a dominant feature, low-dose heparin therapy may be initiated, but this approach requires meticulous monitoring to balance the risk of hemorrhage against thrombus progression. Multidisciplinary collaboration ensures that treatment decisions are tailored to the neonate's condition and response to therapy.

In cases of vitamin K deficiency bleeding (VKDB), rapid correction of coagulopathy is achieved with intravenous or intramuscular administration of vitamin K at a dose of 1–2 mg, which addresses the deficiency and stabilizes the coagulation system. For neonates experiencing severe bleeding, fresh frozen plasma is essential to provide immediate replacement of the deficient clotting factors while the effects of vitamin K take hold. Intracranial bleeding requires urgent neurosurgical evaluation, along with supportive measures such as transfusions and intensive monitoring to prevent further neurological damage. Prevention through prophylactic vitamin K administration at birth is critical to reducing the risk of VKDB.

For thrombotic emergencies such as renal vein or cerebral venous sinus thrombosis, anticoagulation with low molecular weight heparin (LMWH) is the mainstay of therapy. LMWH is preferred for its predictable pharmacokinetics and reduced need for monitoring compared to unfractionated heparin. In rare cases of extensive or life-threatening thrombosis, thrombolytic therapy may be considered, although it carries a significant bleeding risk and must be carefully managed within a multidisciplinary framework. Imaging studies are frequently repeated to monitor thrombus resolution and guide treatment adjustments. Long-term follow-up is necessary to address potential complications and assess the need for ongoing anticoagulation in cases with an identified hereditary thrombophilia.

Management strategies in these emergencies require rapid, precise decision-making and close monitoring to minimize complications and improve neonatal outcomes.

Conclusion

Neonatal hematologic emergencies represent a critical domain of neonatal care, requiring precise diagnostic evaluation and timely intervention. The unique physiological characteristics of the neonatal hematopoietic and hemostatic systems, combined with the immaturity of vital processes, demand an age-specific approach to assessment and management. By understanding the pathophysiology, identifying early clinical signs, and applying evidence-based therapeutic strategies, clinicians can mitigate the morbidity and mortality associated with these complex conditions. A multidisciplinary approach, involving neonatologists, hematologists, and critical care specialists, is essential to optimize outcomes. Continuous research and advancements in neonatal medicine will further enhance our ability to manage these challenging emergencies effectively.

References

Adane, T., Worku, M., Tigabu, A., & Aynalem, M. (2022). Hematological Abnormalities in Culture Positive Neonatal Sepsis. *Pediatric Health, Medicine and Therapeutics*, *13*, 217-225. https://doi.org/10.2147/PHMT.S361188.

Arav-Boger, R., Baggett, H., Spevak, P., & Willoughby, R. (2001). Leukocytosis caused by prostaglandin E1 in neonates. *The Journal of pediatrics*, *138 2*, 263-265. https://doi.org/10.1067/MPD.2001.110304.

Cantor, A. B. (2015). In *Nathan and Oski's Hematology and Oncology of Infancy and Childhood, Eighth Edition* (pp. 128-157).

Christensen, R. D., Henry, E., & Del Vecchio, A. (2012). Thrombocytosis and thrombocytopenia in the NICU: incidence, mechanisms and treatments. *The Journal of Maternal-Fetal & Neonatal Medicine*, *25*(sup4), 7-9.

Davenport, P., & Sola-Visner, M. (2021). Hemostatic challenges in neonates. *Frontiers in Pediatrics*, *9*, 627715.

Garba, N., Ogbenna, A., Adediran, A., & Ib, F. (2016). Coagulation profile in normal full-term neonate in the first week of life in Lagos-Nigeria. *International Journal of Medical Research and Health Sciences*, *5*, 44-48. https://consensus.app/papers/coagulation-profile-in-normal-fullterm-neonate-in-the-garba-ogbenna/2416a81afb78517197c69e1295ae0a43/.

Golomb, O., Schushan-Eisen, I., Maayan-Metzger, A., Elisha, N., Strauss, T., & Mazkereth, R. (2022). The Clinical Significance of Extreme Leukocytosis among Newborns: A Retrospective Cohort Study. *American Journal of Perinatology*, *41*. https://doi.org/10.1055/a-1906-9048.

Gunnink, S. F., Vlug, R., Fijnvandraat, K., Van Der Bom, J. G., Stanworth, S. J., & Lopriore, E. (2014). Neonatal thrombocytopenia: etiology, management and outcome. *Expert review of hematology*, *7*(3), 387-395.

Hochart, A., Pierache, A., Jeanpierre, E., Laffargue, A., Susen, S., & Goudemand, J. (2021). Coagulation standards in healthy newborns and infants. *Archives de Pédiatrie*, *28*(2), 156-158.

Jeon, G. W. (2021). Pathophysiology, classification, and complications of common asymptomatic thrombocytosis in newborn infants. *Clinical and Experimental Pediatrics*, *65*(4), 182.

Katsaras, G. N., Gialamprinou, D., Papacharalampous, E., Chatziioannidis, I., & Mitsiakos, G. (2022). Neonatal bleeding disorders. A practical diagnostic approach. *Journal of Pediatric and Neonatal Individualized Medicine (JPNIM)*, *11*(2), e110231-e110231.

Makatsariya, A., Bitsadze, V., Khizroeva, J., Vorobev, A., Makatsariya, N., Egorova, E., Mischenko, A., Mashkova, T., & Antonova, A. (2020). Neonatal thrombosis. *The Journal of Maternal-Fetal & Neonatal Medicine*, *35*, 1169-1177. https://doi.org/10.1080/14767058.2020.1743668.

Ndour, D. (2017). Vitamin K Deficiency Bleeding: A Case Revealed by Intracranial Haemorrhage. *03*. https://doi.org/10.19080/ajpn.2017.06.555737.

New, H. V., Berryman, J., Bolton-Maggs, P. H., Cantwell, C., Chalmers, E. A., Davies, T., Gottstein, R., Kelleher, A., Kumar, S., & Morley, S. L. (2016). Guidelines on transfusion for fetuses, neonates and older children. *British journal of haematology*, *175*(5).

O'Sullivan, J., & Hunt, B. (2015). Acquired Bleeding Disorders. https://doi.org/10.1002/9780470015902.A0002254.PUB2.

Okoye, H. C., Nwogoh, B., & Odetunde, O. I. (2017). Correlation of hematocrit and Apgar scores in newborns of women with hypertensive disorders in pregnancy. *Journal of Neonatal-Perinatal Medicine*, *10*(4), 387-392.

Ören, H., Koç, A., & Bör, Ö. (2016). *TPHD Eğitim Serisi III Yenidoğan Hematolojisi*. Galenos Yayınevi.

Ostilla, L., Knopoff, K., Myers, P., & Morocco, P. (2024). Disorders of Coagulation in the Newborn. *NeoReviews*, *25*(11), e694-e709.

Perk, Y., Atasay, B., & Çetinkaya, M. (2021). Kan Ürünleri Transfüzyon Rehberi 2021 Güncellemesİ. *Türk Neonatoloji Derneği*

Puckett, R., & Offringa, M. (2000). Prophylactic vitamin K for vitamin K deficiency bleeding in neonates. *The Cochrane database of systematic reviews*, *4*. https://doi.org/10.1002/14651858.CD002776.

Reiquam, C., & Smith, N. J. (1959). Hematologic Disorders in the Newborn. *Postgraduate Medicine*, *26*(2), 123-134.

Roberts, I., & Bain, B. J. (2022). *Neonatal Haematology: A Practical Guide*. John Wiley & Sons.

Roberts, I., & Murray, N. (2003). Neonatal thrombocytopenia: causes and management. *Archives of Disease in Childhood-Fetal and Neonatal Edition*, *88*(5), F359-F364.

Saracco, P., Parodi, E., Fabris, C., Cecinati, V., Molinari, A., & Giordano, P. (2009). Management and investigation of neonatal thromboembolic events: genetic and acquired risk factors. *Thrombosis Research*, *123 6*, 805-809. https://doi.org/10.1016/j.thromres.2008.12.002.

Saxonhouse, M. (2012). Management of neonatal thrombosis. *Clinics in perinatology*, *39 1*, 191-208. https://doi.org/10.1016/j.clp.2011.12.018.

Saxonhouse, M. A., & Manco-Johnson, M. J. (2009). The evaluation and management of neonatal coagulation disorders. Seminars in perinatology,

Shah, J., Balasubramaniam, T., Yang, J., & Shah, P. (2020). Leukopenia and Neutropenia at Birth and Sepsis in Preterm Neonates of <32 Weeks' Gestation. *American Journal of Perinatology*. https://doi.org/10.1055/s-0040-1721133.

Zou, T.-T., & Xu, Y. (2017). The evaluation and management of neonatal coagulation disorders. *International Journal of Anesthesiology and Resuscitation*, *38*, 544-549. https://doi.org/10.3760/CMA.J.ISSN.1673-4378.2017.06.014.

Chapter 22

Neonatal Cardiac Emergencies

Muhammed Yaşar Kılınç*, MD, PhD
Department of Pediatric Cardiology, University of Health Sciences, İzmir, Turkey

Abstract

Neonatal cardiac emergencies represent a critical subset of neonatal pathology, characterized by structural or functional cardiac abnormalities that require immediate recognition and intervention. Although cardiac conditions are relatively uncommon causes of pediatric emergencies, their delayed diagnosis may result in life-threatening complications such as respiratory failure, cardiogenic shock, or circulatory collapse. These emergencies typically present in one of four clinical scenarios: cyanosis, circulatory shock, acute heart failure, or arrhythmias - each often related to ductal-dependent lesions or transitional circulatory changes. The diagnostic process in neonates is particularly challenging due to the limited reliability of physical examination, electrocardiography, and radiographic imaging in this age group. Therefore, clinical suspicion - guided by vital signs, timing of presentation, and characteristic symptom clusters - plays a pivotal role in early identification. Prompt initiation of therapies, such as prostaglandin E1 in suspected ductal-dependent conditions, may be lifesaving prior to confirmatory echocardiography. This chapter provides a systematic approach to recognizing and managing neonatal cardiac emergencies to improve outcomes in this vulnerable population.

Keywords: newborn, cardiac, emergencies

---

* Corresponding Author's Email: drmuhammed007@gmail.com

In: Current Approaches to Newborn Emergencies
Editors: Zuhal Keskin Sarılar and Serap Samut Bülbül
ISBN: 979-8-89530-999-5

Introduction

Approximately 1% of newborns in the world are born with congenital heart disease (CHD), an anomaly with the highest mortality rate [1]. Neonates with cardiac disease may present in acute or critical condition. Although cardiac diseases are not common causes among general pediatric emergencies [2], it is highly important to recognize these causes early and initiate proper treatments, as they need specific and urgent management. Late diagnosis can lead to significant respiratory compromises or circulatory failure in up to 30% of nonsyndromic children born with CHD [3]. Cardiac emergencies in newborns may pose significant diagnostic and therapeutic challenges due to the complexity of possible scenarios. Newborns may present as 'gray babies' in case of cardiogenic shock (due, for instance, to ductal-dependent systemic circulation malformations), as 'blue babies' in ductal-dependent pulmonary circulation malformations, or as 'pink babies' in congestive heart failure (CHF). Furthermore, any number of arrhythmias may present during neonatal life or even during fetal life, requiring early delivery [4]. The etiology of pediatric cardiac emergencies may vary depending on the patient's age and whether the cause of the emergency is congenital or acquired heart disease.

Neonatal cardiac emergencies may represent cardiac structural or cardiac functional abnormalities and can be divided into 2 major categories of presentation: [5].

1. Cyanosis related to:
   i. Ductal-dependent pulmonary blood flow
   ii. Obstructed pulmonary venous drainage
   iii. Transposition physiology.

2. Cardiogenic shock related to:
   i. Ductal-dependent systemic blood flow
   ii. Ventricular dysfunction
   iii. Arrhythmia.

The pathologies are split into four common presentations with the aim of providing a practical approach to cardiac emergencies in newborns: cyanosis, shock/circulatory failure, acute HF, and arrhythmias [6].

The diagnosis of cardiac disease in the neonates is not always straightforward because physical examination, ECG, and CXR are often difficult to interpret in the newborn period compared to older infants or children. Although echocardiography is required to precisely define the anatomical abnormality, it is usually possible to define the functional abnormality on the basis of the clinical and radiographic findings [4].

The timing of presentation and severity depends on

- Nature and severity of defect
- The alteration in cardiovascular physiology secondary to
- the effect of the transitional circulation as
- Closure of ductus/restriction of patent foramen ovale
- (PFO)
- Fall in pulmonary vascular resistance (PVR).

The most important factors in narrowing down the diagnostic possibilities are

- The clinical presentation
- Shock (ductal-dependent systemic circ.) (Grey baby)
- Cyanosis (ductal-dependent pulmonary circ.) (Blue Baby), including severe Ebstein's anomaly
- CHF (shunt lesions) (Pink Baby)
- The timing of the presentation (age)
- Associated noncardiac or genetic anomalies.

So the vital signs and clinical examination in newborns are very important and lead to the right diagnosis: right-sided obstructive lesions (cyanosis), left-sided obstructive lesions (collapse), mixing lesions (cyanosis with CHF), atrial septal defect (ASD)-dependent lesions (cyanosis with CHF), and give a chance to start prostaglandin (PGE1) when there is any suspicion of patent ductus arteriosus (PDA)-dependent lesion (systemic or pulmonary) before the echo [4].

Cyanosis

Cyanotic heart disease is another entity of CHD. The cyanosis results from the presence of deoxygenated hemoglobin more than 5 g/dL. The ability to recognize cyanosis is related to the level of hemoglobin. With higher hemoglobin concentration, we can recognize cyanosis more easily. Cyanosis can be peripheral or central. Central cyanosis involves the whole body, and it is recognizable in the mucosa and conjunctiva and requires a thorough clinical assessment to identify its causes. When a baby presents with cyanosis or desaturation, the physician should look for causes that lead to the presence of deoxygenated hemoglobin in the blood.

In general, this may be due to one of the three causes:

1. Incomplete oxygenation process of blood passing through the lung due to lung pathology leading to intrapulmonary shunt,
2. or due to shunting of deoxygenated blood from the right side of the heart to the left side systemic circulation leading to intracardiac shunt, or
3. due to having abnormal hemoglobin that cannot bind to oxygen.

Examples of the first causes are where the blood does not get fully oxygenated in the lungs, as happens in cases of collapsed lung or in cases of alveolar diseases such as pulmonary edema, respiratory distress syndrome, or severe pneumonia. This type of ventilation/perfusion (V/Q) mismatching is the result of intrapulmonary shunt. The saturation of patients with intrapulmonary shunts may improve with supplemental oxygen and positive pressure ventilation, as it improves V/Q matching. The second type of shunt that can lead to the presence of deoxygenated blood in systemic circulation is an intracardiac shunt that is present when the blood coming from venous circulation (right side of heart) crosses to systemic circulation (left side of heart) through abnormal communication within the heart chamber or great vessels. An example of this intracardiac shunt is Tetralogy of Fallot (TOF), where the venous blood coming to the right side of the heart crosses to the left side through Ventricular Septal Defect (VSD) in association with right ventricle outflow obstruction. When deoxygenated blood is mixed with oxygenated blood, the resulting blood has a lower saturation than normal and may lead to significant central cyanosis. This type of shunt is called an intracardiac shunt. One of the clinical bedside tests that can help differentiate intrapulmonary from intracardiac shunt is by giving 100% FiO2 through an oxygen hood to the affected neonate. The peripheral saturation usually improves in cases of lung diseases associated with intrapulmonary shunt; while on the other hand, the cyanosis, O2 saturation, and PaO2 do not improve in cases of intracardiac shunt due to CHD. The shunt may occur through PDA in cases of persistent pulmonary hypertension of neonates (PPHN), leading to a shunt from the pulmonary artery to the aorta through PDA. In this case, the shunt and saturation may partially improve with supplementing 100% FiO2, which has a vasodilatory effect on the pulmonary vascular bed. Measuring preductal saturation (right arm) and postductal saturation (left leg) may show a significant difference between pre‒ and post‒ductal PaO2, indicating that the blood is shunted at the level of PDA from pulmonary to systemic circulation, as it happens in cases of PPHN [7)

Table 1. Distinction between respiratory and cardiac cyanosis in the neonate [8]

Feature	Respiratory	Cardiac
History	Risk factors, e.g., meconium-stained liquor, prematurity, CNS depression	Suggestive antenatal scan, infant of diabetic mother, syndromes, previous children with CHD, etc.
Onset	At birth	Hours to days after birth
Examination	Respiratory distress tachypnea, grunting, recession	Comfortable unless duct-dependent pulmonary circulation with closing PDA
Auscultation	Lung crackles/wheezes, reduced air entry	Clear lungs, normal air entry, murmur not always present
Blood gas	High pCO_2, low pO_2	Normal/low pCO_2, low pO_2
Hyperoxia test*	'Passed'	'Failed'
Chest X-ray	Lung infiltrates, normal heart size	Clear lung fields, oligemia or plethora, heart normal or enlarged, 'typical' cardiac silhouette**
ECG	Normal	May be abnormal and provide a clue to diagnosis

* Hyperoxia test: measure right radial or brachial arterial pO_2 in 100% O_2 (closed headbox or rebreather mask for 10–15 min); $pO_2 < 150$ mmHg (20 kPa) → cardiac, $pO_2 > 150$ mmHg → respiratory (note: there may be a few exceptions to this rule).

**'Typical' X-ray patterns are only occasionally seen: 'egg on the side' (narrow mediastinum) for transposition, boot heart for tetralogy/pulmonary (and sometimes tricuspid) atresia, 'snowman' sign for supracardiac total anomalous pulmonary venous connection (TAPVC), and cardiomegaly with plethora for truncus arteriosus.

Table 2. The most frequent causes of cyanosis and differential cyanosis and their relationship to the ductus arteriosus

Type of cyanosis	Type of lesion	Ductal-dependent
Cyanosis	HLHS	Yes
	TOF with pulmonary atresia	Yes
	Pulmonary atresia with intact interventricular septum	Yes
	Critical pulmonary stenosis	Yes
	Tricuspid atresia	Yes
	Severe neonatal Ebstein anomaly	Yes
	Transposition of the great arteries	Yes
	Truncus arteriosus	No
	TAPVC	No
Differential cyanosis	Critical aortic stenosis	Yes
	Critical coarctation of the aorta	Yes
	Interrupted aortic arch	Yes

A few pointers are given to assist in distinguishing between respiratory and cardiac causes of cyanosis in the neonate (Table 1), as the former represents the main differential diagnosis, with mention of the more common lesions [8].

The 'five Ts' mnemonic provides a framework for facile recall of prevalent cardiac etiologies contributing to cyanosis in the neonatal period. These encompass dextro-transposition of the great arteries, TOF, truncus arteriosus, TAPVC, and tricuspid valve abnormalities. Other less common malformations that can cause cyanosis are hypoplastic left heart syndrome (HLHS), pulmonary atresia, anomalous systemic venous connection, double outlet right ventricle, or single ventricle [9-10].

The presence of differential cyanosis or reversed differential cyanosis can provide valuable diagnostic insights in a clinical context. Differential cyanosis is characterized by the manifestation of cyanosis in both lower extremities, while the right arm or both arms remain pink. The explanation for this phenomenon is that in patients with pulmonary arterial hypertension and PDA, the deoxygenated blood in the pulmonary artery enters the PDA and travels to the aorta and from there on to the lower half of the body. The color of the left arm depends on where the PDA enters the aorta: if below the left subclavian artery, then the left arm is pink, as it receives blood from the left ventricle (LV), the same as the right arm. If the PDA enters the aorta above the left subclavian artery, then the left arm is cyanotic. Differential cyanosis also appears in persistent pulmonary hypertension of the newborn associated with critical aortic stenosis or coarctation, interrupted or hypoplastic aortic arch [11-12].

Reverse differential cyanosis is encountered in newborns with transposition of the great arteries associated with high pulmonary vascular resistance, coarctation of the aorta, or interrupted aortic arch. In both cases, the descending aorta receives blood from the pulmonary circulation via a PDA; therefore, the legs are pink and the arms are cyanotic [11, 13].

Several ductal-dependent lesions should be suspected whenever differential cyanosis is observed, including critical aortic stenosis, critical coarctation of the aorta, or interrupted aortic arch [11, 12]. Conversely, classical cyanosis may indicate numerous ductal-dependent lesions, such as HLHS, TOF with pulmonary atresia, pulmonary atresia with intact interventricular septum, critical pulmonary stenosis, tricuspid atresia (if there is also severe right ventricular outflow tract obstruction), severe neonatal Ebstein anomaly (in this case a PDA is required to maintain pulmonary blood flow until the PVR diminishes), or transposition of the great arteries. Cyanosis could also be observed in various non-ductal-dependent lesions, such as truncus arteriosus or TAPVC (Table 2) [14].

All cyanotic CHDs are accompanied by central cyanosis. However, several non-cardiac conditions can also cause cyanosis, such as airway obstruction (laryngotracheomalacia or choanal atresia), hemoglobinopathies, neurologic diseases leading to hypoventilation (intraventricular hemorrhage, apnea of prematurity, cerebral infection, neonatal myasthenia gravis, Wernig–Hoffman disease, or phrenic nerve injury), and pulmonary diseases leading to ventilation/perfusion mismatch (pulmonary hypoplasia or hemorrhage, hyaline membrane diseases, emphysema, atelectasis, pleural effusion, or pneumothorax) or impaired alveolar-arterial diffusion (fibrosis or edema) [11, 15]. Therefore, neonates presenting with cyanosis warrant a thorough diagnostic investigation to discern potential major CHDs that necessitate immediate intervention [11].

Shock/Circulatory Failure

Circulatory failure is defined as a state of circulatory dysfunction that leads to a lack of adequate oxygen and nutrients to tissues or organs, resulting in anaerobic respiration. Its etiology is split commonly into four categories [6] (Table 3).

Any newborn presenting with shock should first undergo septic and hypovolemic shock screening, as these are the two most frequent causes of shock during the first month of life [16]. If cardiogenic shock is suspected, the four most frequent causes are congenital heart malformations, arrhythmia, cardiac muscle diseases, or cardiac metabolic disorders, and the baby should be transferred to a pediatric cardiology facility or pediatric intensive care unit [17].

Low cardiac output is the hallmark of cardiogenic shock (of any cause). In this particular clinical context, newborns can exhibit pale or cyanotic skin, diminished peripheral pulse, cold extremities, delayed capillary refill time, the presence of the third or fourth heart sound, tachycardia, diminished urinary output, signs of hepatic or pulmonary congestion, irritability, or lethargy [14, 17]. Clinical presentations in newborns with congenital heart disease in shock are given in Table 4.

Table 3. Types of shock/circulatory failure

Type of Shock	Etiology	Example Pathologies
Distributive	Abnormalities in vessel tone secondary to the release of inflammatory cytokines, problems with endothelial nitric oxide production, or immature neurovascular regulatory pathways	Sepsis, PPHN
Hypovolemic	Loss of fluid from the intravascular space through blood loss or from movement of fluid to extracellular spaces (e.g., third spacing)	Twin-to-twin transfusion, intraventricular hemorrhage, disseminated intravascular coagulation, sepsis, necrotizing enterocolitis
Cardiogenic	Immature or impaired contractility of the heart's myocardium leading to poor cardiac output	Perinatal asphyxia, cardiomyopathy, myositis
Obstructive	A physical obstruction to blood flow from the heart resulting in poor cardiac output	Congenital cardiac lesions, tension pneumothorax, cardiac tamponade

Table 4. Clinical presentations in neonates with congenital heart disease in shock

Duct-dependent systemic circulation and left ventricular outflow tract obstructions	Critical aortic stenosis Interrupted aortic arch Severe coarctation of the aorta HLHS
Rhythm disturbances	Tachyarrhythmias Complete heart block

Table 5. Cause of cardiac tamponade

Classification	Underlying pathology
Iatrogenic	CVC line migration Chest drain misplacement
Cardiac	Hydrops fetalis Myocarditis Infectious pericarditis (viral, bacterial, and fungal) Pericardial tumors, e.g., rhabdomyomas
Respiratory	Pneumopericardium secondary to lung pathology, e.g., pulmonary interstitial emphysema
Metabolic	Disorders of glycosylation Pompe disease

Cardiac tamponade and tension pneumothorax, which are causes of obstructive shock with sudden onset and requiring urgent action, should not be forgotten as neonatal cardiac emergencies [6].

Cardiac tamponade is the accumulation of fluid or air in the pericardial space that causes increased pressure sufficient to impair passive filling of the heart, leading to impaired myocardial contraction and consequent cardiorespiratory decompensation. The most common presentation in a neonate is sudden cardiovascular collapse. Classical features such as distended neck veins or muffled heart sounds are often hard to detect in a newborn baby. However, it can be readily detected on echocardiography via a simple subcostal or apical view [18]. There are numerous causes of pericardial effusions leading to tamponade (Table 5). The most common cause that will present to the neonatologist is secondary to central venous line migration. Thus, cardiac tamponade needs to be considered in any infant with a central venous catheter (CVC) who suddenly clinically deteriorates. The quoted incidence is around 1% of neonates with a CVC and carries a high mortality (50%). This highlights the need to frequently image the position of the CVC in neonatal intensive care to ensure they are in a safe position [19, 20].

A pneumothorax is the progressive increase of an air collection in the pleural space leading to the collapse of lung tissue. It is classified as exhibiting tension when the pneumothorax begins to push the contents of the mediastinum into the contralateral thoracic space. This obstructs the venous return of blood to the heart and cardiovascular collapse. It is estimated to affect up to 2 % of neonates in intensive care and is much more prevalent in neonates with underlying lung pathology (e.g., respiratory distress syndrome) or those who are mechanically ventilated [21]. Infants with a tension pneumothorax exhibit rapid clinical deterioration with tachypnea, pallor, and shock. An early sign of pneumothorax can be a sudden increase in oxygen requirement, especially in newborns on CPAP support. The cardiac impulse is displaced to the contralateral side of the pneumothorax, and there are absent breath sounds with resonant percussion on the affected side. There can also be abdominal distension owing to diaphragmatic distortion, leading to displacement of the liver. Infants will be hypotensive and tachycardic. A blood gas will also show increased partial pressures of CO_2. The affected side will transilluminate with the use of a cold light, and a chest x-ray will make the definitive diagnosis. However, due to the clinical condition of the infant, there is often not enough time to instigate these investigations, and urgent needle thoracocentesis is required [6].

Acute and Congestive Heart Failure

Many of the critical CHDs as well as the arrhythmias discussed in this chapter can present with acute heart failure (HF). The important point is to differentiate HF from respiratory distress due to lung disease or neonatal sepsis, as in older children, useful clues for HF are cardiomegaly and hepatomegaly [8]. In neonates, the history may reveal excessive weight gain owing to the development of peripheral edema and an inability to feed due to breathlessness. Depending on the cause, a cardiac murmur may also be found on examination. Auscultation of the lungs may reveal bilateral crepitations due to pulmonary edema. A chest x-ray can show cardiomegaly with pulmonary venous congestion. When looking at presentations of heart failure at tertiary cardiac centers, literature shows that over 50 % are due to congenital cardiac disease, followed by cardiomyopathies, acquired heart disease, and then arrhythmias. Table 6 outlines the pathologies that may present as acute heart failure in the neonate [22, 23].

Congestive heart failure in the neonate is usually associated with increased pulmonary blood flow and is more common with complex heart defects such as Swiss-cheese-type VSD, double inlet LV (single ventricle), double outlet right ventricle, and tricuspid atresia with a large ventricular septal defect, all without associated pulmonary stenosis [24]. A neonate with septal defects usually presents between 2 and 8 weeks of age with CHF due to pulmonary overcirculation, as there is a fall in PVR causing an increase in pulmonary blood flow. Rarely there can be an early presentation, as in a preterm child where a precipitous fall in PVR occurs, causing a large left-to-right shunt. In any newborn presenting with CHF, one should always look for other causes contributing to heart failure in addition to septal defects, as [25]:

Table 6. Pathologies that may present as acute heart failure in the neonate

Classification	Underlying pathology
Congenital heart disease	VSD ASD Atrioventricular septal defect TOF Coarctation of the aorta HLHS PDA Aortic stenosis TAPVC Truncus arteriosus TGA with VSD
Arrhythmia	Supraventricular tachycardia (SVT) Atrial flutter Atrial fibrillation Third-degree heart block Ventricular tachycardia
Heart muscle disease	Hypertrophic cardiomyopathy Dilated cardiomyopathy
Acquired heart disease	Viral myositis Endocarditis

a. Associated obstructive lesion, especially coarctation of the aorta, interrupted aortic arch, or, rarely, aortic stenosis.
b. Multiple levels of shunts, e.g., at atrial, ventricular, and great artery levels.

Initially, aggressive anti-congestive measures should be instituted. Because most of these defects can't be corrected in the neonatal period despite recent advances in open heart surgery, surgical constriction or banding of the pulmonary artery is useful in this subgroup of patients. Banding not only improves congestive heart failure but also helps achieve normal pulmonary artery pressure so that bidirectional Glenn and Fontan procedures can be safely performed later in the subgroup of patients who have single ventricle physiology. If associated aortic coarctation is present, the aortic obstruction must also be relieved [24].

Acquired ventricular dysfunction can be secondary to myocarditis, dilated cardiomyopathy, septicemia, and metabolic causes (hypoglycemia, hypocalcemia, asphyxia, or arrhythmias) [25].

Arrhythmias

Arrhythmias, though rare, are not uncommon in full-term and preterm newborns. Maternal diabetes, toxemia, and other postnatal conditions, e.g., asphyxia, hypothermia, and metabolic and electrolyte imbalances, all contribute to rhythm disturbances. A high index of suspicion in all neonates with left ventricular dysfunction is necessary to diagnose this condition. A critical evaluation of electrocardiography (ECG) is essential, especially because many of these ECGs may be casually interpreted as sinus tachycardia, which is commonly associated with LV dysfunction. It is not necessary to have a very fast heart rate to diagnose this condition. Suspicion is aroused when

a. The heart rate shows no variability and is fixed between 150 and 180 per minute.
b. Abnormal P wave axis
c. Atrioventricular dissociation
d. Prompt control of heart rate or return to sinus rhythm causes complete return of LV function to normal [25].

Bradyarrhythmias and tachyarrhythmias represent other neonatal cardiovascular emergencies. Commonly seen arrhythmias include junctional ectopic tachycardia, atrial tachycardias and atrioventricular reentrant nodal tachycardia, sinus bradycardia, ventricular premature contractions, ventricular tachycardia, and fibrillation. Children who underwent heart surgery may develop second- or third-degree AV block, right or, less commonly, left bundle branch block, intra-atrial reentrant tachycardia, or sinus bradycardia. An important aspect of arrhythmia prevention relies on normal potassium and magnesium levels. Normal calcium and sodium levels are also desirable. The pH level is also important, as acidosis promotes ventricular arrhythmia [26, 27].

Cardiac arrhythmias in the newborn period most often present as cardiac failure in newborns. They may also present with more subtle signs like persistent tachypnea or difficulty with feeding. When such an arrhythmia has been sustained throughout the antenatal period, the infant may present as hydrops fetalis [28].

The relative immaturity of the conduction systems, neurological regulatory systems, and the myocardium makes arrhythmias common. Identification of the arrhythmia is key in determining its origin and appropriate emergency treatment [6].

The most common neonatal tachyarrhythmias (excluding sinus tachycardia, which usually does not exceed 220/min) are atrioventricular re-entry tachycardia (associated with an accessory AV pathway), followed by atrial flutter. Less likely causes include AV node re-entry tachycardia, ectopic and multifocal atrial tachycardia, and junctional tachycardias. Note that these are all narrow QRS complex tachycardias. Wide complex tachycardias are less commonly seen and, as for older children, merit urgent consultation with a pediatric cardiologist. They are best regarded and treated as ventricular tachycardia rather than SVTs with aberrant conduction [8].

The most common cause of bradycardia in the neonate (defined as a heart rate <70/min) is congenital complete heart block. It is often associated with maternal lupus erythematosus or other connective tissue diseases (which are often asymptomatic in the mother). Less commonly, cases may be isolated or associated with CHD [8].

The pharmacological treatment of acute arrhythmias depends on the arrhythmogenic substrate and type of arrhythmia. Atrial flutter, atrial fibrillation, and atrioventricular nodal reentrant tachycardia may respond to procainamide (10–15 mg/kg loading dose over 30–45 min; infusion 20–40 μg/kg/min). If procainamide proves ineffective, amiodarone should be used (the loading dose of 5 mg/kg IV in 1–2 h in order to prevent acute alpha blockade can be repeated up to three times; infusion 15–20 mg/kg/24 h). Adenosine (50–200 μg/kg rapid bolus) can stop reentrant supraventricular tachycardias but not atrial ectopic tachycardia and junctional ectopic tachycardia. Ectopic atrial foci are better suppressed by esmolol. Verapamil should not be used in newborns [22]. Ventricular arrhythmias usually require lidocaine (1–2 mg/kg loading dose followed by 20–50 μg/kg/min infusion), sotalol (1 mg/kg IV over 60 min), or amiodarone [29]. Cardioversion is also feasible in this age group. Currents of 0.5–1 J/kg are used after adequate analgesia and sedation. The second shock, if required, should have a double intensity. Defibrillation for ventricular fibrillation or pulseless ventricular tachycardia requires higher energies, 2–5 J/kg. Intractable arrhythmias may benefit from extracorporeal membrane oxygenation, ventricular assist device support, or ablation [26, 29].

Management

A list of high-risk fetal or maternal indications generates a direct referral to a fetal cardiologist for fetal echocardiography for CHD screening [30) Otherwise, in most instances, CHD is suspected by the obstetrician or maternal-fetal medicine specialist during the anatomy scan and then confirmed by a fetal cardiologist. Once the diagnosis is made, multiple specialists become involved in prenatal counseling and management [31]. Information from serial fetal monitoring, including ultrasound and echocardiography, is used to modify the birth plan and to prepare for delivery and immediate postnatal care [32]. Specifics of the birth plan, including delivery location, timing, method (vaginal vs. cesarean delivery), presence of additional personnel and resources in the delivery room, and postnatal disposition, are made depending on the likelihood of hemodynamic instability after birth [33].

Birth planning and Neonatal Resuscitation Program (NRP) modifications in complex congenital heart defects are shown in Figure 1 [34].

Any neonatal patient with a cardiovascular emergency must be admitted to a newborn intensive care unit. The monitoring protocol encompasses ECG, temperature assessment, measurement of arterial and central venous pressure, and peripheral saturation. Laboratory tests should include lactate levels, troponin, B-type natriuretic peptide, and other markers of heart failure, myocardial dysfunction, or injury [35].

A chest X-ray is imperative for comprehensive evaluation, capable of revealing not only data concerning the cardiac silhouette but also indicators of oligemia or pulmonary edema. Echocardiography stands as a proficient modality for the discernment of diverse cardiac malformations. It can provide valuable insights into cardiac anatomy, the ejection and shortening fractions, as well as the myocardial performance index [36]. Cerebral and somatic near-infrared spectroscopy is a relatively new monitoring method that relies on the observation that oxygenated and deoxygenated hemoglobin absorb infrared light differently. It can be used to assess adequate tissue oxygen delivery [37].

Alprostadil infusion (PGE1) should be started as soon as a diagnosis is made or even suspected, which helps in keeping the ductus open or reopening a closed ductus. It is administered in doses of 0.05 to 0.1 μgm/kg/min. Complications of alprostadil include apnea, flushing, and hypovolemia. Children who are given prostaglandins may need mechanical ventilation, and if they are to be shifted to a higher center on prostaglandin infusion, they should be electively ventilated [8) Ideally, prostaglandin should be initiated prior to performing an echocardiogram. But if there is no access to echocardiogram or the echocardiogram done is unreliable, prostaglandin should be started on clinical suspicion (38, 39). It is better to start prostaglandin and transfer the child to a higher center, as a stable neonate improves the chances of results of further management (40). Lower doses in the range of 0.01 microgram/kg/min should be used once the duct has opened and continued till definitive surgical repair. With proper monitoring in the ICU for saturations and under echocardiographic guidance (for PDA monitoring), the dose can be reduced to 0.001 microgram/kg/min [41] (Table 7).

Table 7. If no response to prostaglandin infusion (4)

Diagnosis	Management
Transposition of Great Arteries with Intact Ventricular Septum and a Restrictive Interatrial Communication	Needs emergency Balloon Atrial Septostomy
Obstructed TAPVC	Emergency surgery
Noncardiac Diagnosis	Treatment of etiology

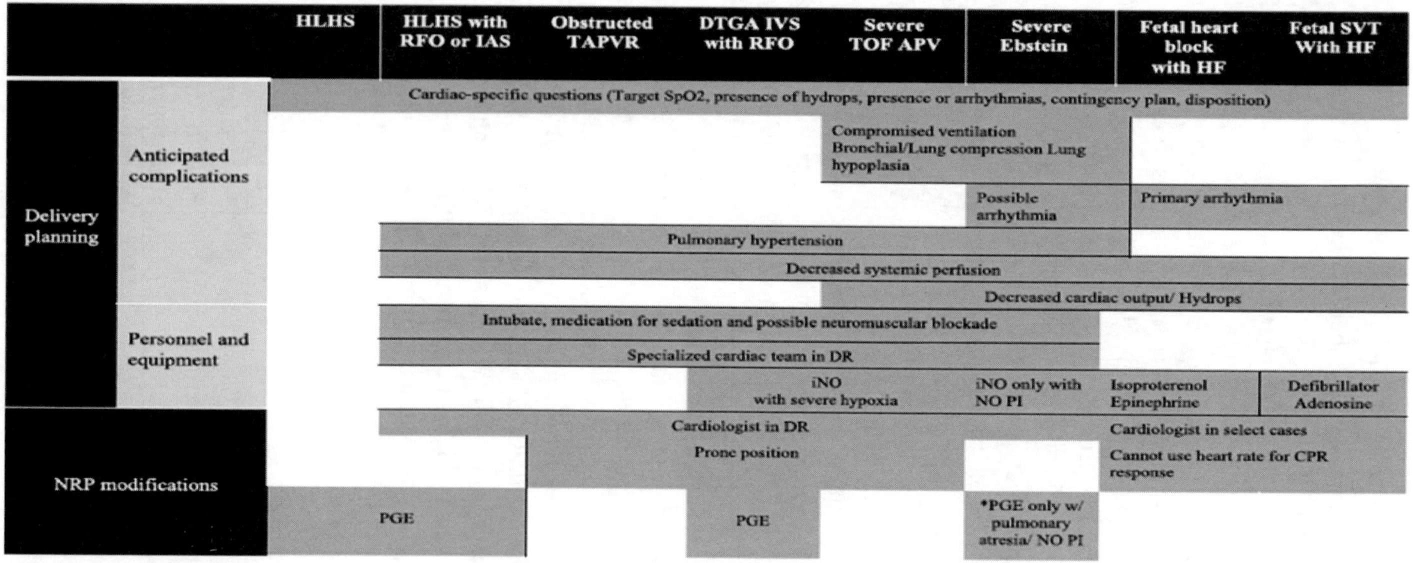

Abbreviations: APV, absent pulmonary valve; DR, delivery room; HF, heart failure; HLHS, hypoplastic left heart syndrome; IAS, intact atrial septum; iNO, inhaled nitric oxide; PGE, prostaglandin; RFO, restrictive foramen ovale; SVT, supraventricular tachycardia; TAPVR, total anomalous pulmonary venous return; TGA, transposition of great arteries; IVS, intact ventricular septum; TOF, tetralogy of Fallot.

Figure 1. Delivery planning and NRP modifications for complex congenital heart defects.

Therapeutic goals in critical patients include improving central and peripheral perfusion and oxygen delivery and consumption. The following therapeutic classes are available for pediatric use: inotropes (dopamine, dobutamine, epinephrine), vasodilators (nitroprusside, nitroglycerin, inhaled nitric oxide, prostaglandins, angiotensin-converting enzyme inhibitors, angiotensin receptor blockers, sildenafil), inodilators (milrinone, levosimendan), chronotropes (isoproterenol), vasoconstrictors (norepinephrine, phenylephrine, vasopressin), and β-adrenergic antagonists (esmolol) [42].

Conclusion

Evaluation and management of CHD in neonates is a crucial part of pediatric care, given the importance and prevalence of this condition. Timely recognition and intervention are essential, as a significant proportion of affected neonates become critically ill shortly after birth. It is essential to develop diagnostic and treatment algorithms for neonatal cardiac emergencies that are accepted across disciplines. Continuous research and clinical developments are essential to improve strategies and optimize care for this patient population.

References

[1] Wu, W., He, J., & Shao, X. (2020). Incidence and mortality trend of congenital heart disease at the global, regional and national level, 1990–2017. *Medicine, 99*(23), e20562.

[2] Meyer, S., Grundmann, U., Reinert, J., & Gortner, L. (2016). Specific aspects of pediatric emergencies in the prehospital setting. *Medizinische Klinik–Intensivmedizin und Notfallmedizin, 111*(1), 65–77.

[3] Watson, T., Kakar, P., Srivastava, S., & Dhanjal, T. S. (2007). Eustachian valve remnant. *Cardiology Journal, 14*(5), 508–509.

[4] Alasrawi, S. (2019). Cardiac emergencies in neonates. *Acta Scientific Health Sciences, 3*(6), 109–113.

[5] Allen, K. Y., Pittsenbarger, Z., & Roben, E. (2018). Neonatal cardiac emergencies. *Clinical Pediatric Emergency Medicine, 19*(4), 340–344.

[6] Mahoney, L., Rojas-Anaya, H., & Rabe, H. (2018). Cardiac emergencies in the newborn. In G. Buonocore, R. Bracci, & M. Weindling (Eds.), *Neonatology* (pp. 1–6). Springer. https://doi.org/10.1007/978-3-319-29489-6_216.

[7] Kabbani, N., Kabbani, M. S., & Al Taweel, H. (2017). Cardiac emergencies in neonates and young infants. *Avicenna Journal of Medicine, 7*(1), 1–6. https://doi.org/10.4103/2231-0770.197506

[8] Comitis, G. A. (2011). Neonatal cardiac emergencies. *Continuing Medical Education, 11*(11), 475–477.

[9] Marino, B., Bird, G., & Wernovsky, G. (2001). Diagnosis and management of the newborn with suspected congenital heart disease. *Clinics in Perinatology, 28*(1), 91–136. https://doi.org/10.1016/S0095-5108(05)70071-3

[10] Izraelit, A., Ten, V., Krishnamurthy, G., & Ratner, V. (2011). Neonatal cyanosis: Diagnostic and management challenges. *ISRN Pediatrics, 2011*, 175931. https://doi.org/10.5402/2011/175931.

[11] Singh, J., & Singh, A. (2013). Differential cyanosis. *American Journal of Medicine, 126*(10), e9. https://doi.org/10.1016/j.amjmed.2013.03.014.

[12] Sharma, A., Parasa, S. K., Gudivada, K. K., & Gopinath, R. (2014). Differential cyanosis and undiagnosed Eisenmenger's syndrome: The importance of pulse oximetry. *Anesthesia: Essays and Researches, 8*(2), 233–235. https://doi.org/10.4103/0259-1162.134518.

[13] Yap, S. H., Anania, N., Alboliras, E. T., & Lilien, L. D. (2009). Reversed differential cyanosis in the newborn: A clinical finding in the supracardiac total anomalous pulmonary venous connection. *Pediatric Cardiology, 30*(3), 359–362. https://doi.org/10.1007/s00246-008-9314-0.

[14] Lee, J. Y. (2010). Clinical presentations of critical cardiac defects in the newborn: Decision making and initial management. *Korean Journal of Pediatrics, 53*(6), 669–679. https://doi.org/10.3345/kjp.2010.53.6.669.

[15] Steinhorn, R. H. (2008). Evaluation and management of the cyanotic neonate. *Clinical Pediatric Emergency Medicine, 9*(3), 169–175. https://doi.org/10.1016/j.cpem.2008.06.006.

[16] Chan, K. H., Sanatani, S., Potts, J. E., & Harris, K. C. (2020). The relative incidence of cardiogenic and septic shock in neonates. *Paediatrics & Child Health, 25*(6), 372–377. https://doi.org/10.1093/pch/pxz078.

[17] Viveiros, E., Aveiro, A. C., Costa, E., & Nunes, J. L. (2013). Cardiogenic shock in a neonate. *BMJ Case Reports, 2013*, bcr2012008440. https://doi.org/10.1136/bcr-2012-008440.

[18] Iyer, V. H. A., Sharma, D. M., Charki, S., & Mohanty, P. K. (2014). Cardiac tamponade in a neonate: A dreadful condition, need for functional echo. *BMJ Case Reports, 2014*, bcr2014207040. https://doi.org/10.1136/bcr-2014-207040.

[19] Warren, M., Thompson, K. S., Popek, E. J., Vogel, H., & Hicks, J. (2013). Pericardial effusion and cardiac tamponade in neonates: Sudden unexpected death associated with total parenteral nutrition via central venous catheterization. *Annals of Clinical & Laboratory Science, 43*(2), 163–171.

[20] Abdellatif, M., Ahmed, A., & Alsenaidi, K. (2012). Cardiac tamponade due to umbilical venous catheter in the newborn. *BMJ Case Reports, 2012*, bcr20126160. https://doi.org/10.1136/bcr-2012-6160.

[21] Apiliogullari, B., Sunam, G. S., Ceran, S., & Koc, H. (2011). Evaluation of neonatal pneumothorax. *Journal of International Medical Research, 39*(7), 2436–2440. https://doi.org/10.1177/147323001103900704.

[22] Nugent, A. W., Daubeney, P. E. F., Chondros, P., Carlin, J. B., Cheung, M., Wilkinson, L. C., Davis, A. M., Kahler, S. G., Chow, C. W., Wilkinson, J. L., & Weintraub, R. G. (2003). The epidemiology of childhood cardiomyopathy in Australia. *New England Journal of Medicine, 348*(17), 1639–1646. https://doi.org/10.1056/NEJMoa021737.

[23] Massin, M. M., Astadicko, I., & Dessy, H. (2008). Epidemiology of heart failure in a tertiary pediatric center. *Clinical Cardiology, 31*(8), 388–391. https://doi.org/10.1002/clc.20262

[24] Rao, P. S. (2008). Neonatal cardiac emergencies: Management strategies. *Neonatology Today, 3*(9), 1–5.

[25] Tomar, M. (2016). Neonatal cardiac emergencies: Evaluation and management. *Journal of Intensive & Critical Care, 2*(2), 1–5.

[26] Ban, J. E. (2017). Neonatal arrhythmias: Diagnosis, treatment, and clinical outcome. *Korean Journal of Pediatrics, 60*(11), 344–352. https://doi.org/10.3345/kjp.2017.60.11.344.

[27] Singh, P., Thakur, A., Garg, P., & Kler, N. (2017). Neonatal arrhythmias. *Current Medicine Research and Practice, 7*(4), 135–145. https://doi.org/10.1016/j.cmrp.2017.04.003.

[28] Wren, C. (2006). Cardiac arrhythmias in the fetus and newborn. *Seminars in Fetal & Neonatal Medicine, 11*(3), 182–190. https://doi.org/10.1016/j.siny.2005.12.001.

[29] Andropoulos, D. B., & Chang, A. C. (2013). *Pediatric cardiovascular intensive care*. Wiley-Blackwell.

[30] Makkar, N., Satou, G., DeVore, G. R., & Sklansky, M. (2022). Prenatal detection of congenital heart disease: Importance of fetal echocardiography following normal fetal cardiac screening. *Pediatric Cardiology, 43*(6), 1203–1211. https://doi.org/10.1007/s00246-022-03032-6.

[31] Davis, J. A. M., Bass, A., Humphrey, L., Texter, K., & Garee, A. (2020). Early integration of palliative care in families of children with single ventricle congenital heart defects: A quality improvement project to enhance family support. *Pediatric Cardiology, 41*(1), 114–122. https://doi.org/10.1007/s00246-019-02231-y.

[32] Udine, M., & Donofrio, M. T. (2023). The role of the neonatologist in fetuses diagnosed with congenital heart disease. *NeoReviews, 24*(9), e553–e568. https://doi.org/10.1542/neo.24-9-e553.

[33] Zloto, K., Hochberg, A., Tenenbaum-Gavish, K., Berezowsky, A., Barbash-Hazan, S., Bardin, R., Hadar, E., & Shmueli, A. (2022). Fetal congenital heart disease: Mode of delivery and obstetrical complications. *BMC Pregnancy & Childbirth, 22*(1), 578. https://doi.org/10.1186/s12884-022-04910-w.

[34] Moisa, S. M., Brinza, C., Floria, M., & Burlacu, A. (2024). Navigating neonatal cardiovascular emergencies: A comprehensive narrative review on assessment and intervention strategies. *Journal of Cardiovascular Emergencies, 10*(1), 1–6.

[35] Kuzin, J. K., Yborra, J. G., Taylor, M. D., Chang, A. C., Altman, C. A., Whitney, G. M., & Mott, A. R. (2007). Family-member presence during interventions in the

intensive care unit: Perceptions of pediatric cardiac intensive care providers. *Pediatrics, 120*(4), e895–e901. https://doi.org/10.1542/peds.2006-294.

[36] Martin, A. C., Rigby, M. L., Penny, D. J., & Redington, A. N. (2003). Bedside balloon atrial septostomy on neonatal units. *Archives of Disease in Childhood. Fetal and Neonatal Edition, 88*(4), F339–F340. https://doi.org/10.1136/fn.88.4.F339.

[37] Rais-Bahrami, K., Rivera, O., & Short, B. L. (2006). Validation of a noninvasive neonatal optical cerebral oximeter in veno-venous ECMO patients with a cephalad catheter. *Journal of Perinatology, 26*(10), 628–635. https://doi.org/10.1038/sj.jp.7211573.

[38] Shivananda, S., Kirsh, J., Whyte, H. E., Muthalally, K., & McNamara, P. J. (2010). Accuracy of clinical diagnosis and decision to commence intravenous prostaglandin E1 in neonates presenting with hypoxemia in a transport setting. *Journal of Critical Care, 25*(1), 174.e1–174.e9. https://doi.org/10.1016/j.jcrc.2009.04.010.

[39] Penny, D. J., & Shekerdemian, L. S. (2001). Management of the neonate with symptomatic congenital heart disease. *Archives of Disease in Childhood. Fetal and Neonatal Edition, 84*(2), F141–F145. https://doi.org/10.1136/fn.84.2.F141.

[40] Jaimovich, D. G., & Vidyasagar, D. (Eds.). (2002). *Handbook of pediatric and neonatal transport medicine* (2nd ed., pp. 93–125). Hanley & Belfus.

[41] Aggarwal, N., Sachdev, M. S., Joshi, R., & Joshi, R. (2011). Neonatal and pediatric cardiac emergencies - Part 1: When to start prostaglandin in neonate. *Office Bearers, 9*, 1–5.

[42] Saengsin, K., Pickard, S. S., & Prakash, A. (2022). Utility of cardiac CT in infants with congenital heart disease: Diagnostic performance and impact on management. *Journal of Cardiovascular Computed Tomography, 16*(4), 345–349. https://doi.org/10.1016/j.jcct.2021.12.004.

Chapter 23

Neonatal Endocrine Emergencies

Ceren Yapar Gümüş*, MD
Department of Pediatrics, Ordu University, Ordu, Turkey

Abstract

Neonatal endocrine emergencies, encompassing conditions such as congenital hypothyroidism, hypoglycemia, hyperglycemia, and congenital adrenal hyperplasia, represent critical challenges in neonatal care. These emergencies arise from hormonal imbalances, congenital anomalies, or acute stress factors, leading to potentially life-threatening complications if not promptly addressed. Early detection through newborn screening programs and accurate diagnostic approaches, such as laboratory evaluations and imaging, is vital for timely intervention. Management strategies focus on hormonal replacement therapy, nutritional adjustments, and supportive care to stabilize acute symptoms while minimizing long-term complications. This chapter highlights the pathophysiology, clinical manifestations, and evidence-based treatment protocols for common neonatal endocrine emergencies, emphasizing the importance of early intervention and tailored therapeutic strategies to optimize outcomes.

Keywords: congenital adrenal hyperplasia, congenital hypothyroidism, endocrine disorders in neonates, hormonal replacement therapy

---

* Corresponding Author's Email: cerenyapar91@gmail.com

In: Current Approaches to Newborn Emergencies
Editors: Zuhal Keskin Sarılar and Serap Samut Bülbül
ISBN: 979-8-89530-999-5

Introduction

The neonatal period, defined as the first 28 days of life, represents a critical timeframe for human development characterized by significant physiological changes and adaptations. During this period, the endocrine system plays an essential role in regulating various metabolic processes necessary for growth, development, and homeostasis. In neonates, the endocrine system is still maturing, rendering them particularly vulnerable to a range of endocrine disorders that, if not promptly recognized and managed, can lead to life-threatening conditions. Neonatal endocrine emergencies encompass a broad spectrum of conditions that can arise from congenital anomalies, hormonal imbalances, or acute stress factors. These emergencies are often life-threatening and, if not addressed promptly, can result in significant morbidity and mortality. For example, congenital hypopituitarism, which has an incidence ranging from 1 in 4,000 to 1 in 10,000 neonates, manifests through nonspecific symptoms such as hypoglycemia, prolonged jaundice, poor weight gain, temperature dysregulation, electrolyte abnormalities, and hemodynamic instability. This condition poses immediate threats to life and can lead to long-term complications (Bautista, 2022; Bosch I Ara et al., 2021). Another critical condition is neonatal hypoglycemia, which can result from various factors, including maternal diabetes, malnutrition, or hormonal deficiencies. Without immediate treatment, neonatal hypoglycemia may lead to irreversible neurological damage, emphasizing the importance of careful monitoring and management of at-risk populations (Parkin et al., 2019). The clinical manifestations of these endocrine emergencies are often nonspecific and may overlap with other clinical conditions, complicating diagnosis and management. Symptoms such as lethargy, feeding difficulties, irritability, and abnormal vital signs may indicate underlying endocrine dysfunction, requiring high clinical suspicion among healthcare providers (Finnegan et al., 2023). Consequently, neonatal screening programs have proven instrumental in early detection and timely initiation of necessary treatments for conditions like congenital hypothyroidism and congenital adrenal hyperplasia (CAH), leading to better outcomes (El-Bakry, 2023; Lee, 2023). However, despite advancements in screening and diagnostic capabilities, many neonates with endocrine emergencies remain undiagnosed until acute symptoms manifest, underscoring the need for continuous education and awareness among clinicians (Kurtoğlu, 2019). In addition to congenital conditions, endocrine emergencies may also result from acquired factors, including infections, metabolic disorders, and environmental stressors. For instance, neonatal sepsis can lead to adrenal insufficiency, complicating the clinical picture and necessitating a multifaceted approach to management (Kanczkowski et al., 2013). The interplay between various systems during the neonatal period underscores the complexity of diagnosing and treating endocrine emergencies, requiring a comprehensive understanding of underlying pathophysiological mechanisms. This section aims to explore the fundamental pathophysiological mechanisms and treatment approaches for neonatal endocrine emergencies, focusing on conditions such as congenital hypothyroidism, neonatal hyperthyroidism, neonatal hypoglycemia, hyperglycemia, neonatal hypocalcemia, hypercalcemia, CAH, and congenital hypopituitarism. Understanding these mechanisms enhances our ability to effectively recognize and manage these emergencies, ultimately improving neonatal outcomes and reducing the risk of long-term complications.

Congenital Hypothyroidism (CH)

Diagnosis of thyroid dysfunction in the neonatal period is often difficult. The first signs and symptoms of the disease are often misleading or vague. To recognize and treat thyroid diseases early, it is necessary to know thyroid physiology well, to be able to evaluate thyroid function tests accurately, and to be alert to emergencies.

General Information

From the 12th week of gestation onward, thyroid-stimulating hormone (TSH), thyroxine (T4), and triiodothyronine (T3) reach detectable levels. Although thyroid activity remains low through mid-gestation, it gradually increases toward term. Postnatally, these hormones undergo rapid and dramatic changes. Within one hour after birth, there is an acute surge in TSH, reaching 60–80 mU/L levels. By the end of the first week of life, TSH levels decrease below 10 mU/L. The rise in TSH triggers significant increases in free T4 (FT4) and T3, peaking on the first day of life and gradually decreasing to infantile levels within the first two weeks (Cornella, 2017, pp. 908–912; translated version). Thyroid hormones critically affect the central nervous system, growth and development, and thermoregulation. Congenital hypothyroidism (CH), characterized by absent or markedly diminished thyroid function at birth, is one of the most common endocrine disorders in neonates, with a prevalence of 1 in 2,000 to 4,000 live births (Yang et al., 2023). It occurs more frequently in females and is significantly more common in infants with Down syndrome. Approximately 15% of cases are hereditary, while 85% are sporadic (Cornella, 2017, pp. 908–912; translated version). The pathophysiology of CH is classified into primary hypothyroidism, secondary hypothyroidism, tertiary hypothyroidism, and hypopituitary hypothyroidism. Primary hypothyroidism occurs due to developmental defects, congenital defects in thyroid hormone synthesis, maternal exposure to radioactive iodine during pregnancy, and antithyroid drug use. Secondary hypothyroidism is associated with TSH deficiency, tertiary hypothyroidism with TRH deficiency, and hypopituitary hypothyroidism with other hormonal deficiencies. The most common cause of congenital hypothyroidism is thyroid dysgenesis, characterized by abnormal thyroid gland development resulting from agenesis, hypoplasia, or ectopia (Rose et al., 2022).

Clinical Findings

Since some of the mother's T4 hormone is passed to the baby through the placenta, most babies with CH have no clinical signs at birth.

Symptoms in Symptomatic Infants

Symptoms are usually absent at birth. However, it may present vague findings in the first weeks of life. Even if the newborn screening test is normal, FT4 and TSH tests should be performed if there is suspicion. Early findings of the disease include a large baby according to gestational age, respiratory distress syndrome, a large fontanelle, umbilical hernia, hypotonia, a tendency to sleep, constipation, hypothermia, feeding difficulties, and prolonged unconjugated hyperbilirubinemia. Late findings usually start after 1.5 months. These findings include crying with a coarse voice, coarse facial appearance, macroglossia, dry coarse skin and hair, palpebral edema, and myxedema (Maniam et al., 2020). In infants with central hypothyroidism, clinical symptoms often develop due to a deficiency of other pituitary hormones. These infants may present with hypoglycemia, micropenis, undescended testes, and hearing loss. The clinical findings associated with congenital hypothyroidism may be nonspecific and overlap with other conditions, making early diagnosis through newborn screening essential. With thyroid hormone replacement therapy, outcomes can significantly improve and prevent the serious consequences of untreated hypothyroidism.

Screening Program

Screening methods can include T4 measurement after TSH measurement, primary T4 level followed by TSH measurement, or T4 and TSH measurement together.

In a healthy newborn, a newborn screening test should be performed by taking heel prick blood on approved filter paper. The ideal timing for this procedure is after the baby has completed 24 hours of life (preferably between 48 and 72 hours) at discharge or before the end of the first week of life, whichever occurs earlier. If any abnormality is detected as a result of screening for congenital hypothyroidism, serum TSH and FT4 levels should be measured as soon as possible. Consultation with a pediatric endocrinologist is recommended, if possible, to support the diagnosis and treatment process.

Assessment of Results

According to the current recommendations of the American Academy of Pediatrics (AAP), the need for urgent follow-up is based on the TSH level measured in the screening program (Rose et al., 2022).

1. If the TSH level is >40 mIU/L in the screening program, levothyroxine (L-T4) treatment (starting dose of 10-15 mcg/kg/day) should be started without waiting for the results after obtaining a confirmatory serum sample.
2. If the TSH level is ≤40 mIU/L in the screening program, repeat the newborn screening, wait for the results of the confirmatory serum sample (preferably within 24 hours), and evaluate the result before starting L-T4 therapy.
    a. If serum TSH is >20 mIU/L and serum FT4 is normal, start L-T4 therapy or continue current therapy.
    b. If serum TSH level is high but ≤20 mIU/L and serum FT4 is normal, L-T4 treatment can be initiated, or serum TSH and FT4 levels can be monitored closely every 1-2 weeks without

treatment. If FT4 is low or TSH levels are above 10 mIU/L after the 4th week of life, L-T4 treatment is recommended.

c. There is insufficient evidence to recommend treatment rather than observation for infants with serum TSH levels >5 mIU/L but ≤10 mIU/L and persisting elevation beyond 4 weeks of age. In these cases, if not already done, consultation with a pediatric endocrinologist is recommended to establish a patient-specific management plan.

d. When the serum TSH level is normal or low and the serum T4 level is low, further testing and evaluation for the possibility of central hypothyroidism is recommended. In this case, T4, FT4, and TSH should be measured as confirmatory serum tests. If T4 is low but FT4 is normal, measurement of thyroxine-binding globulin concentration may be useful to differentiate central hypothyroidism from thyroxine-binding globulin deficiency. Infants with central hypothyroidism should be referred to a pediatric endocrinologist for evaluation of hypothalamic-pituitary dysfunction. Careful attention should be paid to the timing of this evaluation before initiating L-T4 treatment, as such treatment may result in a drop in cortisol levels.

Imaging

Imaging with thyroid ultrasonography or scintigraphy helps establish the etiology of CH but usually does not change the clinical management of the patient before the age of 3 years.

Treatment

CH should be treated with L-T4 given by the enteral route with an initial dose of 10-15 mcg/kg/day once daily (J et al., 2014). The main goal of L-T4 therapy is to support normal neurocognitive development and growth. Achieving the best outcomes, especially in severe cases of CH, depends on initiating adequate L-T4 therapy early (preferably by 2 weeks of age after detection at the first newborn screening) (Aleksander et al., 2018). Rapid normalization of serum FT4 and TSH levels (preferably within 2 to 4 weeks of treatment initiation) contributes to improved neurocognitive outcomes (Salerno et al.,

2002). Late initiation of treatment and delayed normalization of thyroid function are associated with more unfavorable outcomes (Baysal et al., 2017). Treatment aims to keep FT4 levels in the upper half of the age-specific reference range and TSH at the lower limit of normal. Thyroid function, growth, and development should be closely monitored at regular intervals with clinical and laboratory tests to adjust the treatment dose optimally and to assess treatment adherence. The recommended monitoring program for serum TSH and FT4 is as follows (Rose et al., 2022):

1. Follow-up should be performed 1 to 2 weeks after starting L-T4 treatment and every 2 weeks until the serum TSH level reaches normal levels.
2. In the first 6 months of the baby's life, it should be checked every 1 to 2 months.
3. Between 6 months and 1 year every 2 to 3 months
4. Every 3 to 4 months between 1 year and 3 years of age
5. Checks should be performed every 6-12 months until growth is complete.

Evaluation of the Persistence of CH

1. If the patient is found to have thyroid agenesis or an ectopic thyroid gland, CH is a permanent condition.
2. TSH >10 mIU/L after 1 year of age suggests persistence.
3. If TSH increases when treatment is stopped, CH is considered to be persistent.

In the long term, CH can lead to adverse effects on intelligence, cardiovascular function, growth and development, and quality of life. Newborn screening programs have greatly improved neurodevelopmental outcomes in patients with CH, and early diagnosis and adequate treatment prevent the development of severe mental disorders. Individuals with CH who receive adequate L-T4 treatment usually have normal neurocognitive functioning in adulthood (Aleksander et al., 2018). Despite the success of the screening program, doctors should consider this diagnosis when infants show signs of hypothyroidism. In the case of post-screening or acquired hypothyroidism, the possibility of hypothyroidism should not be ruled out in cases where screening was not performed, such as screening errors or some home births. In these cases, serum TSH and FT4 tests should be performed independently of the screening results.

Neonatal Hyperthyroidism

Overproduction of thyroid hormones in newborns is a rare but important endocrine disorder known as neonatal hyperthyroidism. Other autoimmune diseases, including maternal Graves' disease, which is the most common cause, or congenital anomalies of the thyroid gland, can cause this condition. Early recognition and proper management of neonatal hyperthyroidism are crucial to prevent serious complications such as growth retardation and cardiological problems. Graves' hyperthyroidism occurs in about 0.2 percent of pregnant women, and about 1 to 5 percent of babies born to these mothers have neonatal Graves' disease (Alexander et al., 2017). Transplacentally transmitted TSH receptor antibodies (TSHR-Ab) cause this condition. Congenital non-autoimmune hyperthyroidism is associated with mutations activating the TSH receptor and McCune-Albright syndrome.

Clinical Findings

Overproduction of thyroid hormones can lead to a hypermetabolic state in the newborn, affecting multiple systems. Symptoms may start within hours after birth or within the first 10 days. These findings include irritability, hypertension, tachycardia, tremor, decreased weight gain, arrhythmia, pulmonary hypertension, decreased platelet count, hepatosplenomegaly, facial hyperemia, goiter, exophthalmos, craniosynostosis, and eyelid retraction (Farrehi, 1968).

Diagnosis

The diagnosis of neonatal hyperthyroidism is primarily based on clinical findings and laboratory tests. Maternal history of thyrotoxicosis and detection of thyroid-stimulating antibodies in the 3rd trimester of pregnancy affect the development of thyrotoxicosis in the newborn. The patient may be euthyroid or hypothyroid as a result of the tests taken from the baby at birth. However, the presence of goiter in the physical examination of the baby may be the only abnormal finding in addition to the clinical findings of thyrotoxicosis mentioned previously. This shows the importance of history and physical examination in the diagnosis. Elevated serum FT4 and suppressed TSH levels in laboratory tests confirm the diagnosis of neonatal thyrotoxicosis (Benlarbi et al., 2021).

Treatment

Although the disease usually has a self-limiting course, the severity of symptoms is a guiding factor in treatment. Severe forms of the disease are a life-threatening emergency, and treatment should be initiated immediately. In mild disease, only close monitoring will be sufficient. In patients in whom treatment is initiated, appropriate doses of treatment are extremely important to avoid hypothyroidism. Methimazole or propylthiouracil can be used to inhibit thyroid hormone synthesis. The dose of methimazole is 0.5-1 mg/kg/day and is given in 3 divided doses. (Total dose should not exceed 40 mg per day.) The dose of propylthiouracil is 5-10 mg/kg/day in 3 doses (Alexander et al., 2017). Propylthiouracil has more serious side effects, such as hepatotoxicity, than methimazole (Rivkees & Szarfman, 2010). Therefore, methimazole may be preferred as a first-line treatment. A beta-adrenergic blocker such as propranolol, when given at 2 mg/kg/day every eight hours, plays an important role in controlling neuromuscular and cardiovascular hyperactivity. Inhibition of the conversion of T4 to T3 is an advantage of using propranolol over other beta blockers. The disease is usually self-limiting and usually resolves spontaneously within two to four months. The mortality rate in affected newborns is approximately 15% if the disease is not diagnosed and treated. Possible long-term morbidities include advanced bone age, hyperactivity, craniosynostosis, and intellectual impairment (Cornella, 2017, pp. 908–912; translated version).

Neonatal Hypoglycemia

Neonatal hypoglycemia is a critical endocrine emergency that requires early diagnosis and treatment to protect brain development throughout the neonatal period. Low blood glucose levels, especially in the first hours of life, can lead to long-term neurologic complications if not treated promptly. This requires careful monitoring of hypoglycemia with diagnostic thresholds based on the age and clinical status of the newborn. Infants of diabetic mothers, large for gestational age, small for gestational age, and late preterm infants are at risk for hypoglycemia.

Diagnosis

In neonatal hypoglycemia, the diagnostic thresholds for blood glucose vary according to the age and clinical findings of the newborn. The limit value for hypoglycemia is considered to be <40 mg/dL on the first day of life in those with signs of hypoglycemia, <25 mg/dL in the first 4 hours, <35 mg/dL between 4-24 hours, <50 mg/dL after 24 hours, and <60 mg/dL after day 2 in those without signs of hypoglycemia (Aliefendioğlu et al., 2018). These thresholds are defined as critical levels to protect brain development, as low blood glucose levels can cause irreversible damage, especially from a neurodevelopmental point of view. Hypoglycemic newborns often have no obvious symptoms. Symptoms usually occur due to autonomic nervous system activation and neuroglycopenia. Screening for hypoglycemia in symptomatic infants and prompt treatment is important because the presence of symptoms may indicate poor neurodevelopmental outcomes. Therefore, prompt treatment is critical to prevent potential neurologic damage. Symptoms of hypoglycemia include irritability, jitteriness, lethargy, feeding difficulties, apnea, tachypnea, bradycardia, cyanosis, hypothermia, high-pitched crying, abnormal eye movements, hypotonia, convulsions, and coma (Whipple & Frantz, 1935).

Treatment

Neonatal hypoglycemia is a condition that requires rapid intervention to minimize the risk of neurological damage. The treatment goal of hypoglycemia is to prevent brain damage by increasing blood glucose levels to a safe level. Since prolonged or recurrent hypoglycemia can lead to serious neurodevelopmental consequences, newborns in such situations require close monitoring and prompt treatment.

Determining Initial Values and Monitoring

Regular glucose monitoring in the first 24 hours is important in infants at risk of hypoglycemia. The threshold value in the first 24 hours in symptomatic newborns is 40 mg/dL; in asymptomatic newborns, it is 25 mg/dL between 0-4 hours, 35 mg/dL between 4-24 hours, and 50 mg/dL after 24 hours. Treatment should be started immediately in babies with blood glucose levels below these values. Blood glucose levels of babies in the risk group should be checked every 2-3 hours (Aliefendioğlu et al., 2018).

Emergency Treatment and Glucose Infusion

In newborns whose blood glucose level falls below the threshold value and who are especially symptomatic, rapid intervention is required. In the first stage, 2 a mL/kg IV bolus of glucose is given using a 10% dextrose solution. Blood glucose levels are tried to be raised rapidly with this initial bolus. Continuous glucose infusion should then be started at a rate of 6-8 mg/kg/min. Blood glucose levels should be checked every 30 minutes until they reach the target range, and the infusion rate should be increased if necessary (Cornblath et al., 2000).

Glucagon and Other Supportive Treatments

If there is difficulty in establishing an intravenous line or if intravenous therapy is unresponsive, glucagon may be considered as a treatment option. Glucagon raises blood glucose levels by mobilizing liver glycogen stores. However, since glycogen stores are limited, the effect is temporary. The glucagon dose is 0.02-0.30 mg/kg/dose. Hydrocortisone can also be used to overcome cortisol deficiency in cases where there is no response to hypoglycemia. The dose of hydrocortisone is 5 mg/kg/day. Hydrocortisone can reduce the negative effects on the brain by supporting blood glucose levels (Aliefendioğlu et al., 2018; Weston vd., 2016).

Enteral Nutrition and Glucose Stabilization

Enteral nutrition has an important role in controlling hypoglycemia. Frequent breastfeeding can stabilize blood glucose levels in hypoglycemic newborns. In asymptomatic or mildly symptomatic hypoglycemic infants, glucose levels can be normalized by feeding. In cases where enteral nutrition cannot be achieved, intravenous glucose infusion should be continued (Harris et al., 2017). For example, according to the APA recommendation, management of newborns 0-4 hours of age should be as follows (Committee on Fetus and Newborn & Adamkin, 2011):

1. Blood Glucose Level <25 mg/dL:
    - *Treatment:* Nutrition (preferably breast milk or formula) is provided.
    - *Monitoring:* Blood glucose level is rechecked 30 minutes after feeding.
    - If the blood glucose level is still <25 mg/dL, intravenous (IV) glucose infusion is started.

2. Blood Glucose Level ≥25 mg/dL but <40 mg/dL:
    - *Treatment:* Frequent feeding is recommended.
    - *Monitoring:* Blood glucose level is monitored at 2-3 hour intervals.

Management of newborns aged 4-24 hours should be as follows:

1. Blood Glucose Level <35 mg/dL:
    - Treatment: The newborn is fed and rechecked after 30 minutes.
    - If the blood glucose level is still <35 mg/dL, intravenous glucose therapy is started.

2. Blood Glucose Level ≥35 mg/dL but <45 mg/dL:
    - *Treatment:* Glucose stabilization is achieved with nutrition.
    - *Monitoring:* Blood glucose level is monitored at 3-hour intervals.

Advanced Follow-up and Discharge Criteria

Blood glucose levels should be monitored regularly during treatment, and the infusion rate should be reduced slowly when target values are reached. Glucose infusion can be terminated when glucose levels drop to 3-5 mg/kg/min. In cases of persistent hypoglycemia or refractory hypoglycemia, further investigations and long-term follow-up are required. Before discharge, plasma glucose levels are recommended to be at target values after 4-6 hours of fasting before feeding (McKinlay et al., 2015).

When Is Further Investigation Necessary in Hypoglycemia?

Further investigation into neonatal hypoglycemia is important when assessing the risk of persistent hypoglycemia. Such investigations are usually initiated after 48 hours and are recommended in the presence of the following conditions:

1. Failure to Stabilize Blood Glucose Levels:
   - Failure to raise blood glucose levels above 50 mg/dL in the first 48 hours.
   - Failure to maintain blood glucose levels above 60 mg/dL after 48 hours.

2. Severe, Persistent, or Prolonged Hypoglycemia:
   - Inadequate response to treatment or failure to maintain blood glucose levels within the target range.

3. Family History:
   - Family history of congenital hypoglycemia.

4. Syndromic Manifestations:
   - The appearance of dysmorphic features may indicate the possibility of an underlying syndromic hypoglycemia (e.g., abnormalities in facial structure or organ malformations).

In these cases, detailed diagnostic tests and evaluations are performed to determine the underlying causes of hypoglycemia. The aim is to identify the presence of persistent metabolic or endocrine disorders and to determine appropriate long-term treatment strategies.

Laboratory Investigations for Differential Diagnosis

Laboratory investigations for the differential diagnosis of hypoglycemia should be performed with blood samples taken during the episode of hypoglycemia. In enterally fed newborns, a blood sample can be obtained after 6 hours of non-feeding. In infants receiving parenteral glucose infusion, blood samples should be collected at any time when plasma glucose levels fall below 50 mg/dL.

Laboratory parameters to be taken to support the differential diagnosis are as follows:

- *Blood glucose level:* Basic measurement for the diagnosis and management of hypoglycemia.
- *Insulin:* To assess whether hypoglycemia is due to hyperinsulinism.
- *Blood gas, lactate, and pyruvate:* To detect conditions such as metabolic acidosis or lactic acidosis.
- *Beta-hydroxybutyrate and acetoacetate*: To differentiate between ketotic and non-ketotic hypoglycemia.
- *Ammonia level:* To assess metabolic disorders such as urea cycle disorders.
- *Plasma-free fatty acids:* Useful in identifying disorders of fatty acid oxidation.
- *Blood and urine amino acids:* For the detection of metabolic disorders.
- *Acylcarnitine and urinary organic acids:* For the diagnosis of disorders of fatty acid metabolism and other organic acid disorders.
- *Cortisol and C-peptide:* for the differential diagnosis of endocrine disorders.
- These parameters help to elucidate the underlying causes of hypoglycemia, enabling accurate diagnosis and treatment planning (Thornton et al., 2015).

Neonatal Hyperglycemia

Hyperglycemia in neonates can be defined in various ways. The most common definitions are a blood glucose level >125 mg/dL (6.9 mmol/L) or a plasma glucose level >150 mg/dL (8.3 mmol/L). However, these levels may be particularly common in extremely premature infants and neonates receiving glucose infusions and may not always require intervention (Louik et al., 1985). Many neonatologists define clinically significant hyperglycemia as a blood glucose (BG) level above 180-200 mg/dL (10-11.1 mmol/L). This range is generally accepted as the threshold requiring intervention, and these values are taken as the basis in the institutions where the authors work. Hyperglycemia usually occurs as a consequence of immaturity in glucose metabolism, deficient insulin production, or insulin ineffectiveness. It can also be triggered by external factors such as glucose overload and stress response. If left untreated, hyperglycemia can lead to dehydration, electrolyte imbalances, and neurological disorders, with increased morbidity and mortality.

Clinical Findings

The clinical presentation of neonatal hyperglycemia may vary, and many infants may be asymptomatic. However, dehydration, polyuria, feeding difficulties, metabolic acidosis, respiratory distress, and intraventricular hemorrhage may be potential signs and symptoms.

Premature infants, low birth weight, hypoxic, receiving parenteral fluids, receiving medications (dexamethasone, caffeine, diazoxide, phenytoin, aminophylline), and infected infants are at risk for hyperglycemia.

Differential Diagnosis

Neonatal hyperglycemia is usually associated with clinical conditions rather than a specific disorder of glucose metabolism. This is more common in neonates receiving intravenous (IV) glucose infusion. A rare cause of hyperglycemia is neonatal diabetes mellitus, which should be considered under a separate heading. Obtaining blood samples from the IV line or extremity may lead to inaccurate measurements. In addition, in patients with galactosemia, it may be possible for the glucometer to detect galactose as glucose. Therefore, high results obtained on a glucometer must be confirmed with a serum sample.

The following conditions should be considered in the differential diagnosis of true hyperglycemia:

1. *Excessive glucose administration:* In this case, the glucose given to the patient should be reviewed.
2. *Hypoxia:* There is increased production of glucose.
3. *Stress:* Pain, painful stimuli, surgical interventions, necrotizing enterocolitis (NEC), hypoxia, respiratory distress, and intraventricular hemorrhage may lead to hyperglycemia by increasing cortisol secretion.
4. *Infection, sepsis:* This may be the first sign of sepsis. It may occur due to decreased utilization of glucose in peripheral tissues or stress in the body.
5. *Medications*: Use of aminophylline, steroids, caffeine, vasoactive drugs, phenytoin, and maternal use of diazoxide may cause hyperglycemia in the infant.
6. *Glucose metabolization problems:* Occurs secondary to stress or sepsis or in preterm infants.
7. *Disorder of glucose homeostasis:* Occurs because of insulin resistance seen in SGA infants or because of high dextrose IV fluids given to compensate for insensible losses seen in neonates under 1 kg.
8. *Hyperosmolar formula:* It may develop as a result of the preparation of powdered formulas with an inappropriate amount of water.
9. *Neonatal Diabetes:* Neonatal diabetes mellitus (DM) is a rare cause of hyperglycemia. This condition is defined as a persistent hyperglycemia that begins in the first months of life, lasts longer than two weeks, and requires insulin treatment. Neonatal DM is usually a monogenic disorder caused by mutations in genes encoding proteins that affect pancreatic beta cell function.
10. *Idiopathic.*

Evaluation

Medical History and Physical Examination

In the evaluation of a newborn with hyperglycemia, the baby's weight, gestational week, and SGA (small for gestational age at birth) should be questioned. The medications taken by the mother and the treatments taken by the baby should also be evaluated in detail. In addition, attention should be paid to findings such as weight loss and fever. Such symptoms may indicate serious conditions such as sepsis or NEC. Body temperature irregularities should also be examined, and peripheral circulation and gastric aspirate should be checked.

Laboratory Examination

Laboratory evaluation should be done in two steps:

- Step 1:
  - Serum glucose levels should be measured.
  - Serum electrolytes and blood gas analysis should be performed.
  - A hemogram, peripheral smear, and blood culture should be taken to look for signs of infection.

- Step 2:
  - Serum and urine ketone levels should be evaluated.
  - Detailed investigations with insulin, C-peptide, and molecular analyses should be performed. Further investigations are especially important in terms of genetic disorders such as neonatal DM.

Imaging

There is usually no specific imaging method for the evaluation of hyperglycemia. However, a chest X-ray may be needed to assess respiratory distress, and a transfontanel ultrasound may be required to investigate suspected intraventricular hemorrhage.

Treatment

Management of Neonatal Hyperglycemia

Neonatal hyperglycemia is a common metabolic condition, particularly in premature infants receiving parenteral glucose infusion. Management strategies focus on maintaining adequate caloric intake in these infants who depend on parenteral nutrition while bringing blood glucose levels within safe target ranges.

Routine Monitoring

Regular monitoring of blood glucose levels is recommended in all neonates receiving intravenous glucose infusion. Generally, daily measurements are sufficient for most infants; however, more frequent monitoring is necessary in the following situations:

- Extremely low birth weight (ELBW) infants (birth weight <1000 g).
- Infants with critical illness, sepsis, or other stress conditions.
- Infants receiving insulin infusion.

Nutritional Adjustments

Amino Acid and Lipid Infusion

In infants receiving parenteral nutrition, amino acid and lipid infusion is administered to provide substrates for gluconeogenesis and support insulin secretion. This approach can help regulate blood glucose levels without increasing the risk of hypoglycemia.

Enteral Nutrition

Reducing parenteral nutrition and initiating enteral feeding as soon as possible are essential. Enteral feeding enhances pancreatic insulin secretion by stimulating the release of glucose-dependent insulinotropic peptide (GIP) and incretin hormones (GLP-1) from the gastrointestinal system (Shanahan et al., 2018). Enteral feedings play a key role in improving glucose tolerance.

Intervention for Hyperglycemia

In infants with hyperglycemia (blood glucose >180 mg/dL), the following steps are taken:

1. *Review of Medications:* Medications that may contribute to hyperglycemia (e.g., glucocorticoids, phenytoin, beta-adrenergic agents) should be discontinued if possible.
2. *Sepsis Evaluation:* In infants showing signs of sepsis, a blood culture should be obtained, and empirical antibiotic therapy should be initiated.
3. *Reduction of Glucose Infusion Rate (GIR):* In infants with blood glucose levels >180-200 mg/dL, the glucose infusion rate should be reduced to 4-6 mg/kg/min. This is achieved by lowering the dextrose concentration in the fluid, ensuring that the dextrose concentration remains at a minimum of 5%.
4. *Insulin Therapy:* In infants whose hyperglycemia (BG >200 mg/dL) persists despite reducing the GIR, insulin therapy is initiated. Insulin lowers blood glucose levels, enhances caloric intake, and supports growth.

Details of Insulin Therapy

Initial Dose

- Insulin is administered at a concentration of 0.1 units/mL diluted in normal saline. The initial bolus dose is 0.05–0.1 units/kg, given over 15 minutes.
- Blood glucose is monitored regularly, measured every 30–60 minutes.

Continuous Infusion

- In infants with persistent hyperglycemia despite bolus therapy, continuous insulin infusion is initiated at a rate of 0.01–0.1

units/kg/hour. The infusion rate is adjusted to maintain blood glucose levels within the range of 150–200 mg/dL (Tottman et al., 2018).

Monitoring and Discontinuation of Infusion

- When blood glucose levels drop below 150 mg/dL, the infusion rate is gradually reduced, and therapy is discontinued once target levels are achieved. Blood glucose should be closely monitored for 12–24 hours following the cessation of treatment.

Management of Complications

- *Risk of Hypoglycemia:* Hypoglycemia may occur in infants receiving insulin therapy. In such cases, insulin infusion should be stopped, and intravenous dextrose (e.g., 10% dextrose, 2 mL/kg) should be administered.
- *Reduced Caloric Intake:* Prolonged low GIR can negatively impact growth rates. Therefore, transitioning to enteral feeding should be initiated as quickly as possible.

Target Blood Glucose Level

In infants receiving insulin therapy, the target blood glucose level should be maintained within the range of 150–200 mg/dL. Aiming for lower levels increases the risk of hypoglycemia and has not been shown to provide clinical benefits. Strict glycemic control (blood glucose <150 mg/dL) does not offer short- or long-term advantages and poses a higher risk of hypoglycemia (Tottman et al., 2018).

Neonatal hyperglycemia is a common metabolic issue in premature and critically ill infants. Management focuses on carefully adjusting the rate of parenteral glucose infusion, initiating enteral feeding early, and using insulin therapy when necessary. The goal of treatment is to maintain blood glucose levels within a safe range while optimizing growth and neurodevelopmental outcomes.

Neonatal Calcium Disorders

Neonatal Hypocalcemia

Neonatal hypocalcemia is one of the most common metabolic issues encountered in the early stages of life. Disruptions in calcium homeostasis can occur in the neonatal period due to various reasons and may present as symptomatic or asymptomatic. Hypocalcemia is associated with birth weight, gestational age, and underlying conditions. It is defined in neonates as a decrease in serum ionized calcium (iCa) and total serum calcium below specific thresholds:

- In term infants and preterm infants with a body weight >1500 g: iCa <4.4 mg/dL (<1.1 mmol/L) or total serum Ca <8 mg/dL (<2 mmol/L) (Kovacs et al., 1996; Rubin et al., 1991).
- In preterm very low birth weight (VLBW; BW 1000 to <1500 g) and extremely low birth weight (ELBW; BW <1000 g) infants: iCa <4 mg/dL (<1 mmol/L) or total serum Ca <7 mg/dL (<1.75 mmol/L) (Loughead et al., 1988).

Etiology

Hypocalcemia is divided into early hypocalcemia and late hypocalcemia based on the time of onset. Early hypocalcemia occurs in the first week of life, and risk factors include hypoparathyroidism, prematurity, intrauterine growth restriction, perinatal asphyxia, maternal diabetes, congenital anomalies, hypomagnesemia, maternal hyperparathyroidism, and vitamin D deficiency. Late hypocalcemia can occur at any time after the first week of the neonatal period, and risk factors include vitamin D deficiency, high phosphate intake, hypoparathyroidism, and pseudohypoparathyroidism (Teaema & Al Ansari, 2010; Walton et al., 2000).

Clinical Findings

Symptomatic hypocalcemia may present with irritability, tremor, jitteriness, hyperreflexia, clonus, tetany, laryngospasm, apnea, or seizure (Thomas et al., 2012). Asymptomatic cases are usually detected during screening tests.

Diagnosis and Evaluation

The preferred method for diagnosing hypocalcemia is iCa measurement. Total serum Ca measurements may be affected by hypoalbuminemia or acid-base disturbances. Additional evaluations are performed to determine the underlying cause of hypocalcemia: phosphate level, as levels may be high in late hypocalcemia; parathormone (PTH) and vitamin D levels for hypoparathyroidism and vitamin D deficiency; serum magnesium levels should be measured as it may impair the release and effect of PTH.

Treatment

Most newborns with asymptomatic early hypocalcemia improve with nutritional support alone. Therefore, the management plan aims to ensure adequate Ca intake by starting feeding as early as possible. In babies requiring parenteral nutrition, 10% calcium gluconate (500 mg/kg, 50 mg/kg elemental Ca) is added to the solution daily and administered as a continuous infusion. (Asghar et al., 2021). If parenteral calcium infusion lasts longer than 48 hours, additional phosphate supplementation may be necessary based on serum phosphate levels. If there is an underlying disease during the treatment process, interventions should be planned accordingly. Symptomatic hypocalcemia requires acute treatment: Within the scope of acute treatment, intravenous calcium gluconate is administered as a 10% solution (100 mg/mL) at a rate of 1 mL/kg over 10 minutes, and each milliliter contains 9,3 mg of elemental calcium. After acute treatment, calcium gluconate 50-75 mg/kg is added to the maintenance fluid. In case of hypomagnesemia accompanying hypocalcemia, a 50% magnesium sulfate solution is administered intravenously at 25-50 mg/kg, and treatment is continued until serum magnesium levels rise above 1.5 mg/dL. Additionally, in cases of hypocalcemia associated with high phosphate intake, diets low in phosphate and high in calcium are recommended. Breast milk is a preferred food source in such cases; where this is not possible, formulas with low phosphate content can be used. In the treatment of late hypocalcemia, 400 IU/day vitamin D3 supplementation is recommended. In more severe cases, calcitriol (0.08-0.1 mcg/kg) can be added to the treatment to increase the gastrointestinal absorption of calcium. Following parenteral calcium treatment, if the baby can tolerate enteral nutrition, it is recommended to continue treatment with oral calcium supplements. This approach aims to maintain long-term calcium balance and prevent recurrence of hypocalcemia. Neonatal hypocalcemia is a condition that can be managed with early diagnosis and appropriate treatment. Recognizing clinical signs and correct interpretation of iCa measurements are critical to the success of treatment. Additionally, treating underlying causes is important in improving long-term outcomes.

Neonatal Hypercalcemia

Hypercalcemia in the neonatal period is a very rare condition and usually occurs due to iatrogenic reasons. Hypercalcemia is defined as a serum Ca level >11 mg/dl or an iCa level > 1.35 mmol/L. An increase in the calcium level to >14 mg/dl may lead to a serious, life-threatening situation and require urgent intervention.

Etiology

Neonatal hypercalcemia usually results from iatrogenic causes or rare genetic and metabolic disorders. Iatrogenic causes include high doses of vitamin D or Ca intake and hypophosphatemia due to insufficient phosphate intake, especially in premature babies. Genetic causes include Williams syndrome, hypophosphatasia, and familial hypocalciuric hypercalcemia (FHH), while endocrine causes include hyperparathyroidism. Additionally, granulomatous diseases and rare malignancies can also cause hypercalcemia.

Diagnosis

After taking a detailed anamnesis for etiology, the diagnosis is made by evaluating serum Ca, phosphorus, total protein, albumin, PTH, vitamin D, thyroid hormones, alkaline phosphatase, creatinine, urine Ca and phosphorus levels, and blood gas analysis. Low alkaline phosphatase should first bring to mind the diagnosis of hypophosphatasia. Elevated PTH and low serum phosphorus levels accompanying hypercalcemia suggest hyperparathyroidism.

Treatment

If there is an iatrogenic cause, this cause should be eliminated first in the treatment. In the treatment of acute symptomatic hypercalcemia, hydration is first provided with physiological saline, and then calcium excretion is increased by using furosemide. In severe cases of hypercalcemia, if the condition cannot be controlled despite treatment, hemodialysis may be required. In cases of chronic hypercalcemia, medications such as calcitonin, glucocorticoids, and bisphosphonates are among the treatment options.

Congenital Adrenal Hyperplasia (CAH)

CAH is a group of autosomal recessive diseases that occur due to deficiencies in enzymes involved in cortisol biosynthesis. Multiple causes of CAH include 21-hydroxylase, 11-hydroxylase, 17-alpha-hydroxylase, 20-22 lyase enzyme deficiencies, and 3-beta-hydroxysteroid dehydrogenase defects. The most common form is 21-hydroxylase deficiency, accounting for more than 90% of cases (Draznin et al., 2022). CAH can occur in classical and non-classical forms; the classical form is divided into salt-wasting and simple virilizing types. Early diagnosis and treatment are critical to preventing life-threatening adrenal crises and reducing long-term complications.

Clinical Findings

While the salt-wasting form of classical CAH manifests itself with ambiguous genital structure (clitoromegaly, posterior labial fusion) in female babies, normal genital structure is observed at birth in male babies; however, symptoms such as vomiting, dehydration, and weight loss occur in the first weeks of life. Systemic findings of this form include hyponatremia, hyperkalemia, hypoglycemia, and growth failure. In the simple virilizing form, milder virilization symptoms are observed in female babies, while early virilization symptoms, such as early puberty and rapid growth, are noted in boys. The non-classical form usually occurs at a later age and is characterized by premature puberty, hirsutism, or menstrual irregularities in girls.

Diagnosis

Newborn screening programs are implemented by measuring 17-hydroxyprogesterone (17-OHP) levels in heel blood samples. Screening results are evaluated by gestational age and birth weight because baseline 17-OHP levels are higher in premature infants, and age-specific reference ranges are required. High 17-OHP levels are confirmed by LC-MS/MS (lipid chromatography-mass spectrometry). A serum 17-OHP level >300 ng/dl indicates severely affected cases. In addition, increased adrenal androgen levels (androstenedione, testosterone) and low cortisol levels are guiding in the diagnosis. Adrenocorticotropic hormone (ACTH) stimulation testing supports the diagnosis by revealing an exaggerated increase in 17-OHP. It is important to detect mutations in the CYP21A2 gene to confirm the diagnosis and determine carrier status (Speiser & White, 2003).

Adrenal Crisis

Adrenal crisis is a life-threatening condition in newborns and requires urgent intervention. Clinically, it may occur with hypotension, dehydration, hypoglycemia, and electrolyte imbalances. The primary goal of treatment is to correct cortisol deficiency, treat hypotension and dehydration, and correct electrolyte imbalances. In the treatment approach, fluid replacement with 0.9% saline solution and dextrose is applied. Especially in the case of hypoglycemia, a 10% dextrose solution can be applied as 5-10 mL/kg (Bornstein et al., 2016). A blood sample should be taken to evaluate steroid hormone levels; a 17-OHP test should be performed, especially to determine 21-hydroxylase deficiency. Then, treatment should be started with a hydrocortisone stress dose. First, a 50 to 100 mg/m² IV bolus of hydrocortisone should be administered (a 25 mg dose is usually used for neonates). Then, treatment should be continued with IV hydrocortisone doses of 50-100 mg/m² at six-hour intervals. These stress doses must be maintained until the patient becomes stable and resumes a normal diet. Hyperkalemia usually resolves with the mineralocorticoid effect of hydrocortisone, but in cases of severe hyperkalemia, insulin and glucose therapy may be required. Electrolyte levels and blood pressure should be monitored closely.

Long-Term Treatment and Follow-Up

In babies diagnosed with CAH, hydrocortisone is usually started at a dose of 20-30 mg/m²/day and administered in three equal doses per day. For mineralocorticoid replacement, fludrocortisone is used at a dose of 0.1 mg/day. Sodium supplementation is also often necessary during the first year of life. Regular monitoring is required to monitor electrolytes, hormone levels (17-OHP, androstenedione), and growth during treatment. Excessive glucocorticoid replacement should be avoided during treatment, and doses should be adjusted so as not to suppress growth. The treatment and follow-up plan should be closely managed by the pediatric endocrinologist.

Congenital Hypopituitarism

Congenital hypopituitarism is a rare condition characterized by a deficiency of one or more pituitary hormones. It occurs due to developmental abnormalities of the pituitary gland or genetic mutations. Diagnosis of this condition may be difficult with nonspecific symptoms such as hypoglycemia, jaundice, hypothermia, and failure to thrive, which are frequently encountered in the neonatal period. Early diagnosis and treatment are critical to prevent life-threatening complications.

Etiology and Clinical Findings

The main causes of congenital hypopituitarism include genetic mutations (such as PROP1, POU1F1, and HESX1) and structural abnormalities such as hypoplasia or dysplasia of the pituitary gland. Ectopic posterior pituitary (EPP) and pituitary stalk anomalies are common structural findings. Clinically, it may occur in newborns with symptoms such as hypoglycemia, prolonged jaundice, hypothermia, inadequate weight gain, and micropenis. Babies with ACTH deficiency may develop cholestasis in the first weeks, and this is associated with cortisol deficiency impairing bile flow (Di Iorgi et al., 2012; Mehta et al., 2009).

Diagnosis

Laboratory evaluation and imaging methods are important in the diagnosis of congenital hypopituitarism. Measurement of serum cortisol, growth hormone (GH), thyroid hormones (free T4 and TSH), ACTH, and insulin-like growth factor 1 (IGF-1) levels is a critical starting point. However, as hormone levels in newborns may vary physiologically, caution should be exercised in interpreting laboratory results (Bosch I Ara et al., 2021; Mehta et al., 2009). Structural anomalies of the pituitary gland (hypoplasia or ectopy) can be detected with Magnetic Resonance Imaging (MRI). Pituitary Stalk Interruption Syndrome (PSIS), especially characterized by pituitary stalk anomaly and ectopic posterior pituitary, is common in cases of severe hypopituitarism. Detection of PROP1, POU1F1, and other mutations through genetic analysis can confirm the diagnosis and guide treatment (Di Iorgi et al., 2012). Treatment of congenital hypopituitarism involves replacing missing hormones and focuses primarily on treating life-threatening hormone deficiencies in newborns:

1. *Corticosteroid Replacement:* Hydrocortisone treatment in newborns with ACTH deficiency is started with an initial dose of 9-12 $mg/m^2/day$, and the dose is divided into 3-4 equal parts. In case of adrenal crisis, intramuscular hydrocortisone (25 mg for <1 year) should be given urgently (Bosch I Ara et al., 2021; Mehta et al., 2009).

2. *Levothyroxine:* A 10-15 µg/kg/kg/day starting dose is recommended in babies with TSH deficiency. Before beginning treatment, it is important to exclude cortisol deficiency, as levothyroxine can increase cortisol metabolism and trigger the risk of adrenal crisis. (Bosch I Ara et al., 2021).
3. *Growth Hormone Replacement:* Subcutaneous recombinant human growth hormone (rhGH) treatment is applied to newborns with GH deficiency. The starting dose is usually 0.16-0.24 mg/kg per week and supports the rate of treatment enhancement (Ogilvy-Stuart, 2003).
4. *Desmopressin:* Although fluid therapy is prioritized in the presence of diabetes insipidus (DI), low-dose desmopressin can be applied in severe cases.

Monitoring and Follow-Up

In the long-term follow-up of neonates with congenital hypopituitarism, regular laboratory tests should be conducted to assess the effectiveness of hormonal replacement therapy. Growth, metabolic parameters, and neurodevelopmental outcomes should be closely monitored. Genetic counseling is recommended, particularly for families associated with identified genetic mutations. Follow-up may also be necessary for other structural anomalies based on MRI findings.

Conclusion

Neonatal endocrine emergencies require prompt recognition and effective management to mitigate life-threatening risks and prevent long-term complications. Early screening, accurate diagnosis, and evidence-based treatment protocols are essential to improving survival and neurodevelopmental outcomes. Ongoing research and education are crucial for advancing diagnostic tools and management strategies to ensure better care for neonates with endocrine disorders.

References

Aleksander, P. E., Brückner-Spieler, M., Stoehr, A.-M., Lankes, E., Kühnen, P., Schnabel, D., Ernert, A., Stäblein, W., Craig, M. E., Blankenstein, O., Grüters, A., & Krude, H. (2018). Mean High-Dose l-Thyroxine Treatment Is Efficient and Safe to Achieve a Normal IQ in Young Adult Patients With Congenital Hypothyroidism. *The Journal of Clinical Endocrinology and Metabolism*, *103*(4), 1459-1469. https://doi.org/10.1210/jc.2017-01937.

Alexander, E. K., Pearce, E. N., Brent, G. A., Brown, R. S., Chen, H., Dosiou, C., Grobman, W. A., Laurberg, P., Lazarus, J. H., Mandel, S. J., Peeters, R. P., & Sullivan, S. (2017). 2017 Guidelines of the American Thyroid Association for the Diagnosis and Management of Thyroid Disease During Pregnancy and the Postpartum. *Thyroid: Official Journal of the American Thyroid Association*, *27*(3), 315-389. https://doi.org/10.1089/thy.2016.0457.

Aliefendioğlu, D., Çoban, A., Hatipoğlu, N., Ecevit, A., Arısoy, A. E., Yeşiltepe, G., Baş, F., Bideci, A., & Özek, E. (2018). Management of hypoglycemia in newborn: Turkish Neonatal and Pediatric Endocrinology and Diabetes Societies consensus report. *Turk Pediatri Arsivi*, *53*(Suppl 1), S224-S233. https://doi.org/10.5152/TurkPediatriArs.2018.01820.

Asghar, I., Khan, I. A., & Hassan, F. (2021). Effect of head covering on phototherapy induced hypocalcemia in term neonates with hyperbilirubinemia: A randomised controlled study. *Journal of Neonatal-Perinatal Medicine*, *14*(2), 245-251. https://doi.org/10.3233/NPM-200442.

Bautista, G. (2022). Overview of Congenital Hypopituitarism for the Neonatologist. *NeoReviews*, *23*(5), e300-e310. https://doi.org/10.1542/neo.23-5-e300.

Baysal, B. T., Baysal, B., Genel, F., Erdur, B., Ozbek, E., Demir, K., & Ozkan, B. (2017). Neurodevelopmental Outcome of Children with Congenital Hypothyroidism Diagnosed in a National Screening Program in Turkey. *Indian Pediatrics*, *54*(5), 381-384. https://doi.org/10.1007/s13312-017-1111-5.

Benlarbi, H., Simon, D., Rosenblatt, J., Dumaine, C., de Roux, N., Chevenne, D., Storey, C., Poidvin, A., Martinerie, L., Carel, J.-C., & Léger, J. (2021). Prevalence and course of thyroid dysfunction in neonates at high risk of Graves' disease or with non-autoimmune hyperthyroidism. *European Journal of Endocrinology*, *184*(3), 427-436. https://doi.org/10.1530/EJE-20-1320.

Bornstein, S. R., Allolio, B., Arlt, W., Barthel, A., Don-Wauchope, A., Hammer, G. D., Husebye, E. S., Merke, D. P., Murad, M. H., Stratakis, C. A., & Torpy, D. J. (2016). Diagnosis and Treatment of Primary Adrenal Insufficiency: An Endocrine Society Clinical Practice Guideline. *The Journal of Clinical Endocrinology and Metabolism*, *101*(2), 364-389. https://doi.org/10.1210/jc.2015-1710.

Bosch i Ara, L., Katugampola, H., & Dattani, M. T. (2021). Congenital Hypopituitarism During the Neonatal Period: Epidemiology, Pathogenesis, Therapeutic Options, and Outcome. *Frontiers in Pediatrics*, *8*. https://doi.org/10.3389/fped.2020.600962.

Committee on Fetus and Newborn, & Adamkin, D. H. (2011). Postnatal glucose homeostasis in late-preterm and term infants. *Pediatrics*, *127*(3), 575-579. https://doi.org/10.1542/peds.2010-3851.

Cornblath, M., Hawdon, J. M., Williams, A. F., Aynsley-Green, A., Ward-Platt, M. P., Schwartz, R., & Kalhan, S. C. (2000). Controversies regarding definition of neonatal hypoglycemia: Suggested operational thresholds. *Pediatrics*, *105*(5), 1141-1145. https://doi.org/10.1542/peds.105.5.1141.

Cornella, T. J. (Ed.). (2017). *Neonatology* (Translated by A. Çoban & Z. İnce). Istanbul Medical Publishing. (Original work published by McGraw Hill Education, ISBN: 978-0-07-176801-6).

Di Iorgi, N., Allegri, A. E. M., Napoli, F., Bertelli, E., Olivieri, I., Rossi, A., & Maghnie, M. (2012). The use of neuroimaging for assessing disorders of pituitary development. *Clinical Endocrinology*, *76*(2), 161-176. https://doi.org/10.1111/j.1365-2265.2011.04238.x.

Draznin, M., Borgohain, P., & Kanungo, S. (2022). Newborn Screening in Pediatric Endocrine Disorders. *Endocrines*, *3*(1), Article 1. https://doi.org/10.3390/endocrines 3010010.

El-Bakry, N. M. (2023). Newborn Screening for Congenital Hypothyroidism and Congenital Adrenal Hyperplasia in Egypt. *Annals of Neonatology*, *5*(1), 17-27. https://doi.org/10.21608/anj.2022.276380.

Farrehi, C. (1968). Accelerated maturity in fetal thyrotoxicosis. *Clinical Pediatrics*, *7*(3), 134-137. https://doi.org/10.1177/000992286800700304.

Finnegan, P., Tierney, E., Rafferty, S., Neylon, O., & Sadlier, M. (2023). Congenital panhypopituitarism unmasked by PHACE screening. *JAAD Case Reports*, *39*, 118-121. https://doi.org/10.1016/j.jdcr.2023.07.003.

Harris, D. L., Gamble, G. D., Weston, P. J., & Harding, J. E. (2017). What Happens to Blood Glucose Concentrations After Oral Treatment for Neonatal Hypoglycemia? *The Journal of Pediatrics*, *190*, 136-141. https://doi.org/10.1016/j.jpeds.2017.06.034.

Kanczkowski, W., Alexaki, V.-I., Tran, N., Großklaus, S., Zacharowski, K., Martinez, A., Popovics, P., Block, N. L., Chavakis, T., Schally, A. V., & Bornstein, S. R. (2013). Hypothalamo-pituitary and immune-dependent adrenal regulation during systemic inflammation. *Proceedings of the National Academy of Sciences*, *110*(36), 14801-14806. https://doi.org/10.1073/pnas.1313945110.

Kovacs, C. S., Lanske, B., Hunzelman, J. L., Guo, J., Karaplis, A. C., & Kronenberg, H. M. (1996). Parathyroid hormone-related peptide (PTHrP) regulates fetal-placental calcium transport through a receptor distinct from the PTH/PTHrP receptor. *Proceedings of the National Academy of Sciences of the United States of America*, *93*(26), 15233-15238. https://doi.org/10.1073/pnas.93.26.15233.

Kurtoğlu, S. (2019). Neonatal Hypopituitarism: Approaches to Diagnosis and Treatment. *Journal Of Clinical Research In Pediatric Endocrinology*, *11*(1), 4-12. https://doi.org/10.4274/jcrpe.galenos.2018.2018.0036.

Lee, H. J. (2023). Diagnosis and treatment of congenital hypothyroidism. *Journal of the Korean Medical Association*, *66*(3), 191-197. https://doi.org/10.5124/jkma.2023.66.3.191.

Léger, J., Olivieri, A., Donaldson, M., Torresani, T., Krude, H., van Vliet, G., Polak, M., & Butler, G. (2014). European Society for Paediatric Endocrinology consensus guidelines on screening, diagnosis, and management of congenital hypothyroidism.

The Journal of Clinical Endocrinology and Metabolism, *99*(2). https://doi.org/10.1210/jc.2013-1891.

Loughead, J. L., Mimouni, F., & Tsang, R. C. (1988). Serum ionized calcium concentrations in normal neonates. *American Journal of Diseases of Children (1960)*, *142*(5), 516-518. https://doi.org/10.1001/archpedi.1988.02150050054030.

Louik, C., Mitchell, A. A., Epstein, M. F., & Shapiro, S. (1985). Risk factors for neonatal hyperglycemia associated with 10% dextrose infusion. *American Journal of Diseases of Children (1960)*, *139*(8), 783-786. https://doi.org/10.1001/archpedi.1985.02140100045025.

Maniam, G., Dean, R., Pungwe, P., Batson, A., Tijani, S., & Adesanya, O. (2020). Term Neonate with Respiratory Distress Syndrome Secondary to Congenital Hypothyroidism. *International Journal of Integrative Pediatrics and Environmental Medicine*, *5*, 30-33. https://doi.org/10.36013/ijipem.v5i1.84.

McKinlay, C. J. D., Alsweiler, J. M., Ansell, J. M., Anstice, N. S., Chase, J. G., Gamble, G. D., Harris, D. L., Jacobs, R. J., Jiang, Y., Paudel, N., Signal, M., Thompson, B., Wouldes, T. A., Yu, T.-Y., Harding, J. E., & CHYLD Study Group. (2015). Neonatal Glycemia and Neurodevelopmental Outcomes at 2 Years. *The New England Journal of Medicine*, *373*(16), 1507-1518. https://doi.org/10.1056/NEJMoa1504909.

Mehta, A., Hindmarsh, P. C., Mehta, H., Turton, J. P. G., Russell-Eggitt, I., Taylor, D., Chong, W. K., & Dattani, M. T. (2009). Congenital hypopituitarism: Clinical, molecular and neuroradiological correlates. *Clinical Endocrinology*, *71*(3), 376-382. https://doi.org/10.1111/j.1365-2265.2009.03572.x.

Ogilvy-Stuart, A. L. (2003). Growth hormone deficiency (GHD) from birth to 2 years of age: Diagnostic specifics of GHD during the early phase of life. *Hormone Research*, *60*(Suppl 1), 2-9. https://doi.org/10.1159/000071219.

Parkin, K., Kapoor, R., Bhat, R., & Greenough, A. (2019). Genetic causes of hypopituitarism. *Archives of Medical Science*, *16*(1), 27-33. https://doi.org/10.5114/aoms.2020.91285

Rivkees, S. A., & Szarfman, A. (2010). Dissimilar hepatotoxicity profiles of propylthiouracil and methimazole in children. *The Journal of Clinical Endocrinology and Metabolism*, *95*(7), 3260-3267. https://doi.org/10.1210/jc.2009-2546.

Rose, S. R., Wassner, A. J., Wintergerst, K. A., Yayah-Jones, N.-H., Hopkin, R. J., Chuang, J., Smith, J. R., Abell, K., LaFranchi, S. H., Section On Endocrinology Executive Committee, & Council On Genetics Executive Committee. (2022). Congenital Hypothyroidism: Screening and Management. *Pediatrics*, *151*(1), e2022060419. https://doi.org/10.1542/peds.2022-060419.

Rubin, L. P., Posillico, J. T., Anast, C. S., & Brown, E. M. (1991). Circulating levels of biologically active and immunoreactive intact parathyroid hormone in human newborns. *Pediatric Research*, *29*(2), 201-207. https://doi.org/10.1203/00006450-199102000-00020.

Salerno, M., Militerni, R., Bravaccio, C., Micillo, M., Capalbo, D., Di, M. S., & Tenore, A. (2002). Effect of different starting doses of levothyroxine on growth and intellectual outcome at four years of age in congenital hypothyroidism. *Thyroid: Official Journal of the American Thyroid Association*, *12*(1), 45-52. https://doi.org/10.1089/105072502753451968.

Shanahan, K. H., Yu, X., Miller, L. G., Freedman, S. D., & Martin, C. R. (2018). Early Serum Gut Hormone Concentrations Associated With Time to Full Enteral Feedings in Preterm Infants. *Journal of Pediatric Gastroenterology and Nutrition*, *67*(1), 97-102. https://doi.org/10.1097/MPG.0000000000001987.

Speiser, P. W., & White, P. C. (2003). Congenital Adrenal Hyperplasia. *New England Journal of Medicine*, *349*(8), 776-788. https://doi.org/10.1056/NEJMra021561.

Teaema, F. H., & Al Ansari, K. (2010). Nineteen cases of symptomatic neonatal hypocalcemia secondary to vitamin D deficiency: A 2-year study. *Journal of Tropical Pediatrics*, *56*(2), 108-110. https://doi.org/10.1093/tropej/fmp063.

Thomas, T. C., Smith, J. M., White, P. C., & Adhikari, S. (2012). Transient neonatal hypocalcemia: Presentation and outcomes. *Pediatrics*, *129*(6), e1461-1467. https://doi.org/10.1542/peds.2011-2659.

Thornton, P. S., Stanley, C. A., De Leon, D. D., Harris, D., Haymond, M. W., Hussain, K., Levitsky, L. L., Murad, M. H., Rozance, P. J., Simmons, R. A., Sperling, M. A., Weinstein, D. A., White, N. H., Wolfsdorf, J. I., & Pediatric Endocrine Society. (2015). Recommendations from the Pediatric Endocrine Society for Evaluation and Management of Persistent Hypoglycemia in Neonates, Infants, and Children. *The Journal of Pediatrics*, *167*(2), 238-245. https://doi.org/10.1016/j.jpeds.2015.03.057.

Tottman, A. C., Alsweiler, J. M., Bloomfield, F. H., Gamble, G., Jiang, Y., Leung, M., Poppe, T., Thompson, B., Wouldes, T. A., Harding, J. E., & PIANO Study Group. (2018). Long-Term Outcomes of Hyperglycemic Preterm Infants Randomized to Tight Glycemic Control. *The Journal of Pediatrics*, *193*, 68-75.e1. https://doi.org/10.1016/j.jpeds.2017.09.081.

Walton, D. M., Thomas, D. C., Aly, H. Z., & Short, B. L. (2000). Morbid hypocalcemia associated with phosphate enema in a six-week-old infant. *Pediatrics*, *106*(3), E37. https://doi.org/10.1542/peds.106.3.e37.

Weston, P. J., Harris, D. L., Battin, M., Brown, J., Hegarty, J. E., & Harding, J. E. (2016). Oral dextrose gel for the treatment of hypoglycaemia in newborn infants. *The Cochrane Database of Systematic Reviews*, *5*, CD011027. https://doi.org/10.1002/14651858.CD011027.pub2.

Whipple, A. O., & Frantz, V. K. (1935). Adenoma Of Islet Cells With Hyperinsulinism: A Review. *Annals of Surgery*, *101*(6), 1299-1335. https://doi.org/10.1097/00000658-193506000-00001.

Yang, L., Sato, M., Saito-Abe, M., Miyaji, Y., Sato, C., Nishizato, M., Kumasaka, N., Mezawa, H., Yamamoto-Hanada, K., Ohya, Y., & the Japan Environment and Children's Study Group. (2023). Congenital hypothyroidism and thyroid function in a Japanese birth cohort: Data from The Japan Environment and Children's Study. *Clinical Pediatric Endocrinology*, *32*(4), 213-220. https://doi.org/10.1297/cpe.2022-0068.

Chapter 24

Neonatal Metabolic Emergencies

Safiye Elif Uzlu*, MD

Department of Pediatrics, Division of Neonatology,
Giresun Maternity and Children Training and Research Hospital, Giresun, Turkey

Abstract

Metabolic diseases such as sepsis and congenital heart diseases should be considered in the etiology of sudden deterioration and severe clinical disorders in newborn babies with good appearance and mostly without postnatal problems. Metabolic disorders often present with nonspecific findings. These include hypoglycemia, metabolic acidosis, impaired liver function tests, lethargy, vomiting, and seizures. After baseline tests for etiology are performed, rapid removal of toxic metabolites such as ammonia, appropriate caloric support, administration of appropriate fluids, and use of proper cofactors may be life-saving.

Keywords: metabolic diseases, toxic metabolites, nonspecific symptoms

Introduction

Metabolic disorders can lead to an emergency that may result in various morbidities and death. Therefore, metabolic disorders should be considered in any severe illness of unknown etiology in neonates (Sharma et al., 2008). Metabolic diseases are typically characterized by acute metabolic deterioration that occurs after a period of well-being. Some metabolic

---

* Corresponding Author's Email: drseuzlu@hotmail.com

In: Current Approaches to Newborn Emergencies
Editors: Zuhal Keskin Sarılar and Serap Samut Bülbül
ISBN: 979-8-89530-999-5

disorders can be successfully recognized and treated early through screening programs. Some neonates are diagnosed when life-threatening emergencies occur in the first days of life. However, in some patients, the diagnosis is confirmed months or years later when decompensation occurs (Fleisher et al., 2006).

Metabolic disorders are rare diseases characterized by a single gene defect and can be inherited as autosomal recessive, X-linked, or autosomal dominant and may also occur due to mitochondrial DNA mutations (Martins, 1999). Some of the metabolic diseases are asymptomatic. In general, their clinical classification can be analyzed in 3 main groups. Intoxication-type metabolic diseases are characterized by the accumulation of toxins. Therefore, after a symptom-free period, it manifests clinically with symptoms such as lethargy, vomiting, and elevated liver enzymes. The second group is metabolic diseases that develop from energy deficiency. In this group, it can be caused by the lack or use of a product required for energy. It is possible to see symptoms of hypoglycemia, elevated lactic acid, myopathy, or cardiac pathologies. In the third group, chronic accumulation of complex molecules secondary to defective catabolism in organelles such as lysosomes and peroxisomes may result in progressive symptoms in which metabolic compensation mechanisms are ineffective (Ezgu, 2016). The three main groups of metabolic diseases according to their clinical classification are shown in Table 1 (Brunetti-Pierri, 2023).

Table 1. Clinical classification of metabolic diseases

Intoxication Type	Energy Deficiency	Chronic Accumulation of Complex Molecules
Aminoacid Metabolism Disorders	Mitochondrial Respiratory Chain Disease	Lysosomal Storage Diseases
Ure Cycle Defects	Krebs Cycle Defects	Peroxisomal Disorders
Organic Acidurias	Fatty Acid Oxidation Defects	Congenital Glycosylation Defects
Galactosemia, Hereditary Fructose Intolerance	Glycogen Storage Disease	

Clinical Presentation and Emergencies

The occurrence of an acute life-threatening condition in a neonate without an underlying cause should always suggest the possibility of metabolic disease. It often presents with nonspecific symptoms. These include persistent vomiting, lethargy, seizures, vomiting, respiration due to severe metabolic acidosis, acute liver failure, and hypothermia. Anamnesis should be taken carefully; consanguineous marriage and family history of sudden infant death should be questioned (Clarke, 2006).

Gastrointestinal Presentation

Recurrent vomiting, dehydration, and growth failure are more common in amino acid disorders, organic acidemias, and urea cycle defects. Liver failure may be seen in galactosemia, tyrosinemia, or neonatal hemochromatosis. The association of cholestatic jaundice and liver failure may be seen in disorders of bile acid or cholesterol metabolism, as well as in peroxisomal diseases and Niemann-Pick Type C disease (Ezgu, 2016; Leonard & Morris, 2006).

Neurological Presentation

Cerebral edema may be seen in diseases causing hyperammonemia and hypoglycemia, such as organic acidemias, urea cycle defect, and MSUD (maple syrup urine disease).

Lethargy and coma may be seen in amino acid metabolism disorders, urea cycle defects, fatty acid oxidation defects, mitochondrial diseases, and carbohydrate metabolism diseases.

Seizures can be seen in all metabolic disorders. This is usually due to hypoglycemia or toxic metabolite accumulation due to the existing disease. However, it should be kept in mind that pyridoxine dependent seizures can be the only etiology; therefore pyridoxine should be considered in the treatment of refractory convulsions (Cleary & Green, 2005; Sharma et al., 2008).

Respiratory Presentation

Urea cycle defects and hyperammonemia may cause hyperpnea and consequently respiratory alkalosis with respiratory system stimulation. This condition is caused by cerebral edema due to the accumulation of ammonia, glutamine, and other metabolites (Butterworth, 1998). Causes such as organic acidemia leading to metabolic acidosis may cause Kussmaul respiration. Neurologic dysfunction and consequent apnea may be seen in deep acidosis.

Some metabolic diseases, such as amino acid metabolism disorders, organic acidemias, fatty acid oxidation defects, and mitochondrial diseases, are also involved in the etiology of SIDS (sudden infant death syndrome) and ALTE (apparent life-threatening event) (Olpin, 2004).

Cardiovascular Presentation

Cardiomyopathies can be seen in glycogen storage disease type 2 and metabolic diseases such as fatty acid oxidation defects (Sharma et al., 2008).

Laboratory Emergencies

Hypoglycemia

Hypoglycemia in the neonatal period, especially if it occurs in the first few days, is usually caused by hyperinsulinism or sepsis. However, metabolic diseases may also cause severe and refractory hypoglycemia. Plasma and urine ketone levels should be seen immediately to clarify the etiology. Low plasma and urine ketone levels accompany hypoglycemia in fatty acid oxidation defects and hyperinsulinism, glycogen storage disease type 1, and fructose 1-6 diphosphatase deficiency. High ketone levels can be seen in glycogen storage diseases except type 1. Lactate, pyruvate, triglycerides, and uric acid levels are typically elevated in these diseases. Hypoglycemia and ketosis may be associated with organic acidemias and maple syrup urine disease (Enns & Packman, 2001).

Hyperammonemia

Ammonia levels need to be performed in every patient with a severe neurologic clinic, such as lethargy or acute encephalopathy. Hyperammonemia is a life-threatening condition. It is recognized by ammonia elevation seen in uric acid defects, ammonia elevation seen in organic acidemia and fatty acid oxidation defects, and the absence of ketoacidosis. Normal ammonia level is <150 mol/l in newborns. If this value is >200 mol/l, it should be a warning for metabolic diseases. Measurement of blood amino acid levels and urine organic acid levels is necessary to elucidate the etiology (Enns & Packman, 2001; Häberle et al., 2019).

Metabolic Acidosis

In metabolic diseases, they are usually associated with an increased anion gap because there are causes, such as lactic acid elevation, ketosis, and organic acid elevation, that cause metabolic acidosis. However, metabolic acidosis accompanied by a normal anion gap is seen in renal bicarbonate loss, such as renal tubular acidosis, or bicarbonate loss from the gastrointestinal tract, such as diarrhea or mineralocorticoid deficiencies. Urine pH measurement is a simple method that can give an idea about the differential diagnosis. Generally, if pH<5, more metabolic causes are considered in etiology, whereas renal tubular acidosis may be considered if pH>5. Among metabolic diseases, ketoacidosis, hyperammonemia, and bi-cytopenia are seen in organic acidemia. Urine organic acid and blood acylcarnitine profiles should be performed for the diagnosis. Fatty acid oxidation deficiency may also be associated with ammonia elevation. In this case, hypoglycemia, elevated creatine kinase, cardiac symptoms, and liver failure may also accompany (Enns & Packman, 2001).

Lactic Acidosis

When elevated lactic acid is observed in the neonate, causes such as hypoxia, sepsis, and congenital heart disease are generally considered. Among metabolic disorders, pyruvate metabolism disorders, mitochondrial fatty acid oxidation disorders, mitochondrial respiratory chain defects, gluconeogenesis, and carbohydrate disorders are the ones that generally cause energy metabolism disorders. Simultaneous examination of lactate and pyruvate values and their ratio to each other issuggestive of the diagnosis. A high lactate/pyruvate ratio is a warning sign for pyruvate carboxylase deficiency, and a low lactate/pyruvate ratio is a warning sign for gluconeogenesis defects (Enns & Packman, 2001).

Respiratory Alkalosis

Respiratory alkalosis is usually caused by hyperpnea caused by elevated ammonia. This is seen in urea cycle defects.

Investigations

Baseline investigations should be performed immediately in every infant with clinically suspected metabolic disease in terms of treatable diseases. Baseline investigations are shown in Table 2 (Brunetti-Pierri, 2023; Gupta et al., 2024).

Table 2. Baseline investigations

Urine	Smell, color PH, density Electrolytes Ketone Reducing agent
Blood	Complete blood count Liver function tests Kidney function tests Ketoacids Arterial blood gas Ammonia Uric acid Coagulation profile Coombs test Lactate/Pyruvate level Albumin Fractionated bilirubin
Others	Lumbar puncture Chest X-ray ECG, Echocardiography Cerebral ultrasound EEG

ECG, electrocardiogram; EEG, electroencephalogram.

Secondary tests result in a longer period. These are diagnostic tests such as blood amino acids, urine amino acids, urine organic acids, tandem mass spectrometry, enzyme assay, genetic tests, plasma very long chain fatty acid levels, magnetic resonance spectroscopy, etc. Although baseline tests seem to be lifesaving in acute situations, it is important to take baseline tests in every infant with suspected metabolic disease and, if possible, to take secondary tests simultaneously for diagnosis in the following days because diagnostic test results may be affected by blood transfusion and various medical interventions.

Management

Emergency intervention should be initiated immediately after baseline investigations are performed in a critically ill patient with suspected metabolic disease. Treatment should be planned as supportive pretreatment, removal of toxins, provision of high-energy nutrition to stop catabolism, and transition to a specific treatment.

Supportive Care

In these patients, airway support should be provided first, and the patient should be intubated if necessary. Patients with signs of dehydration should be given fluid support with an appropriate amount of saline, taking into account their serum electrolyte status. The use of Ringer's lactate should be especially avoided as it may increase lactic acidosis. In addition, hypotonic solutions should not be given because they may cause brain edema. Anticonvulsive treatment should be initiated in a convulsing infant, and pyridoxine should be given in resistant cases. However, sodium valproate should be avoided because it may increase ammonia levels (Sharma et al., 2008).

Antibiotherapy should be initiated in cases of sepsis. Especially, galactosemia and organic acidemia predispose to neutropenia and sepsis.

Fresh-frozen plasma may be necessary in patients with liver failure and consequent coagulopathy (Fleisher et al., 2006).

Elimination of Toxic Metabolites and Nutrition

Enteral and parenteral nutrition should be stopped as a first priority. Electrolyte imbalance and dehydration should be focused on. Because there may be an increase in toxic metabolites in amino acid metabolism disorders or carbohydrate metabolism disorders. High caloric support can be provided with fats after high glucose utilization and fatty acid oxidation defects have been ruled out. Protein-free caloric support can be applied in the first two days.

Elevated ammonia is a neurotoxic protein breakdown product. It may cause irreversible brain damage and death. Although it is also seen in organic acidemias, if the blood ammonia level is >400 umol/l, urea cycle defects should be considered as the primary diagnosis. In this case, ammonia should be rapidly removed from the blood by hemodialysis or medical methods. In medical treatment, it is aimed to achieve nitrogen excretion by conjugation with glycine and glutamine through the use of sodium benzoate IV (intravenous) or orally (loading dose 250 mg/kg, initial dose 400 mg/kg/day in 4 divided doses), sodium phenylbutyrate (loading dose 250 mg/kg/day, initial dose 250-500 mg/kg). The conjugation products formed are water-soluble forms and are excreted in the urine. Therefore, renal function tests are important. L-arginine and carbamylglutamate can be used in N-acetylglutamate deficiency or organic acidemia. It should be prepared for hemodialysis, especially when the ammonia level is >500 umol/l (Häberle et al., 2019; Sharma et al., 2008).

Correction of Metabolic Acidosis

Sodium bicarbonate may be required in the treatment of metabolic acidosis. Bicarbonate infusion should be used when $pH < 7.10$ and $HCO_3 < 10$ mmol/L, especially in severe ketoacidosis. However, it should be kept in mind that rapid and aggressive treatment may cause hypernatremia, cerebral edema, and intracranial hemorrhage (Fleisher et al., 2006).

Hypoglycemia Treatment

Hypoglycemia should be treated as fast as possible. An intravenous glucose infusion rate of 8-10 mg/kg/min should be provided. In cases accompanied by neuroglycopenic symptoms, a 2 ml/kg minibolus of 10% dextrose solution may be given. In hypoglycemia accompanied by hyperinsulism, higher glucose concentrations may be needed, and therefore central venous access may be required. Gluconeogenesis defects should be considered in fasting hypoglycemia accompanied by high lactic acidity. Hypoglycemia with liver failure may be observed in galactosemia. In these cases, dietary intake of galactose should be avoided (Ogier de Baulny, 2002).

Hyperlactatemia Treatment

It can be seen in lactic acidosis, glycogen storage diseases, organic acidemias, fatty acid oxidation defects, and congenital lactic acidosis. In addition to the treatment of acidosis, biotin, thiamine, and riboflavin may be used in treatment (Brunetti-Pierri, 2023; Ogier de Baulny, 2002).

Cofactor Treatments

Vitamin B12 (cobalamin): 1 mg subcutaneously or intramuscularly can be used in methylmalonic acidemia and homocystinuria.

Pyridoxine-100 mg IV or pyridoxal phosphate (activated form of pyridoxine) - 10 mg/kg IV should be used in seizures not responding to antiseizure treatments. If the seizure does not stop despite pyridoxine, leucovorin (2.5 mg IV) should be used.

Biotin: In recurrent convulsions, 10 mg can be given enterally in terms of multiple carboxylase deficiency.

Riboflavin In multiple acyl-CoA dehydrogenase deficiency and riboflavin transport deficiency, 150 mg/kg/day in three divided doses IV can be considered.

Carnitine: 100 mg/kg/day in three divided doses orally may be considered in organic acidemias, fatty acid oxidation defects, and primary carnitine deficiencies (Chakrapani et al., 2001; Sharma et al., 2008).

Conclusion

In case of acute deterioration after the well-being period in neonates, although diagnoses such as sepsis and cardiovascular disease are considered in the foreground, metabolic diseases should be evaluated. Some of the metabolic emergencies are treatable when recognized early in newborns and may protect the infant from severe morbidity, permanent neurologic damage, or even death. Basal emergency metabolic tests should be performed in every suspected infant, and secondary tests should be performed simultaneously if possible.

References

Brunetti-Pierri, N. (2023). Inborn Metabolic Diseases, Jean-Marie Saudubray, Matthias R. Baumgartner, Angeles Garcia-Cazorla, John H. Walter Eds, 7th edition, Springer, Berlin, Germany, 2022. *Journal of Inherited Metabolic Disease*, *46*(3), 536-536. https://doi.org/https://doi.org/10.1002/jimd.12611.

Butterworth, R. F. (1998). Effects of hyperammonaemia on brain function. *J Inherit Metab Dis*, *21 Suppl 1*, 6-20. https://doi.org/10.1023/a:1005393104494.

Chakrapani, A., Cleary, M. A., & Wraith, J. E. (2001). Detection of inborn errors of metabolism in the newborn. *Arch Dis Child Fetal Neonatal Ed*, *84*(3), F205-210. https://doi.org/10.1136/fn.84.3.f205.

Clarke, J. T. R. (2006). *A clinical guide to inherited metabolic diseases* (3rd ed.). Cambridge University Press. Publisher description http://www.loc.gov/catdir/enhancements/fy0665/2006273396-d.html.Table of contents only http://www.loc.gov/catdir/enhancements/fy0665/2006273396-t.html.

Cleary, M. A., & Green, A. (2005). Developmental delay: when to suspect and how to investigate for an inborn error of metabolism. *Arch Dis Child*, *90*(11), 1128-1132. https://doi.org/10.1136/adc.2005.072025.

Enns, G. M., & Packman, S. (2001). Diagnosing Inborn Errors of Metabolism in the Newborn: Clinical Features. *NeoReviews, 2*(8), e183-e191. https://doi.org/10.1542/neo.2-8-e183.

Ezgu, F. (2016). Inborn Errors of Metabolism. *Adv Clin Chem, 73*, 195-250. https://doi.org/10.1016/bs.acc.2015.12.001.

Fleisher, G. R., Ludwig, S., Henretig, F. M., Ruddy, R. M., & Silverman, B. K. (Eds.). (2006). *Textbook of pediatric emergency medicine* (5th ed.). Lippincott Williams & Wilkins.

Gupta, R., Joshi, S., Asghar, A., & Gray, M. M. (2024). Metabolic emergencies in the NICU. *Semin Perinatol, 48*(8), 151987. https://doi.org/10.1016/j.semperi.2024.151987.

Häberle, J., Burlina, A., Chakrapani, A., Dixon, M., Karall, D., Lindner, M., Mandel, H., Martinelli, D., Pintos-Morell, G., Santer, R., Skouma, A., Servais, A., Tal, G., Rubio, V., Huemer, M., & Dionisi-Vici, C. (2019). Suggested guidelines for the diagnosis and management of urea cycle disorders: First revision. *J Inherit Metab Dis, 42*(6), 1192-1230. https://doi.org/10.1002/jimd.12100.

Leonard, J. V., & Morris, A. A. (2006). Diagnosis and early management of inborn errors of metabolism presenting around the time of birth. *Acta Paediatr, 95*(1), 6-14. https://doi.org/10.1080/08035250500349413.

Martins, A. M. (1999). Inborn errors of metabolism: a clinical overview. *Sao Paulo Med J, 117*(6), 251-265. https://doi.org/10.1590/s1516-31801999000600006.

Ogier de Baulny, H. (2002). Management and emergency treatments of neonates with a suspicion of inborn errors of metabolism. *Semin Neonatol, 7*(1), 17-26. https://doi.org/10.1053/siny.2001.0084.

Olpin, S. E. (2004). The metabolic investigation of sudden infant death. *Ann Clin Biochem, 41*(Pt 4), 282-293. https://doi.org/10.1258/0004563041201473.

Sharma, S., Kumar, P., Agarwal, R., Kabra, M., Deorari, A. K., & Paul, V. K. (2008). Approach to inborn errors of metabolism presenting in the neonate. *Indian J Pediatr, 75*(3), 271-276. https://doi.org/10.1007/s12098-008-0058-x.

Chapter 25

Neonatal Gastrointestinal Emergencies

Gökçe Çıplak*, MD

Department of Pediatrics, Division of Neonatology, Sivas Cumhuriyet University, Sivas, Turkey

Abstract

Gastrointestinal emergencies in neonates and infants can be life-threatening and require prompt recognition and intervention. These emergencies encompass a wide range of conditions, including both upper and lower gastrointestinal disorders, each presenting distinct challenges in diagnosis and management. Conditions such as esophageal atresia, hypertrophic pyloric stenosis, duodenal atresia, malrotation, meconium ileus, Hirschsprung disease, anorectal malformations, necrotizing enterocolitis, and intussusception are commonly encountered in neonatal care. This article reviews the pathophysiology, clinical presentation, diagnostic approaches, and surgical and medical management strategies for these conditions, emphasizing the importance of early intervention in preventing morbidity and mortality.

Keywords: neonate, upper gastrointestinal emergencies, lower gastrointestinal emergencies, congenital malformations

---

* Corresponding Author's Email: gokchech@gmail.com

In: Current Approaches to Newborn Emergencies
Editors: Zuhal Keskin Sarılar and Serap Samut Bülbül
ISBN: 979-8-89530-999-5

Introduction

Gastrointestinal emergencies in neonates and infants are critical conditions that demand immediate medical attention. These emergencies often present as obstructive, malformative, or inflammatory disorders of the gastrointestinal tract and may lead to severe complications, including dehydration, sepsis, and intestinal perforation. Early recognition of symptoms such as vomiting, abdominal distension, feeding intolerance, and failure to pass meconium is essential for effective management. Neonatal gastrointestinal emergencies, such as esophageal atresia, infantile hypertrophic pyloric stenosis, and necrotizing enterocolitis, can significantly affect the neonate's physiological stability and require rapid intervention, often through surgical means. Timely and accurate diagnosis is essential to avoid life-threatening consequences, with management strategies focusing on surgical correction, supportive care, and nutritional support.

Upper Gastrointestinal Emergency

Esophageal Atresia

Esophageal atresia (EA) is a congenital condition characterized by the absence of a portion of the esophagus, which may result in the formation of one or more fistulas between the malformed esophagus and the trachea. There are five distinct classifications of tracheoesophageal anomalies: Type A, which involves a tracheoesophageal fistula (TEF) without the presence of a tracheoesophageal fistula (10%); Type B, which includes a TEF with a fistula located in the proximal esophageal segment (<1%); Type C, in which the TEF is located in the distal esophageal segment (85%); Type D, where a TEF occurs in both the proximal and distal esophageal segments (<1%); and Type E, which refers to a TEF without a fistula (4%). In prenatal diagnosis, the absence of visualization of the polyhydramnios and/or the stomach, or the presence of a small stomach, are key indicators that raise suspicion for esophageal atresia. Newborns affected by EA typically exhibit symptoms shortly after birth, such as excessive secretions, which lead to respiratory distress and an inability to feed. Furthermore, in infants with EA, the orogastric catheter will often be unable to be passed beyond approximately 10 to 15 cm during insertion. This observation can be confirmed through an anteroposterior chest radiograph, which will show the catheter curving within the upper esophageal pouch. The treatment for EA is surgical intervention (Baldwin & Yadav, 2023; Clark, 1999).

Infantile Hypertrophic Pyloric Stenosis

Infantile hypertrophic pyloric stenosis (IHPS) is a condition characterized by the hypertrophy of the pylorus in young infants, which may lead to near-complete obstruction of the gastric outlet, resulting in nonbilious projectile vomiting. It typically manifests between 3 and 5 weeks of age, with very few cases occurring after 12 weeks. The incidence ranges from approximately 1 to 3.5 per 1,000 live births, although rates and trends can vary significantly by region. The exact etiology remains unclear, though a combination of genetic predisposition and environmental factors is believed to contribute (El-Mefleh, 2025; Rich 6 Dolgin, 2021).

The disorder commonly presents with sudden, projectile vomiting after feeding in infants aged 2 to 6 weeks, with the vomit being nonbilious. As the condition progresses, the symptoms may worsen, leading to weight loss and potentially severe electrolyte imbalances. The most notable electrolyte disturbance is hypokalemic, hypochloremic metabolic alkalosis, resulting from the loss of gastric hydrochloric acid. On physical examination, the hypertrophic pylorus can often be palpated as an "olive"-shaped mass. The preferred imaging technique for definitive diagnosis is ultrasonography. Treatment for IHPS is primarily surgical. In addition to surgery, it is crucial to maintain normal serum electrolyte levels and administer appropriate parenteral fluid therapy. Laparoscopic pyloromyotomy is a safe and effective surgical intervention. Following successful surgery, long-term outcomes are typically favorable, with no significant physiological deterioration observed (Aspelund & Lange, 2007; Gürkan et al., 2024).

Duodenal Atresia

Duodenal atresia and stenosis are the most commonly observed forms of intestinal obstruction identified during prenatal screening. There are three recognized types of duodenal atresia. Type 1, which is the most prevalent (69%), involves membranous mucosal atresia with an intact muscular wall. Type 2 is characterized by a short fibrous cord connecting the two ends of the atretic duodenum. Type 3, the most severe form, involves complete separation of the two duodenal segments and is frequently associated with biliary tract anomalies. Neonates with duodenal atresia typically exhibit gastric distension and vomiting, which is often nonbilious. In some cases, meconium may be expelled. This condition is found to be associated with malrotation in approximately 10-20% of instances. Prenatal ultrasonography may reveal suggestive signs of obstruction, including polyhydramnios and dilation of the intestinal loop. Postnatal diagnosis is confirmed through direct radiography and ultrasonography. The hallmark radiologic feature is the "double bubble" sign, indicative of dilatation in both the stomach and proximal duodenum, with an absence of gas in the distal segment. A contrast radiography study is typically used to confirm the diagnosis. Surgical intervention is required for treatment (Sigmon et al., 2023; Treider et al., 2023).

Further investigations should be conducted to assess potential associations with Trisomy 21, vertebral anomalies, and renal abnormalities (Atiyat et al., 2024).

Malrotation and Midgut Volvulus

Malrotation results from a disruption in the normal rotation of the embryonic intestine. Intestinal malrotation is rare after the first year of life, with approximately 30% of cases occurring within the first month. This condition can be associated with various congenital anomalies, including congenital diaphragmatic hernia, omphalocele, gastroschisis, congenital heart disease, and certain syndromes. The primary clinical manifestations include vomiting with bile, hemodynamic instability due to hypovolemia and/or septic shock, abdominal distension, peritonitis, and the presence of bloody stools. In infants suspected of having volvulus, serial radiographs of the upper gastrointestinal tract are considered the gold standard for diagnosis. The hallmark diagnostic feature is the abnormal positioning of the duodenojejunal junction. Treatment involves parenteral fluid support, hemodynamic stabilization, and urgent surgical intervention to address the underlying issue (Kedoin et al., 2024).

Lower Gastrointestinal Emergency

Jejunoileal Atresia

Jejunoileal atresia is an acquired condition resulting from vascular abnormalities that lead to ischemia-induced necrosis of a portion of fetal intestinal tissue. This disorder is categorized into four distinct types based on its anatomical features. Type I is characterized by obstruction caused by an intact diaphragm or membrane that covers the lumen, mucosa, and submucosa. Type II involves a short fibrous band connecting the proximal and distal intestinal segments. In Type IIIa, a gap similar to that seen in Type II exists within the intestinal structure, but without a tissue connection between the blind ends. Type IIIb presents with atresia of the proximal small intestine, the absence of the middle small intestine (which is typically supplied by the distal superior mesenteric artery), and a significant gap in the mesentery of the small intestine. This type is the most prevalent. Finally, Type IV involves multiple atresias, with the bowel being shortened anteriorly (Osuchukwu & Rentea, 2023).

Jejunoileal atresia typically manifests with symptoms of intestinal obstruction, including abdominal distension and vomiting. The absence of meconium output is a common sign, which varies based on the level of the obstruction, although it is generally considered nonspecific. Vomiting usually begins within the first 24 to 48 hours following birth. Fewer than 5% of neonates with jejunoileal atresia present with associated chromosomal abnormalities. Diagnosis is confirmed by direct radiography, which reveals dilated intestinal loops and air-fluid levels, a hallmark feature of jejunal or ileal atresia. In infants with distal small bowel atresia, bowel distension is more pronounced. The condition is treated surgically (Schmedding et al., 2021).

Meconium Ileus

Meconium ileus (MI) is a condition characterized by the obstruction of the small intestine due to the accumulation of meconium at the level of the terminal ileum. In infants with MI, meconium passage is typically absent within the first 72 hours of life, although this may not always be accompanied by abdominal distension or vomiting. Plain abdominal radiography commonly reveals dilated intestinal loops and the presence of calcification. If no signs of perforation are present, the diagnosis is confirmed through hyperosmotic contrast enema radiography (Parikh et al., 2023; Sellouti et al., 2024). Meconium ileus is classified into two forms: simple and complicated. The complicated form is characterized by the presence of intestinal perforation, accompanied by additional gastrointestinal pathologies such as meconium peritonitis, atresia, or volvulus. In contrast, the simple form does not involve these associated gastrointestinal conditions (Sellouti et al., 2024).

Meconium Plug Syndrome

Meconium plug syndrome is a condition that occurs in approximately 1 in 500 live births, resulting from colonic dysmotility or abnormal meconium consistency. Diagnosis and treatment are often achieved through contrast enema, which serves both diagnostic and therapeutic purposes. It is important to consider Hirschsprung's disease in neonates presenting with meconium plug syndrome, as it may present with similar symptoms (Yasir et al., 2023).

Meconium Peritonitis

Meconium peritonitis (MP) is an aseptic chemical inflammation caused by intrauterine intestinal perforation. These perforations may arise due to conditions such as mesenteric ischemia, intestinal atresia, volvulus, intussusception, meconium plug syndrome, inguinal hernia, Hirschsprung's disease, and meconium ileus, often associated with cystic fibrosis. Diagnostic features of MP may include abdominal calcifications, ascites, polyhydramnios, meconium pseudocysts, echogenic masses, and dilated bowel or intestinal obstruction, as observed on prenatal ultrasonography. Clinical outcomes and treatment strategies are dependent on the underlying cause of the perforation. Management also varies depending on the presence or absence of concurrent gastrointestinal pathologies (Zheng et al., 2024).

Hirschsprung' Disease

Hirschsprung's disease (HD) is a motor disorder of the colon that results from the incomplete migration of neural crest cells (which are the precursors of enteric ganglion cells) during fetal intestinal development. This failure of migration leads to an aganglionic segment of the colon, which cannot relax, causing functional obstruction. The incidence of HD is approximately 1 in 5,000 live births, and it is often associated with chromosomal abnormalities. The majority of HD cases are diagnosed during the neonatal period, with affected infants presenting with symptoms of distal intestinal obstruction, such as bile-containing vomiting, abdominal distension, and delayed passage of meconium or stool (Lotfollahzadeh et al., 2023).

Diagnosis is typically made based on delayed passage of the first meconium, and rectal biopsy remains the gold standard for confirming the diagnosis. A common clinical sign in newborns with HD is the explosive expulsion of gaseous and liquid stools following a digital rectal examination. In some infants, typical clinical features, such as poor feeding, abdominal distension, and constipation, may first become apparent when transitioning from breast milk to formula. HD can also present with sepsis-like symptoms, including vomiting, diarrhea, abdominal distention, and enterocolitis - a potentially life-threatening condition that may progress to toxic megacolon (Penaloza et al., 2024).

A rare complication of HD is volvulus, most often affecting the sigmoid colon or less frequently, the transverse colon and cecum. HD may also be associated with neonatal appendicitis and appendiceal perforation. Additionally, meconium ileus (MI) should raise suspicion for cystic fibrosis in all infants, and appropriate diagnostic testing should be performed to confirm the diagnosis (Penaloza et al., 2024; Rogu et al., 2024).

Anorectal Malformation

Anorectal malformation is a condition that arises from abnormal separation of the hindgut from the urogenital tract during embryonic development. Approximately two-thirds of affected individuals have associated congenital anomalies, often as part of the VACTERL association (vertebral defects, anal atresia, cardiac defects, tracheoesophageal fistula, renal anomalies, and limb abnormalities), while the remaining third presents as an isolated anomaly. The spectrum of malformations can range from an isolated imperforate anus to a persistent cloaca. These malformations are classified into two categories: "high" supralevator lesions, which terminate above the levator sling and are typically associated with fistulas, and "low" infralevator lesions, which terminate below the levator sling and are generally not associated with fistulas. Management and treatment strategies depend on the specific nature and severity of the anomaly (Smith & Avansino, 2023; Tonni, 2023).

Necrotizing Enterocolitis

Necrotizing enterocolitis (NEC) is a critical gastrointestinal emergency in neonates, particularly affecting preterm infants, with a mortality rate that can reach as high as 50%. The pathophysiology of NEC involves intestinal inflammation, which facilitates bacterial invasion, leading to cellular damage and necrosis of the intestinal tissue. Advanced cases of NEC can progress to peritonitis, sepsis, and intestinal perforation. The signs and symptoms of NEC are often nonspecific, including feeding intolerance, vomiting, lethargy, and abdominal tenderness, all of which should raise suspicion for the condition. Laboratory findings also tend to be non-specific, with metabolic acidosis, hyponatremia, and hypoalbuminemia commonly observed in advanced stages of the disease. Diagnostic confirmation is typically achieved through plain abdominal radiography, which may show dilated intestinal loops, pneumatosis intestinalis (air within the intestinal wall), and gas in the portal vein. Pneumatosis intestinalis is considered pathognomonic for NEC, while gas in the portal vein is associated with a poor prognosis. Free air in the abdomen may also be present in cases of intestinal perforation (Ginglen & Butki, 2023; Walsh & Kliegman, 1986; Su et al., 2023).

Management of NEC focuses on stabilizing the infant's vital signs. Enteral nutrition should be discontinued, and total parenteral nutrition should be provided. In cases where the infant's condition deteriorates, or if there is a lack of response to medical treatment or presence of intestinal perforation, surgical intervention is required (Hulscher et al., 2024).

Intussusception

Intussusception, though rare in the newborn period, is the most common cause of gastrointestinal obstruction in children under the age of 2. The exact etiology remains unknown, but the condition requires urgent surgical intervention. Delays in diagnosis and treatment can lead to increased morbidity and mortality. Intussusception occurs when a segment of the intestine folds into an adjacent section, causing obstruction and compromising blood supply, which can result in ischemia, necrosis, and perforation if left untreated (Mullis et al., 2019).

Conclusion

Gastrointestinal emergencies in neonates are a major cause of morbidity and mortality in this vulnerable population. Effective management relies on early identification of symptoms and prompt intervention, often through surgical procedures, to correct anatomical anomalies or relieve obstructive processes. The understanding of conditions such as malrotation, necrotizing enterocolitis, and Hirschsprung disease, among others, is vital for neonatologists and pediatricians in order to reduce the risk of long-term complications and improve survival rates. Multidisciplinary approaches involving neonatologists, pediatric surgeons, and radiologists are critical to providing the best outcomes for these infants. With timely diagnosis and appropriate management, the prognosis for most neonatal gastrointestinal emergencies can be significantly improved.

References

Aspelund, G., & Langer, J. C. (2007). Current management of hypertrophic pyloric stenosis. *Seminars in Pediatric Surgery, 16*(1), 27–33. https://doi.org/10.1053/j.sempedsurg.2006.10.004.

Atiyat, D. K., Al-Nusair, D. A., Alhajahjeh, A., Al-Awadi, M. Y., & Aborajooh, E. (2024). Global prevalence of duodenal atresia in trisomy 21: A systematic review and meta-analysis. *European Journal of Pediatric Surgery, Advance online publication.* https://doi.org/10.1055/a-2471-6435.

Baldwin, D. L., & Yadav, D. (2023). Esophageal atresia. In *StatPearls*. StatPearls Publishing.

Clark, D. C. (1999). Esophageal atresia and tracheoesophageal fistula. *American Family Physician, 59*(4), 910–920.

El-Mefleh, N. (2025). Recurrent hypertrophic pyloric stenosis: Neonatal age and pyloric canal length as risk factors. *Pediatrics and Neonatology, 66*(1), 2–6. https://doi.org/10.1016/j.pedneo.2024.10.009.

Ginglen, J. G., & Butki, N. (2023). Necrotizing enterocolitis. In *StatPearls*. StatPearls Publishing.

Gürkan, Ö. E., Öztürk, H., Kaya, C., Kaya, N. G., Bozbulut, N. E., Can, A., Ceylan, K., Aksu, A. Ü., Düztaş, D. T., Sarı, S., Dalgıç, B., Kapısız, A., Coşkun, D., Emmez, G., İnan, G., Akdulum, İ., Pampal, H. K., Eryılmaz, N. C., Erel, S., Şıvgın, V., & Sönmez, K. (2024). A classification for gastric outlet obstruction in childhood: Extending beyond infantile hypertrophic pyloric stenosis. *Turkish Journal of Gastroenterology, 35*(3), 255–261. https://doi.org/10.5152/tjg.2024.23202.

Hulscher, J., Irvine, W., Conforti, A., Di Cesare, A., Ichino, M., Sfeir, R., Madadi Sanjanig, O., Strohm, J., Hukkinen, M., Moschino, L., Norsa, L., Kokešová, A., Bakx, R., Kooi, E., Obermann-Borst, S., Palleri, E., Vermeulen, M., Spruce, M., Rolle, U., Miserez, M., & Burgos, C. M. (2024). European Reference Network for Inherited and Congenital Anomalies evidence-based guideline on surgical aspects of necrotizing enterocolitis in premature neonates. *Neonatology*, 1–9. Advance online publication. https://doi.org/10.1159/000542540.

Kedoin, C., Muto, M., Nagano, A., Matsui, M., Sugita, K., Baba, T., Miyoshi, K., Masuya, R., Murakami, M., Yano, K., Onishi, S., Harumatsu, T., Yamada, W., Yamada, K., Matsukubo, M., Kawano, T., Kuda, M., Nakame, K., Torikai, M., & Ieiri, S. (2024). Notable clinical differences between neonatal and post-neonatal intestinal malrotation: A multicenter review in Southern Japan. *Journal of Pediatric Surgery, 59*(4), 566–570. https://doi.org/10.1016/j.jpedsurg.2023.11.020.

Lotfollahzadeh, S., Taherian, M., & Anand, S. (2023). Hirschsprung disease. In *StatPearls*. StatPearls Publishing.

Mullis, S., Keesee, A. B., & Newberry, D. (2019). Intussusception in the neonate: A case study. *Neonatal Network, 38*(4), 199–205. https://doi.org/10.1891/0730-0832.38.4.199.

Osuchukwu, O. O., & Rentea, R. M. (2023). Ileal atresia. In *StatPearls*. StatPearls Publishing.

Parikh, N. S., Ibrahim, S. Y., & Ahlawat, R. (2023). Meconium ileus. In *StatPearls*. StatPearls Publishing.

Penaloza, C. S. Q., Barreto, A. C., Ortolan, E. V. P., Zani, A., & Lourenção, P. L. T. A. (2024). Management of Hirschsprung's disease: A survey with Brazilian pediatric surgeons. *Children, 11*(11), 1405. https://doi.org/10.3390/children11111405.

Rich, B. S., & Dolgin, S. E. (2021). Hypertrophic pyloric stenosis. *Pediatrics in Review, 42*(10), 539–545. https://doi.org/10.1542/pir.2020-003277.

Rogu, P. J., Colalillo, E., Rogu, N., & Rogu, G. (2024). Atypical presentation of Hirschsprung's disease in an infant: Challenges in early diagnosis and management of recurrent enterocolitis. *Cureus, 16*(11), e73862. https://doi.org/10.7759/cureus.73862.

Schmedding, A., Hutter, M., Gfroerer, S., & Rolle, U. (2021). Jejunoileal atresia: A national cohort study. *Frontiers in Pediatrics, 9,* 665022. https://doi.org/10.3389/fped.2021.665022.

Sellouti, M., Agadr, A., & Abilkassem, R. (2024). Complicated meconium ileus in a male neonate with cystic fibrosis: Case report. *Radiology Case Reports, 20*(1), 187–190. https://doi.org/10.1016/j.radcr.2024.09.098.

Sigmon, D. F., Eovaldi, B. J., & Cohen, H. L. (2023). Duodenal atresia and stenosis. In *StatPearls*. StatPearls Publishing.

Smith, C. A., & Avansino, J. (2023). Anorectal malformations. In *StatPearls*. StatPearls Publishing.

Su, Y., Xu, R. H., Guo, L. Y., Chen, X. Q., Han, W. X., Ma, J. J., Liang, J. J., Hao, L., & Ren, C. J. (2023). Risk factors for necrotizing enterocolitis in neonates: A meta-analysis. *Frontiers in Pediatrics, 10,* 1079894. https://doi.org/10.3389/fped.2022.1079894.

Tonni, G., Koçak, Ç., Grisolia, G., Rizzo, G., Araujo Júnior, E., Werner, H., Ruano, R., Sepulveda, W., Bonasoni, M. P., Lituania, M., & International Perinatology Research Group (IPRG). (2023). Clinical presentations and diagnostic imaging of VACTERL association. *Fetal and Pediatric Pathology, 42*(4), 651–674. https://doi.org/10.1080/15513815.2023.2206905.

Treider, M., Granheim, S., Engebretsen, A. H., Pripp, A. H., Røkkum, H., Skari, H., Sæter, T., & Bjørnland, K. (2023). Congenital duodenal obstruction: National trends in management and outcomes during the last quarter of a century in Norway. *European Journal of Pediatric Surgery, 33*(6), 503–509. https://doi.org/10.1055/a-2003-1920.

Walsh, M. C., & Kliegman, R. M. (1986). Necrotizing enterocolitis: Treatment based on staging criteria. *Pediatric Clinics of North America, 33*(1), 179–201. https://doi.org/10.1016/s0031-3955(16)34975-6.

Yasir, M., Kumaraswamy, A. G., & Rentea, R. M. (2023). Meconium plug syndrome. In *StatPearls*. StatPearls Publishing.

Zheng, X. Q., Wu, D. M., Chen, X., Lin, J. X., Wang, X. C., Ren, K. H., Liu, H. Q., Xu, R. L., & Yan, J. Y. (2024). Analysis of the clinical diagnosis and treatment of fetal meconium peritonitis. *The Journal of Maternal-Fetal & Neonatal Medicine, 37*(1), 2250045. https://doi.org/10.1080/14767058.2023.2250045.

Index

A

B

C

D

E

N

O

P